An Introduction to Orthopaedic Nursing

FOURTH EDITION

Authors

Nora Bass, MSN, MBA, ONC®
Orthopaedic Nurse Practitioner
Providence Hospital & Medical Centers
Southfield, Michigan

Maureen P. Cooper, MSN, RN, CS, ONC®
Clinical Nurse Specialist
William Beaumont Hospital
Royal Oak, Michigan

Cathleen E. Kunkler, MSN, RN, ONC®
Assistant Professor, Nurse Education
Orthopaedic and Sports Medicine Center
Corning, New York

Nancy S. Morris, PhD, APRN
Associate Professor
University of Massachusetts, Graduate School
of Nursing
Worcester, Massachusetts

Cathy A. Murray, MSN, RN, OCNS-C®
Clinical Nurse Specialist, Orthopaedics
Ball Memorial Hospital – A Clarian Health Partner
Muncie, Indiana

Lisa A. Olds, BSN, RN, ONC®
Orthopaedic Spine Nurse Clinician
Oakland Orthopaedic Surgeons
Royal Oak, Michigan

Mary Catherine Rawls, BSN, RN-BC, MS, ONC®
Clinical Nurse Specialist, Surgery and
Surgical Specialties
Dartmouth-Hitchcock Medical Center
Lebanon, New Hampshire

Dottie Roberts, MSN, MACI, RN, CMSRN, OCNS-C®
Nursing Instructor
South University
Columbia, South Carolina

Cathy D. Trame, MS, RN, CNS, BC
Perioperative Pain Coordinator/Clinical Nurse
Specialist, Pain Services
Miami Valley Hospital
Dayton, Ohio

Anita C. Summerville, BS, PTA, PAS, CSCS
Director/ Personal Trainer
Mind & Body Fitness Systems, LLC
Lake Orion, Michigan

Conflict of Interest

Each author and reviewer has been asked to disclose if he/she has received something of value (in excess of $500) from a commercial company or institution which relates directly or indirectly to writing and reviewing of this book. Those have been indicated with an asterisk (*) all others have no conflict of interest. NAON does not view the existence of these disclosed interests or commitments as necessarily implying bias or decreasing the value of the author or reviewers participation in our product.

Reviewers

Kayla R. Dieball, BSN, CNOR, CRNFA, MSN, FNP-BC, ONP-C®
Orthopaedic Nurse Practitioner
Orthopaedic and Sports Medicine Center
Manhattan, Kansas

Linda Hansen, MSN, RN, ONC®
Clinical Nurse Specialist, Orthpaedic Services
Spectrum Health
Grand Rapids, Michigan

Carol V. Harvey, MSN, APRN, ACNS, ONC®
Professor of Nursing / Orthopaedic Clinical
Nurse Specialist
Cypress College Department of Registered Nursing
Cypress, California

Matt Janes, PT, DPT, MHS, OCS, CSCS*
National Orthopedic Specialist
Gentiva Health Services
Louisville, Kentucky

Cariann Johnson-Huber, MSN, RN
Advanced Practice Nurse - Nursing Education
and Informatics
UPMC St. Margaret
Pittsburgh, Pennsylvania

Barbara J. Levin, BSN, RN, ONC®, LNCC
Clinical Scholar Orthopaedics/Trauma Unit
Massachusetts General Hospital
Boston, Massachusetts

Pati Ludovici, MSN, RN, CCM, CPHQ, ONC®
Coordinator, Joint Replacement Center
Broward General Medical Center
Ft. Lauderdale, Florida

Bev Morris, RN, CNP, MBA
Researcher, Author
University of California, San Diego Medical Center
San Diego, California

Carolyn Vitale, MSN, RN, ONC®
Director of Organizational Development
North Suburban Medical Center
Thornton, Colorado

Editor

Cindi M. Mosher, MSN, RN, ANP, ONC®
Nurse Practitioner
Oakland Orthopaedic Surgeons, PLLC
Royal Oak, Michigan

Preface

Orthopaedic conditions affect millions of Americans and their families at some point in their lifetimes. Nurses are called upon to address orthopaedic afflictions not only in their work, but in their everyday lives. *An Introduction to Orthopaedic Nursing* is intended to provide an overview of basic musculoskeletal anatomy, common adult orthopaedic conditions, and appropriate nursing assessment and care. Whether the reader is a novice to orthopaedic nursing, or a seasoned practitioner, the book comprehensively addresses common pathologies, complications, and surgical techniques.

An Introduction to Orthopaedic Nursing is presented in nine chapters. Each chapter is based on learning objectives. Key terms and definitions as well as references are identified for each chapter. An index is provided for easy location of subject matter within the book. The online post tests for each chapter assess the reader's learning and can be submitted for contact hour credit.

Thank you to all authors and reviewers of this 4th edition of *An Introduction to Orthopaedic Nursing*. Best wishes to all readers as you learn more about care of the patient with orthopaedic conditions.

Cindi Mosher, MSN, RN, ANP, ONC®

Editor, *An Introduction to Orthopaedic Nursing (4th ed.)*

Contact Hour Instructions

New to this edition: Now you can earn 12.4 contact hours online.

Step 1: Read through each section of the book.

Step 2: Go online to **www.orthonurse.org** and select Online Store.

Step 3: Purchase the post-test for all 9 chapters (a total of 95 questions in four separate tests) for only $75.

Step 4: Answer all of the post-test questions and with a passing result receive your contact hours online.

For assistance or further questions, please contact NAON at **naon@smithbucklin.com** or **800.289.6266**.

Chapter 1

Musculoskeletal Anatomy and Neurovascular Assessment

Cathleen E. Kunkler, MSN, RN, ONC®

Objectives

- Describe the micro/macroscopic structure, function, and types of bone.

- Identify the peripheral vascular and peripheral neurological components of a comprehensive neurovascular assessment.

- Identify nursing assessment parameters for neurovascular assessment.

- Describe potential patient outcomes that may occur secondary to abnormal neurovascular findings.

Key Terms

Blanching: to lose color; to assess the integrity of the circulation performed by applying and then quickly releasing pressure to a fingernail or toenail.

Cancellous bone: a type of structural organization of woven bone; characterized by a spongy or lattice-like structure.

Capillary refill: amount of time it takes a blanched nailbed to return to a normal pink appearance; generally 2 to 3 seconds.

Compact bone: dense or cortical bone.

Cortex: the dense bone that forms the external surface of a bone.

Diaphysis: the central part of the shaft of a long tubular bone.

Endosteum: the membrane lining the medullary cavity of a bone.

Epiphyses: the ends of a bone that lie between the joint surface on one side and the epiphyseal plate on the other.

Epiphyseal plate: the zone of cartilage between the epiphysis and the metaphysis responsible for the longitudinal growth of bones (also known as the physis or growth plate).

Flat bone: a bone that is in the form of a plate with broad, curved surfaces for muscle attachments, (i.e. scapula, ribs, pelvis, and parietal bones).

Haversian system: the functional unit of mature cortical bone also known as an osteon.

Innervation: nerve supply to a specific body part.

Ischemia: temporary deficiency of blood flow to an organ or tissue.

Irregular bone: a bone with varied shapes and many surface features for muscle attachment or articulations (i.e. vertebrae).

Long bone: an elongated bone of the extremities that consists of a diaphyseal shaft and wider epiphyseal, articulating ends (i.e. tibia).

Medullary cavity: a marrow-filled space within the diaphysis of a long bone, also known as the marrow cavity or intramedullary cavity.

Metaphysis: the widened end of the long bone shaft between the diaphysis and epiphysis.

Osteoblast: the basic cell that forms all bones.

Osteoclast: a large, multinucleated bone cell that reabsorbs mineralized bone matrix, thus breaking down bone.

Osteocyte: a mature bone cell derived from the osteoblast.

Osteogenic cells: cells that differentiate into osteoblasts and osteoclasts; found between the periosteum and bone in the medullary cavity.

Osteoid: the organic matrix formed by the osteoblast that becomes bone when mineralized.

Paresthesia: abnormal or unpleasant sensation that results from injury to one or more nerves, often described by patients as numbness or a prickly, stinging, or burning feeling.

Periosteum: a specialized connective tissue membrane that covers bone surfaces except for the points of tendon and ligament attachments and the articular surfaces.

Pulse points: palpable pulses of the body where there is throbbing caused by the regular contraction and alternate expansion of an artery as the wave of blood passes through the vessel.

Sesamoid bone: an ovoid nodule of bone that develops within a tendon (i.e. patella).

Short bone: a cube-shaped bone nearly equal in length and width to a thin layer of compact bone covering cancellous bone (i.e. carpals).

Trabeculae: the name given to the latticework structures of cancellous bone.

Introduction

The musculoskeletal system affords flexibility and protection to the human body.

Our hectic daily life gives little thought or attention to the human body's ability to function automatically in order to accomplish the simplest of functions. Vital organs such as the brain, heart, lungs, and abdomen are protected by the body's musculoskeletal system, a system composed of muscles, tendons, ligaments, bones, and joints.

Osseous tissue, because of its unique composition and structure, is perhaps the most distinctive form of connective tissue in the body. As in other connective tissues, it consists of cells, fibers, and intercellular material or matrix. Bone is highly vascular, metabolically active, and supplied with nerves. Its function is interdependent with other tissues and structures which are part of the musculoskeletal system such as muscles, nerves, blood vessels, cartilage, ligaments, and tendons, allowing appropriate responses and adaptation to the environment.

Musculoskeletal system injuries may not always be life-threatening; however, they are often limb-threatening because potential ischemia, deformity, or loss of function may lead to disability or the need for amputation. The onset of abnormal neurovascular findings may develop gradually or in a rapidly changing situation, therefore, all measures to reduce insult to the musculoskeletal system during the acute injury phase are vital.

Peripheral vascular structures and nerves are close to bone and are often traumatized simultaneously. Nerves perform the functions of transmitting messages to generate motor responses, translate sensory information, as well as manage thoughts, emotions and complex information (Urden, Stacey, & Lough, 2006). Nerves are particularly vulnerable to changes in local blood flow. Patients who present with musculoskeletal injury or for elective orthopaedic surgery require ongoing neurovascular monitoring—the foundation of orthopaedic nursing assessment. Nurses must be knowledgeable of the basic anatomy and physiology of the musculoskeletal system to provide astute neurovascular assessment and positive patient outcomes. It is important to

Figure 1-1
Anatomy of a Long Bone

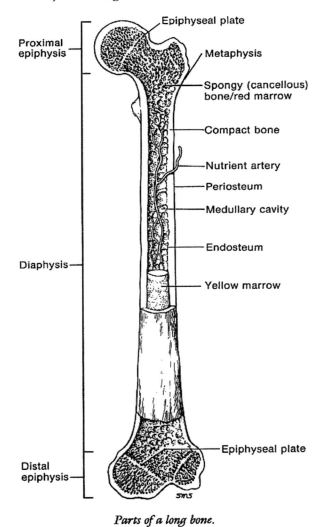

Parts of a long bone.

Reprinted with permission from Mott, S.R., James, S.R., & Sperhac, A.M. (1990). *Nursing Care of Children and Families* (p.1554). Upper Saddle River, NJ: Pearson.

note that neurovascular assessment encompasses motor and sensory function, as well as nerve and vascular assessment.

Organization

The skeletal system can be divided into two principle divisions. The axial skeleton is comprised of 80 bones, 74 of which form the perpendicular axis. The remaining 6 are the auditory ossicles (stapes, incus, and malleus) found in each middle ear. In the appendicular skeleton, 126 bones form the extremities that attach to the axial skeleton.

Bone Structure

All bones contain two types of tissue: compact (dense) and cancellous (porous, spongy) tissue (see Figure 1-1). Living bone cells occupy space in each type of bone, refuting the idea that bone is lifeless. Compact bone is the hard, outer layer of bone called the cortex. Cancellous bone, below the compact layer, appears spongy or web-like and contains many spaces (see Figure 1-1). Cancellous or trabecular bone is found in metaphyses and epiphyses of bone (Altizer, 2007).

Bones can be grouped into 4 types according to shape, each with a specific function (see Table 1-1). Long bones, which are longer than they are wide, have a diaphysis, expand into the epiphyses, and act as levers (i.e. the femur). Short bones transfer forces of movement (i.e. the carpals). Broad, curved

Table 1-1
Types of Bones

Type	Examples
Long	Humerus, radius, ulna, metacarpals, femur, tibia, fibula, metatarsals, phalanges
Short	Carpals, tarsals
Flat	Skull, (frontal, parietal, temporal, occipital), ribs, scapula,
Irregular	Vertebrae, pelvis, facial bones, bones of the inner ear, hyoid
Sesamoid	Patella

Reprinted with permission from Van De Graaff, K. (2002). Skeletal system: Introduction and the axial skeleton. In *Human Anatomy* (6th ed., pp. 131-171). New York: McGraw-Hill.

surfaces of flat bones allow for muscle attachments and offer protection to underlying organs (i.e. the sternum or pelvis). Irregular bones (i.e. the vertebrae, inner ear bones), which have peculiar and varied surface features, allow for muscle attachment or movement. (Van DeGraff, 2002). The sesamoid bone is the least common type and is a unique irregular bone found enclosed in a tendon near a joint. The patella is a sesamoid bone and provides extra leverage to the muscles moving the knee joint (Murray, 2010).

Figure 1-2
Enlarged Aspect of Haversian Systems in Compact Bone

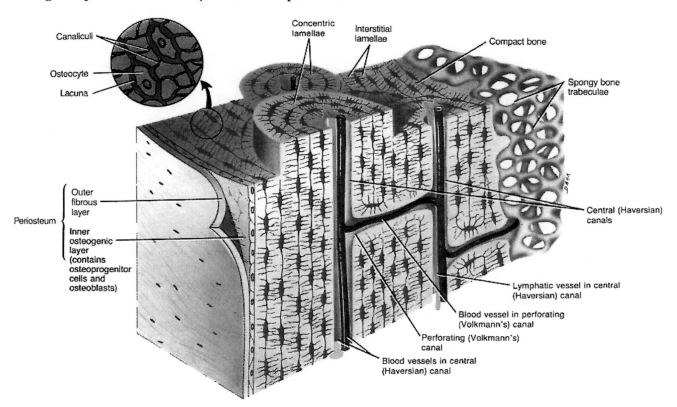

Reprinted with permission from Tortora, G.J., & Anagnostakos, N.P. (1990). *Principles of anatomy and physiology* (6th ed., p.145). New Jersey: John Wiley & Sons.

Figure 1-3
Left: Enlarged Aspect of Several Trabeculae of Spongy Bone; Right: Details of a Section of a Trabecula

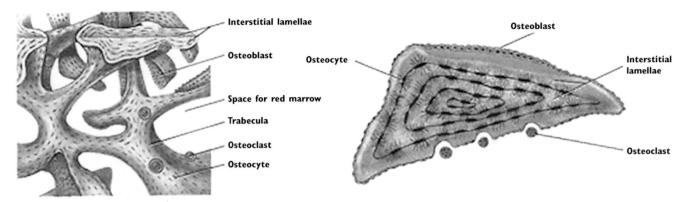

Reprinted with permission from Tortora, G.J., & Anagnostakos, N.P. (1990). *Principles of anatomy and physiology* (6th ed., p.146). New Jersey: John Wiley & Sons.

Histology

A typical long bone (see Figure 1-1) contains a diaphysis, epiphysis, medullary cavity, and periosteum (Patterson, 2010). The flared area between the epiphysis and diaphysis is the metaphysis. The epiphyseal line (plate), eventually replacing the physis or epiphyseal plate at skeletal maturity, separates the epiphysis and metaphysis. Protuberances found on the exterior of bones serve as attachments for other structures such as tendons and ligaments. Compact bone lies below the periosteum and contains yellow bone marrow within the medullary cavity. Yellow bone marrow, responsible for fat storage, is an important source of energy. Endosteum is the name given to the membranous tissue lining the medullary cavity. The epiphyses are formed of cancellous bone containing red bone marrow, a site of blood cell production. Articular cartilage covers the ends of the epiphyses. A joint is formed where separate bones meet. Cartilage provides a friction-free surface and acts as a cushion during joint motion.

Compact bone, although appearing very hard and dense, is not solid. The structural unit of cortical, compact bone is the Haversian system (Murray, 2010). Viewing a Haversian system under a microscope (Figure 1-2) displays vertical, interconnected, column-like structures that resemble rings on a tree trunk. These structures contain central canals for blood, lymphatic vessels, nerves, and spaces where confined osteocytes live and function to maintain healthy bone tissue. Refer to Figure 1-2 for a description of the remaining parts of the Haversian system.

In cancellous or spongy bone, Haversian systems do not exist. Instead, trabeculae form the structural framework (see Figure 1-3). Within the trabeculae are lacunae, each containing an osteocyte and communicating canaliculi extending in all directions. Filling the spaces between the trabeculae is red bone marrow, a site of hematopoiesis.

Bone Cells

Osteogenic cells line the periosteum and endosteum. Osteoblasts are bone-building cells found in the endosteum and beneath the periosteum. A characteristic of osteoblasts is the production of type I collagen and noncollagenous protein osteocalcin or osteoid (Brinkley, Harris, & Wraa, 2010). Bone strength will depend upon the matrix-mineralization deposits of calcium, phosphate, and other minerals. Osteocytes are isolated and confined in the lacunae of mineralized bone matrix. By delivering oxygen and nutrition, and removing waste products, osteocytes assist in the constant maintenance of healthy bone tissue and the regulation of blood calcium levels. Osteoclasts are important in the growth, maintenance, and repair of bone. Through enzymatic action and under hormonal influence, they resorb or break down bone to release calcium, magnesium, and other minerals to the blood when serum levels are deficient (see Figures 1-2 and 1-3).

Bone Health

Long after bones finish growing, bone tissue formation and resorption continue. The importance of adopting a lasting healthy lifestyle is essential. During the aging process, bone resorption exceeds the rate of bone formation and deposition, predisposing to weakened bones. Proper nutritional intake is necessary to maintain optimum bone health. Without adequate intake of vitamins C and D and the minerals calcium, phosphorous, and magnesium, bone composition is compromised.

Additionally, certain hormones influence normal physiologic bone growth and maintenance. Growth hormone (pituitary gland) and thyroxine (thyroid gland) work synergistically at the growth plate allowing a bone to grow to its proper length. Androgens and estrogens exert an influence on bone development during the adolescent growth spurt.

A delicate balance exists between calcitonin (thyroid gland) and parathyroid hormone (parathyroid gland) to maintain balanced calcium levels in the blood. Blood, which is low in calcium, passes through the parathyroid gland, stimulating osteoclasts to initiate breakdown of bone matrix thereby returning calcium levels to normal. If the thyroid gland detects high blood calcium levels, osteoclast activity is inhibited

(Brinkley et al., 2010). This reciprocal interchange takes place many times a day to maintain calcium homeostasis.

Bones remain strong and healthy when they are subjected to stress and load through regular weight-bearing activity. Walking and jogging are excellent forms of weight-bearing exercise. Inactivity and lack of exercise increase calcium release from bone and eventually lead to osteoporosis and the risk of fracture. Loss of calcium and bone density is a natural consequence of aging. In females, this process leading to osteoporosis is accelerated due to the withdrawal of estrogen during the menopausal years. During menopause, women should take vitamin D and calcium to offset bone density loss. Osteoporosis can occur in males but is usually seen later in life due to naturally higher levels of bone density and the production of androgen and estrogen throughout their lives. Women over the age of 35 and men over 55 have a decrease in bone mineral density of 1% per year (Maher, Salmond, & Pellino, 2002); therefore, it is important at any age to maintain regular exercise and proper nutrition to assure quality bone health.

Throughout the life span, the human body is at risk for injury to the musculoskeletal system. Injuries sustained by children on a playground, risky behavior by young adults, falls in the elderly, or elective procedures can result in potential injury to the musculoskeletal system with possible neurovascular compromise.

Musculoskeletal System Compromise

Nurses must be aware of patients at risk for neurovascular compromise. Whether working in a trauma intensive care unit, an ambulatory surgery unit, or a dedicated orthopaedic in-patient unit, nurses must understand the essential components of neurovascular compromise, demonstrate competency in performing and documenting a peripheral neurovascular assessment, and make clinical decisions related to the findings. Baseline bilateral neurovascular assessment is critical for guiding future assessment, subsequent critical thinking, and decision-making. In the trauma victim, early neurovascular assessment is important as baseline data to help differentiate the cause of neurovascular impairment: the injury itself or later interventions or complications.

Patient-Centered Assessment

Initial preparation to assess the musculoskeletal system of the patient includes the removal of nail polish, dirt, blood, or surgical antiseptics, as well as the removal of clothing from the distal extremities to be examined. The neurovascular assessment should be conducted with a good source of daylight or diffused overhead lighting. Nurses should not hesitate to turn on overhead lighting to conduct a thorough assessment during nighttime hours. The use of a flashlight should be avoided, as this distorts the color and appearance of the nail bed. The unaffected extremity should be assessed first, followed by the affected extremity, as the assessment of the unaffected extremity serves as a baseline for the patient.

Peripheral Vascular Assessment

Assessment of the peripheral vascular system consists of an inspection of the arms and legs. The following discussion examines the components of color, temperature, capillary refill, peripheral pulses, and the presence or absence of edema. For a comparison of venous and arterial insufficiency, see Table 1-2.

Color

Scales to grade skin color (Table 1-3) provide a baseline assessment; however, what is normal for one individual may be significantly altered by the variations in individual skin tone. Once again, comparison of skin color in the affected versus unaffected extremity is assessed to determine adequate arterial and vascular blood flow. Pale or blanched appearance of the skin, coolness to touch, and a slow or absent capillary refill may indicate arterial insufficiency (Table 1-3). Mottled or cyanotic discoloration, engorgement, and warmth to the touch may indicate inadequate venous return (Yantis, O'Toole, & Ring, 2009).

Temperature

The dorsum (back) of the nurse's hand is placed on the extremity to assess the warmth or coldness of the affected and unaffected extremity. The temperature of the extremity becomes cool just distal to an arterial occlusion. Cool temperature indicates inadequate arterial supply. Symmetrical coolness usually indicates peripheral vasoconstriction, and asymmetrical coolness may represent arterial insufficiency (Fahey, 2004). A warm temperature suggests venous congestion.

Temperature assessment is the least reliable sign of vascular compromise, yet combined with other components of the peripheral vascular assessment, it supports critical information. Environmental factors which may influence the patient's skin

Table 1-2
Peripheral Vascular Assessment Parameters

	Normal	Inadequate Arterial Supply	Inadequate Venous Return
Color	Pink	Pale/white	Blue/cyanotic, mottled
Temperature	Warm	Cool	Hot
Capillary Refill	1-2 seconds	>2 seconds	Immediate
Tissue Tugor	Full	Hollow/prune-like	Distended/tense

Adapted from Sermeus, S.M. (1984). Reconstructive surgery; High-tech, high-touch nursing. *Orthopaedic Nursing, 3*(2), 12.

Table 1-3
Skin Color Variations

Color	Condition	Cause	Assessment Location
Blue (cyanosis)	Increased amount of deoxygenated hemoglobin, associated with hypoxia.	Heart or lung disease, cold environment.	Nail beds, lips, mouth, skin (severe cases).
Pallor (decrease in color)	Reduced amount of oxyhemoglobin. Reduced blood flow. Congenital or autoimmune condition causing lack of pigment.	Anemia, shock. Vitiligo.	Face, skin, nail beds, conjunctivae, lips. Skin, nail beds, conjunctivae. Patchy areas on skin.
Yellow-orange (jaundice)	Increased deposition or bilirubin in tissues.	Liver disease, destruction of red blood cells.	Sclerae, mucous membranes, skin.
Red (erythema)	Dilation of blood vessels or increased blood flow.	Fever, direct trauma, blushing, alcohol intake.	Face, area of trauma.
Tan-brown	Increased amount of melanin.	Suntan, pregnancy, endocrine disorder.	Areas exposed to sun, face, areolas, nipples.

Reprinted with permission from Elsevier, from Perry, A.G., & Potter, P.A. (Eds.) (1998). *Clinical nursing skills and techniques* (4th ed.). St. Louis: Mosby.

temperature include the room temperature, the environment in which the injury occurred, the time spent in the operating and post-anesthesia recovery areas, the application of heat or ice, the bed linens, or the recent application of a cast.

Capillary Refill

Assessing capillary refill evaluates the arterial blood flow to the small peripheral vessels, the capillary bed being the farthest portion of the vascular system from the heart. Thus, capillary refill evaluates peripheral perfusion and cardiac output. Capillary filling is determined by measuring the time it takes for color to return to a nail bed that has been blanched. Capillary refill is measured by squeezing a nail bed for 2 to 3 seconds until it blanches, then releasing and

observing the time required for the nail bed to regain color. Normal capillary refill occurs within 3 seconds or less (McConnell, 2002; Judge, 2007). If a blanched nail bed does not return to its pre-blanched color by the time the nurse thinks or says "capillary refill," the patient is considered to have abnormal capillary filling. When there is an appreciable amount of venous congestion in the extremity, capillary refill may be inadequate, which is indicative of inadequate venous return. See Table 1-2 for capillary refill related to arterial or venous insufficiency.

Peripheral perfusion is important to obtain pulse oximetry readings. Hypotension, hypothermia, and vasoconstriction reduce arterial blood flow, and finger movements interfere with accurate interpretation of oxygen saturation.

During the nurse's initial assessment of the patient, information regarding medications, supplements, and lifestyle habits can be helpful in identifying potential peripheral perfusion problems. Certain medications such as aspirin, non-steroidal anti-inflammatories, and warfarin can increase the risk of bleeding. Smoking is a potent vasoconstrictor and should be considered for the patient with a history of tobacco use.

Figure 1-4
Dorsalis Pedis Pulse

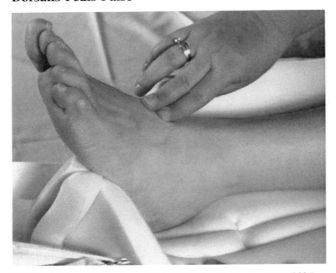

Reprinted with permission from *An introduction to orthopaedic nursing* (2004). C. Mosher (Ed.), (3rd ed., p. 17). Chicago, IL: National Association of Orthopaedic Nurses.

Peripheral Pulses

Palpation of the peripheral vessels is conducted to assess the flow of blood at pulse points throughout the body. Palpation of pulses allows assessment for presence, rate, equality, regularity, and strength. Palpation is accomplished by applying easy pressure to the pulse point using the pad of the index and middle fingers. Pulse volume or amplitude may be documented using a 0 to 4 grading scale. While there are variations, the following scale is generally accepted (Cooper & Osborn, 2010):

0 = no palpable pulse
1+ = weak, barely palpable or easily obliterated
2 + = palpable
3+ = strong, easily palpable
4+ = bounding

Nonpalpable pulses must be assessed using an ultrasonic doppler, a hand-held device that provides an audible evaluation of the blood flow where a palpable assessment cannot be obtained. Dopplers are sensitive to arterial blood flow signals in vessels at only 20 mmHG pressure, where pulses are palpable at 70 mmHG (Fahey, 2004). Dopplers are simple to use, relatively inexpensive, and noninvasive; however, their reliability is directly related to the skill of the examiner. Once the pulse point is located, an "X" can be marked on the skin to aid in future assessment.

Eight major pulse points are included in the peripheral vascular assessment. In the upper extremity, the axillary, brachial, ulnar, and radial pulses are assessed; the lower extremity assessment includes the femoral, popliteal, posterior tibial, and dorsalis pedis pulses. Intact pulses may be present even in the presence of arterial damage. It is also important to note that compromise of the microvascular structures caused by compartment syndrome does not initially affect the peripheral pulses. Loss of arterial pulsations is not a part of normal aging and demands careful evaluation. Diminished or absent pulses indicate the presence of an arterial stenosis or occlusion proximal to the site being assessed, whereas abnormally strong pulses may suggest an occlusion distal to the assessed site or the presence of an aneurysm (Fahey, 2004).

Patients most likely to develop peripheral artery occlusion are those with coronary conditions that predispose them to thrombus formation: certain arrhythmias (such as atrial fibrillation), myocardial infarction, or valvular disease. Peripheral artery disease from atherosclerosis and lower-extremity bypass grafting also increases the risk of occlusion (Lewis, 1999).

The axillary pulse is found in the upper medial arm, in the groove between the triceps and biceps muscles. With the forearm supinated, the brachial pulse can be palpated on the medial aspect of the antecubital fossa above the elbow. The ulnar pulse is located on the inner surface (volar) of the wrist on the side of the fifth digit (little finger). The radial pulse is palpated on the thumb side of the volar surface of the wrist over the distal radius. Upper extremity circulation is generally considered sufficient if the brachial and radial pulses are palpable, as the ulnar pulse may be difficult to palpate due to its anatomic location (Fahey, 2004).

Assessment of the lower extremity pulses begins with palpation of the femoral pulse in the groin. The femoral artery and vein arise from within the external iliac artery and vein in the pelvis. These vascular structures become the popliteal artery and vein and vascularize the knee joint. The popliteal pulse is difficult to palpate, since it lies deep in the popliteal fossa behind the knee. Flexing the patient's knee and using both hands to palpate may be easier. Eventually the popliteal artery bifurcates into the anterior tibial artery, which becomes the dorsalis pedis artery and the posterior tibial artery. If the dorsalis pedis pulse is present in the foot, omission of popliteal pulse palpation is acceptable.

The posterior tibial pulse is located behind and just above the medial malleolus of the ankle. The dorsalis pedis pulse is located on the mid-dorsum of the foot aligned with the second and third digits (Figure 1-4). Due to anatomic variations, the posterior tibial and dorsalis pedis pulse may be absent in 10% of the population (Fahey, 2004).

Figure 1-5
Pitting Edema

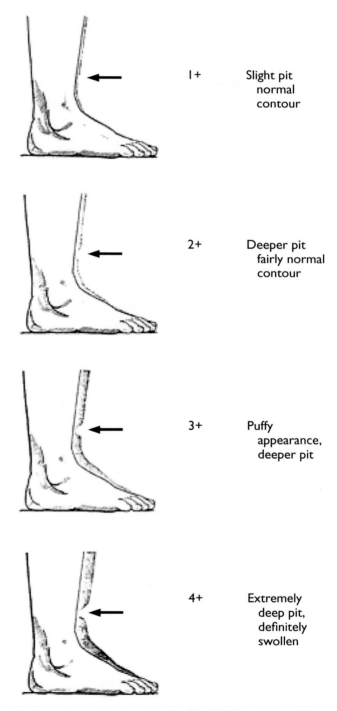

1+   Slight pit normal contour

2+   Deeper pit fairly normal contour

3+   Puffy appearance, deeper pit

4+   Extremely deep pit, definitely swollen

Reprinted with permission from Judge, R. et al. (1982). *Clinical diagnosis* (4th ed.). Philadelphia: Lippincott, Williams, & Wilkins.

Figure 1-6
Fracture Blister

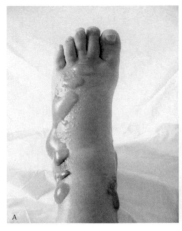
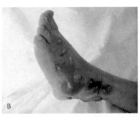
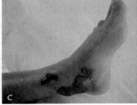

Clinical pictures demonstrating blisters associated with lower-extremity fracture. The patient was a 36-year-old male who sustained a trimalleolar ankle fracture during a motor vehicle accident. Surgical fixation of the fracture was performed 10 days after the injury (a surgical delay of 6 days secondary to the presence of the fracture blisters).

Reprinted with permission from Strauss, E., Petrucelli, G., Bong, M., Koral. K.J., Egol, K.A. et al. *Blisters associated with lower-extremity fracture: Results of a prospective treatment protocol* (p. 619). Philadelphia: Lippincott, Williams, & Wilkins.

The nurse must document the presence of diminished pulses and altered capillary filling. Following six to eight hours of ischemia, revascularization of the distal extremity is difficult to achieve. Therefore, astute assessment of pulses and early detection of abnormalities are paramount to optimal outcomes.

Edema

Edema may result as a physiologic response to injury or surgery. Increasing edema in a confined space threatens neurovascular functioning and heightens the risk of compartment syndrome. Compartment syndrome is due to either increased contents or decreased size within a muscle compartment and is an emergency requiring surgical decompression. See Chapter 8, *Complications Associated with Orthopaedic Conditions and Surgeries*, for an in-depth discussion of compartment syndrome. As ischemia progresses, so does the accompanying edema, creating venous congestion, taut skin, declining sensory and motor ability, along with pallor and pain. The indentation that remains after pushing on the skin over the foot or tibia for five seconds is known as pitting edema. Figure 1-5 uses the gradation scale of 0 (absent), 1+ (barely detectable), 2+ (depression, 5 mm), 3+ (depression of 5 to 10 mm) and 4 + (depression > 1 cm). Pitting edema can also be graded according to the length of time it takes to return the skin to baseline position or according to the depth of the indentation: mild (0 to 1/4 inch), moderate (1/4 to 1/2 inch), severe (1/2 inch to 1 inch) or very severe (> 1 inch) (L'ecuyer, 2010). The nurse must remember to determine if the patient has preexisting bilateral edema due to cardiac disease or unilateral edema due to chronic venous or lymphatic obstruction.

Fracture Blisters

Fracture blisters (Figure 1-6) result from dermal-epidermal separation that occurs in the skin during initial fracture deformity. A major factor in fracture blister formation is injury to the dermal-epidermal junction that results from exposure to elevated shear forces in the skin during bony displacement. Blood-filled blisters have complete separation of the dermis from the epidermis. Clear fluid-filled blisters have partial epidermal separation, with a few scattered areas of retained epithelial cells on the dermis. Accurate neurovascular assessment of the edema present at fracture sites is imperative and must accompany meticulous wound care. Strauss, Petrucelli, Bong, Koval, and Egol (2006) in a study on care of fracture blisters, determined that unroofing clear-filled and blood-filled blisters and treating the blister beds with silver sulfadiazine (Silvadene) was successful in minimizing wound and skin complications, except in patients with comorbid diabetes mellitus.

Electrolyte Monitoring

With significant post-injury or surgical interstitial fluid shift, fluid and electrolyte levels must be monitored. Shifts in sodium chloride and potassium may significantly impact the overall homeostasis of the patient. Edema is caused by inflammatory mediators that are released by a variety of cells which in turn cause nearby blood vessels to dilate and leak plasma resulting in swelling of the tissues. Sodium is the major extracellular fluid determinant of osmolality, whereas potassium is the major intracellular fluid determinant. Equilibrium is maintained by the free exchange of these electrolytes across the cell membrane.

Isotonic fluid volume deficit occurs as a result of capillary leak syndrome (third spacing of intravascular fluids) due to the trauma and damage to the capillary membranes that permit the flow of water, solutes, and plasma proteins into the interstitial (third) space (Holcomb, 2009). Fluid shifts can cause circulatory collapse and death due to hypovolemia. During initial resuscitation following an injury, strict attention to urinary output and serum electrolyte levels is required to prevent hypotonic or hypertonic dehydration from occurring. Rapid physiologic responses from the patient, combined with interventions on the part of the health care team, can culminate in a severe electrolyte imbalance crisis (Table 1-4).

Patients at risk for compartment syndrome must also be assessed for rhabdomyolosis (myoglobinuric renal failure). Altered renal perfusion may compound fluid imbalances experienced by the patient with multi-system injuries.

Peripheral Neurologic Assessment

Neurologic injury can begin within 30 minutes of inadequate blood supply and become functionally irreversible within 4 to 6 hours. If compressed, stretched, or lacerated, peripheral nerves decrease or cease functioning, and the muscles they normally innervate weaken or fail to contract, producing the sensation of numbness or tingling. An assessment of the peripheral neurologic function consists of checking the sensation and motor function of the tissues of the extremities, comparing the affected extremity to the unaffected extremity.

Table 1-4
Electrolyte Considerations in Neurovascular Assessment

Electrolyte Imbalances	Signs and Symptoms
Hyponatremia	• Symptoms variable • Usually don't appear until serum sodium falls below 125 mEq/liter • Common complaints include headache, nausea, abdominal cramps, muscle tremors, twitching, and weakness • Mild hyponatremia can cause confusion in the elderly • Severe hyponatremia can cause confusion, seizures, and coma
Hypovolemia	• Orthostatic hypotension, poor skin turgor, dry mucous membranes, a slight temperature elevation, and tachycardia • Elderly patients may become lethargic and confused
Hypervolemia	• Elevated BP, irritative cough, shortness of breath, jugular vein distension, and crackles on lung auscultation

Adapted from Schmidt, T. (2000). Assessing a sodium and fluid imbalance. *Nursing, 30*(1),18.

The upper extremity is evaluated primarily for deficits of the radial, median, or ulnar nerves. Lower extremity assessment includes the femoral, sciatic, peroneal, and tibial nerves.

Musculoskeletal injury management often requires the use of orthotics, braces, casts, splints, immobilizers, external fixation devices, continuous passive motion machines, or a HALO apparatus. Each therapeutic modality requires astute neurovascular assessment and documentation of findings.

Sensation

Ask the patient to close his or her eyes prior to initiating assessment of sensory function. Lightly touch the patient's extremity along the course of a nerve, and ask, "Where am I touching you?" rather than "Do you feel this?" Then ask the patient to describe the sensation to determine if paresthesia is present. Figure 1-7 depicts the area of sensory assessment of the median, radial, and ulnar nerves. Normal sensory innervation of the tibial and peroneal nerves is illustrated in Figure 1-8.

The major nerves supplying the lower extremity are the sciatic nerve, which divides into the common peroneal nerve and tibial nerve, and the femoral nerve. The peroneal nerve bifurcates into the superficial and deep peroneal nerves which innervate the anterior aspect of the lower leg and foot. The tibial nerve supplies the posterior aspect of the lower leg and foot. The femoral nerve turns into the saphenous nerve and supplies most of the anterior muscles of the thigh.

Motor Function

Peripheral neurologic assessment of motor function focuses on the patient's ability to perform normal movement of the muscles along the course of a nerve's innervations, the strength of movement against resistance, and the presence of pain associated with passive motion. Motor function of the median, ulnar, radial, tibial, and peroneal nerves are illustrated in Figures 1-7 and 1-8. Impairment of the radial nerve results in wrist drop, while impairment of the ulnar nerve results in claw hand or Volkman's contracture. Foot drop, the result of impairment of the peroneal nerve, will affect an individual's gait pattern and may require bracing and/or use of assistive devices for ambulation. Reduced sensory and motor function accompanying foot drop places

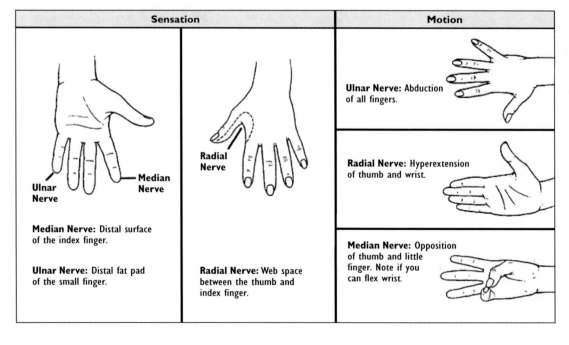

Sensation

Median Nerve: Distal surface of the index finger.

Ulnar Nerve: Distal fat pad of the small finger.

Radial Nerve: Web space between the thumb and index finger.

Motion

Ulnar Nerve: Abduction of all fingers.

Radial Nerve: Hyperextension of thumb and wrist.

Median Nerve: Opposition of thumb and little finger. Note if you can flex wrist.

Figure 1-7
Sensory and Motor Function of the Median, Ulnar, and Radial Nerves

Reprinted with permission from the National Association of Orthopaedic Nurses (1990). Poster: *Neurovascular Assessment.* Chicago, IL.

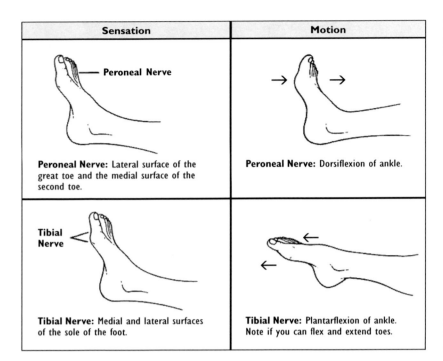

Sensation	Motion
Peroneal Nerve: Lateral surface of the great toe and the medial surface of the second toe.	Peroneal Nerve: Dorsiflexion of ankle.
Tibial Nerve: Medial and lateral surfaces of the sole of the foot.	Tibial Nerve: Plantarflexion of ankle. Note if you can flex and extend toes.

Figure 1-8
Sensory and Motor Function of the Tibial and Peroneal Nerves

Reprinted with permission from the National Association of Orthopaedic Nurses (1990). Poster: *Neurovascular Assessment.* Chicago, IL.

individuals at risk for falls and heightens the need to be aware of safety issues. In addition, wrist drop or foot drop can significantly impede the ability to work and has consequences related to body image perception.

Accurate nursing assessment and careful attention to subtle changes in the patient's motor and sensory function are critical. A peripheral neurologic assessment is best accomplished with an alert, cooperative patient. In the unresponsive patient, motor and sensory assessment must be based upon responses to painful stimuli as demonstrated through reflex motions or other expressions of pain. In addition, patients should be taught the components of neurovascular assessment as part of discharge instructions. Patients and significant others need to be aware of the potential alterations in normal neurovascular status that may indicate an impending complication.

Common Nerve Motor/Sensory Injuries

Injuries involving the elbow must be thoroughly assessed for neurovascular integrity. Prevention of edema and subsequent neurovascular compromise is integral to prevent Volkman ischemic contracture (Volkman, 2007), which occurs when ischemia of the forearm muscles follows an elbow injury, causing muscle necrosis and permanent elbow, wrist, and hand contractures. Postoperative shoulder surgeries require assessment for brachial plexus or musculocutaneous nerve impairment (Brown, 2008).

Brachial plexus injury can range from neuropraxia (stretch injury) to severe avulsion of the nerve root and can affect both motor and sensory innervation. The nerves which control hand, wrist, elbow, and shoulder function can be damaged by pressure, stretching, or surgical incisions. Injuries can range from minor to severe disability, and are dependent upon the age of the individual, and the type, severity, and location of the injury. Most frequently, trauma from motor vehicle accidents, sports injuries, falls, or childbirth (Erb's palsy) precipitate brachial plexus injury. Ongoing neurovascular assessment focuses on presence of edema, pain, vascular integrity, weakness (limp or paralyzed upper extremity), and paresthesia commensurate with the level of injury (Brown, 2008). Assuring the patient's arm and wrist are kept in neutral alignment following injury or surgery and that shoulder brace straps are not applied tightly can decrease the risk of brachial plexus injury.

Injury to the femoral nerve is thought to be rare (0.5 % to 2.0 %) because of the nerve's relatively protected position between the iliac and psoas muscles as it exits the pelvis deep to the inguinal ligament (Rue, Inoue, & Mont, 2004). Sciatic nerve palsy associated with an acetabular fracture has an estimated prevalence ranging from 10% to 36%. Sciatic nerve palsy most commonly affects the peroneal division following an acetabular fracture or a posterior hip

Table 1-5
Nursing Diagnoses for Neurovascular Assessment

Nursing Diagnoses for Neurovascular Assessment
Fluid Volume, Excess
Infection, Risk for
Mobility: Physical, Impaired
Neurovascular Dysfunction: Peripheral, Risk for Pain, Acute
Skin Integrity, Impaired
Tissue Integrity, Impaired
Tissue Perfusion, Ineffective, Peripheral

dislocation. Peroneal nerve palsy may occur as a result of injury or surgical intervention in the lower extremity. Foot drop and paresthesia may result from supracondylar fracture, promixal tibia fracture, or knee dislocation injuries. Positioning of the lower extremity in the operating room or incorrect use of abduction devices may cause pressure on the peroneal nerve resulting in transient paresthesia and motor deficits. Additionally, casts, skin, or skeletal traction applied to the lower extremity can also be attributed to peroneal nerve injury. The patient must be assessed to assure the lower extremity is in neutral alignment and that abduction device straps are not applied too tightly. Patient reports of pain, numbness, or motor deficits must be assessed and reported to the surgeon (Colegate-Stone & Hussain, 2008).

Serial electromyographic examinations can be helpful in evaluating the patient who has a longer-than-expected delay in the return of clinically apparent nerve function. Farrell, Spring, Haidkewych, and Morrey's (2005) retrospective study of 27,004 primary total hip arthroplasties identified 47 patients (0.17%) with identified postoperative motor nerve dysfunction. The data indicated that the majority of the 47 patients with nerve palsy, whether complete or incomplete, never fully recovered preoperative strength.

Documentation

Initial documentation of neurovascular assessment for the trauma victim begins at the time of injury or in the emergency department. Elective surgical patients need to be assessed during their preadmission screening and during their postoperative recovery. A flow sheet is a valuable tool for ongoing documentation of neurovascular status and can visually demonstrate 'trending' patterns of declining or improving neurovascular assessments.

Once a patient is discharged from PACU, vital signs are often measured every 15 minutes times four, every 30 minutes times four, every 2 hours times four, then every 4 hours for 24-48 hours if the patient's condition is stable (Chard, 2010). Ongoing postoperative neurovascular assessments are performed at the same time the vital signs are checked (Ignatavicius & Murray, 2010). In addition, the frequency of assessment must be based upon an index of suspicion for those at high risk of developing neurovascular compromise. The minimum frequency is every 2-4 hours (Cooper & Osborn, 2010). If a new treatment modality is initiated, such as continuous passive motion (CPM), casting, or traction, assessment frequency should be increased until the patient's stability is assured.

Table 1-5 identifies selective nursing diagnoses applicable to care of the patient requiring neurovascular assessment.

Summary

The nurse who is thoroughly familiar with the musculoskeletal system components and underlying scientific rationale of the neurovascular assessment can provide care competently and quickly. The nurse is responsible for ongoing neurovascular assessment, documenting accurate patient data, and communicating assessment findings to other members of the health care team. Thorough assessment and communication can prevent or detect signs and symptoms of potential or developing complications.

References

Altizer, L. (2007). Anatomy and physiology. In the National Association of Orthopaedic Nursing *NAON's core curriculum for orthopaedic nursing* (6th ed., pp. 15-36). Boston: Pearson.

Brinkley, K., Harris, J., & Wraa, C. (2010). Caring for the patient with musculoskeletal disorders. In K. Osborn, C. Wraa, & A.Watson (Eds.), *Medical-surgical nursing preparation for practice* (pp. 1729-1775). Upper Saddle River, NJ: Pearson.

Brown, F. (2008). Nursing care after a shoulder arthroplasty. *Orthopaedic Nursing, 27*(1), 3-9.

Chard, R. (2010). Care of postoperative patients. In D. Ignatavicius, & M. Workman (Eds.), *Medical-surgical nursing patient-centered collaborative care* (6th ed., pp. 285-303). St. Louis: W.B. Saunders.

Colegate-Stone, T., & Hussain, S. (2008). Iatrogenic sciatic nerve palsy following hemiarthroplasty of the hip. *European Journal of Trauma and Emergency Surgery, 34*(2), 171–172.

Cooper, K., & Osborn, K. (2010). Caring for the patient during musculoskeletal surgical procedures. In K. Osborn, C. Wraa, & A. Watson (Eds.), *Medical-surgical nursing preparation for practice* (pp. 1802-1832). Upper Saddle River, NJ: Pearson.

Fahey, V. (2004). *Vascular nursing* (4th ed.). St. Louis: W.B. Saunders.

Farrell, C., Spring, B., Haidkewych, G., & Morrey, B. (2005). Motor nerve palsy following primary total hip arthroplasty. *The Journal of Bone & Joint Surgery, 87*-A(12), 2619-2625.

Holcomb, S. (2009). Third-spacing: When body fluid shifts. *Nursing Critical Care, 4*(2), 9-12.

Ignatavicius, D., & Murray, C. (2010). Care of patients with arthritis and other connective tissue diseases. In D. Ignatavicius, & M. Workman (Eds.), *Medical-surgical nursing patient-centered collaborative care* (6th ed., pp. 322-361). St. Louis: W.B. Saunders.

Judge, N. (2007) Neurovascular assessment. *Nursing Standard, 21*(45), 39-44.

L'ecuyer, K. (2010). Nursing assessment of patients with cardiovascular disorders. In K. Osborn, C.Wraa, & A.Watson (Eds.), Medical-surgical nursing preparation for practice (pp. 1052-1073). Upper Saddle River, NJ: Pearson.

Lewis, A. (1999). Orthopedic and vascular emergencies! *Nursing, 29*(12), 54-57.

Maher, A., Salmond, S., & Pellino, T. (2002). *Orthopaedic nursing* (3rd ed., p. 173). Philadelphia: W.B. Sanders

McConnell, E. (2002). Assessing neurovascular status in a casted limb. *Nursing, 32*(9), 20.

Murray, C. (2010). Assessment of the musculoskeletal system. In D. Ignativicus, & M.Workman, (Eds.), *Medical-surgical nursing patient-centered collaborative care* (pp. 1140-1151). St. Louis: W.B. Saunders.

Patterson, M. (2010). Caring for the patient with musculoskeletal trauma. In K. Osborn, C. Wraa, & A. Watson (Eds.), *Medical-surgical nursing preparation for practice* (pp. 1776-1801). Upper Saddle River, NJ: Pearson.

Rue, J., Inoue, N., & Mont, M. (2004). Current overview of neurovascular structures in hip arthroplasty: Anatomy, preoperative evaluation, approaches, and operative techniques to avoid complications. *Orthopedics, 27*(1), 73-81.

Strauss, E., Petrucelli, G., Bong, M., Koval, K., & Egol, K. (2006). Blisters associated with lower-extremity fracture: Results of a prospective treatment protocol. *Journal of Orthopaedic Trauma, 20*(9), 618-622.

Urden, L., Stacey, K., & Lough, M. (2006). Neurologic anatomy and physiology. In Thelan's *Critical care nursing* (5th ed., pp. 691-719). St. Louis: Mosby Elsevier.

Van De Graaff, K. (2002). Skeletal system: Introduction and the axial skeleton. In *Human anatomy* (6th ed, pp. 131-171). New York: McGraw Hill.

Volkmann, R. (2007). THE CLASSIC: Ischaemic muscle paralyses and contractures. *Clinical Orthopaedics & Related Research, 456*, 20-21.

Yantis, M., O'Toole, K., & Ring, P. (2009). Leech therapy. *American Journal of Nursing, 109*(4), 36-42.

Chapter 2

Care of the Patient with Upper Extremity Problems

Nora Bass, MSN, MBA, ONC®

Objectives

- Identify common shoulder conditions and associated clinical findings and the implications relative to caring for those patients.

- Discuss common orthopaedic conditions affecting the elbow, wrist, and hand, defining nursing assessment and care as it relates to those problems.

- Describe surgical and non-surgical care for common upper extremity disorders.

Key Terms

Acromioplasty: Surgical resection of the undersurface of the acromion, done arthroscopically or by open surgery.

Active assisted ROM: Active muscle contraction, muscle stretch, and joint range of motion facilitated by an outside force, usually the physical therapist.

Arthroscopic surgery: Interior joint examination with a fiberoptic scope and small tools, with or without cutting, grinding, or suturing.

Bankart lesion: Detachment of the anterior inferior labrum from the glenoid, which often causes the shoulder to dislocate.

Fibrosis: Formation of pathologic fibrous tissue, often in response to inflammation.

Hill-Sachs lesion: Impaction fracture of the posterior humeral head caused during a dislocation; the back of the humeral head hits the front rim of the socket.

Isometric exercises: Muscle contraction without joint motion.

Mumford procedure: Removal of the distal articular segment of the clavicle.

Passive ROM: An outside force is used to move the joint or stretch the muscle.

Pendulum exercises: Commonly used after shoulder surgery to mobilize the shoulder without resistance; performed by leaning forward and gently swinging the arm.

Reverse total shoulder arthroplasty: Glenoid is resurfaced with a humeral head shaped component and the humeral component is socket shaped. Implants are reverse shapes of traditional total shoulder arthroplasty.

Rotator cuff: Collective term referring to the supraspinatus, infraspinatus, teres minor, and subscapularis muscles.

Shoulder hemiarthroplasty: Humeral head replacement without glenoid resurfacing.

SLAP lesion: Superior Labral Anterior-Posterior disruption or tear.

Total shoulder arthroplasty: Humeral head replacement with glenoid resurfacing.

The upper extremity is comprised of the shoulder and associated structures, the elbow, and the hand. All of these structures together are critical to the patient's performance of activities of daily living. Consider eating, bathing, toileting, and even mobility when understanding the implications of upper extremity injuries and their impact upon a patients' daily routine, especially when the dominant upper extremity is involved. Significant disability can result both short term and long term due to associated nerve injuries, deformities, and lost range of motion. The goal of nursing care will initially be pain management, post surgical care, cast/splint monitoring, and neurovascular assessments. Later interventions will focus on preserving function with therapy and range of motion. Occupational therapy can assist with compensatory devices and strategies for accomplishing daily work.

The shoulder is a dynamic structure of bony, ligamentous, and muscular tissues, interfacing and allowing greater range of motion than any other joint in the body. There are three primary bones and their processes, a number of muscle-tendon units, and five articulations present in each shoulder unit (Jobe, 1998). The ligaments connect bone to bone to maintain the osseous relationships. The tendons are soft tissue structures that link muscle to bone, allowing the muscles to work in unity with the bone structures. The shoulder has an extreme range of motion. This ability unfortunately creates an ideal environment for injury because of trauma or the stress of motion beyond normal limits. Shoulder conditions can be acute and chronic and can affect both osseous and soft tissues. Injuries about the shoulder can result in pain, stiffness, weakness, and lost motion. Typically, pain is ultimately why most patients seek health care (Cofield et al., 2001), in the face of acute and/or chronic problems.

Figure 2-1
Anterior View of the Left Shoulder

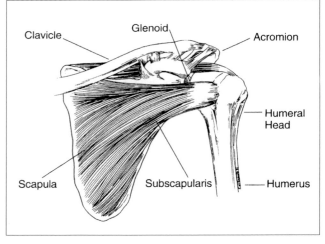

Illustration by Kristen Wienandt. Reprinted with permission from Deuschle, J.A., & Romeo, A.A. (1998). Understanding shoulder arthroplasty. *Orthopaedic Nursing, 17*(5), 8.

Beyond the shoulder is the elbow joint which is made up of the distal humerus, the proximal radius, and the proximal ulna. Injuries to the elbow can create significant physical disability. Lindenhovius, Buijze, Kloen, & Ring (2008) demonstrated that physical disability correlated with patient's self reports of disability as it related to specific tasks such as changing light bulbs, placing items on over-the-head shelves, blow drying hair, turning a key, or opening a tight jar. Injuries can include soft tissue or the osseous anatomy. Fractures and fracture dislocation injuries can be catastrophic, but tendonitis can be as problematic for the average patient.

More distal to the elbow joint is the wrist which interfaces the distal radius and ulna at the base of the hand. Patients may present with complaints of acute or chronic injuries. Like the shoulder, nursing care will be focused on swelling, neurovascular compromise in the face of acute injuries, and pain management strategies. In more chronic conditions of the elbow, wrist, or hand, such as arthritis or tendonitis, interventions will focus on adaptation strategies to eliminate activities that aggravate the condition.

The Shoulder

The shoulder consists of significant anatomy, providing for the five articulations, or joints, within the shoulder. These joints are cartilage-covered structures surrounded by muscles, tendons, and ligaments, allowing for the frictionless and fluid motion that is normally seen. The glenohumeral joint is the largest articulation within the shoulder. It is made up of the head of the humerus and the glenoid socket which comes off the most lateral aspect of the scapula (Figure 2-1).

The humerus is the long bone of the upper extremity that lies between the axilla and the forearm (see Figure 2-1). The proximal humerus has a rounded hemispheric head. Where it interfaces with the glenoid, it is referred to as the glenohumeral joint. The glenoid has a shallow fossa or cavity with a similar radius of curvature. The shoulder joint is shallow and can be likened to a golf ball on a tee. The glenoid labrum is a fibrous structure forming a rim from the bone, effectively deepening the glenoid for improved stability. The structures are completely enclosed by synovial tissue and a fibrous joint capsule. The cartilage of the head of the humerus is thicker at the center and thinner toward the periphery. The glenoid fossa has opposite features, in that it is thinner at the center and thicker toward the periphery. These properties effectively contribute to the stability of the shallow joint, deepening the socket by 50 percent (McMahon & Skinner, 2003).

Within the shoulder there are several ligaments: the inferior, middle, and superior glenohumeral ligaments (Musgrave & Rodosky, 2001). Together with the biceps and coracoacromial and coracoclavicular ligaments, these soft tissues provide for added constraints to enhance the stability of the glenohumeral joint. Injuries to these structures can contribute to instability and result in added injury.

The scapula is a large, flat, triangular-shaped bone, articulating with the posterior-lateral chest wall. It serves mainly for

Figure 2-2
The Shoulder: Rotator Cuff Muscles

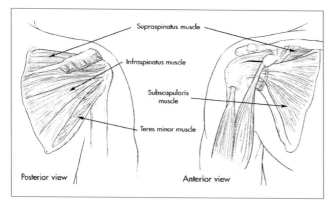

Supraspinatus muscle

Infraspinatus muscle

Subscapularis muscle

Teres minor muscle

Posterior view

Anterior view

Reprinted with permission from Rockwood, C., & Matsen, F. (1990). *The shoulder*. Philadelphia: W.B. Saunders.

muscle attachment (Jobe, 1998). The scapula overlaps the second to seventh ribs. Its concave undersurface glides over the muscles of the posterior thorax, accommodating and increasing the motion of the upper extremity by rotating. The scapular spine is a bony ridge that ends distally with the acromion process. The clavicle meets the acromion process to make up the acromioclavicular joint.

The coracoid process comes off of the scapula as well and serves as an attachment of muscles, tendons, and ligaments. The coracoid process is the attachment site of the short head of the biceps and coracobrachialis tendons, the pectoralis minor muscle, and the coracoacromial, coracohumeral, and coracoclavicular ligaments.

The clavicle, or collarbone, runs horizontally from the sternum to the acromion (Figure 2-1). The clavicle articulates with the manubrium of the sternum and the cartilage of the first rib on its medial border to form the sternoclavicular joint. The lateral aspect articulates with the acromion. The shaft of the collarbone is serpentine-shaped and easily palpated anterior and superior to the chest wall. Clavicular injuries are the most common bony injury resulting from trauma to the shoulder (Schoen, 2000).

The glenohumeral joint is deep within the axilla. The tendons of 4 different muscles reinforce the glenohumeral joint capsule. Together, these structures are referred to as the rotator cuff (RC), as seen in Figure 2-2. They can be remembered as the "SITS" muscles: the Supraspinatus, which runs above the joint; the Infraspinatus and Teres minor, which cross the joint posteriorly and insert on the greater tuberosity of the humerus; and the Subscapularis, which arises from the anterior scapula and crosses the joint anteriorly to insert on the lesser tuberosity of the humerus (Jobe, 2003). The RC muscles unite within the subacromial space which is beneath the acromion process. As the shoulder moves, the common tendon unit glides beneath the acromion process. These motions are cushioned because of the overlying bursa.

The role of the RC is to stabilize the humeral head on the glenoid. The RC muscles facilitate shoulder motion by working with the deltoid to produce active motion, especially abduction and external rotation. The cuff is musculotendinous and can undergo degenerative changes with age and rupture in areas of wear or thinning. The cuff can also tear in the face of acute trauma. Not a part of the rotator cuff, the deltoid is the largest muscle of the shoulder. It possesses three heads originating off the clavicle, the acromion, and the scapula. It fully encapsulates the shoulder anteriorly, posteriorly, medially, and laterally.

Common conditions affecting the shoulder can be categorized as either acute or chronic. Acute conditions of the shoulder and upper arm include fractures, shoulder joint dislocations (glenohumeral), acromioclavicular separations, tendon ruptures (biceps or RC), and labral tears, which are actually cartilage tears in the shoulder. Chronic conditions also include RC tears, as well as glenohumeral and/or acromioclavicular arthritis, shoulder instability and/or recurrent dislocation, and adhesive capsulitis or "frozen shoulder". Shoulder conditions can be quite painful and debilitating, as the shoulder is critical to moving the upper extremity in all the directions to perform activities of daily living (ADLs).

The Elbow

The elbow joint is comprised of the distal humerus and the proximal radius and ulna. The humerus consists of the rounded medial and lateral condyles which interface with the radial head and the olecranon, the more proximal aspect of the ulna. The olecranon is the bony prominence felt at the elbow joint; bursitis and tendonitis can either be acute or chronic in this region. Fractures can arise within each of the condyles above, below, and between. The radius and the olecranon can also fracture with trauma and are especially suspect in the face of dislocations. Dislocations of the elbow are common childhood injuries and are commonly associated with a fall on an outstretched hand (Orflay, 2001).

The Wrist

The distal radius and head of the ulna meet the carpals of the hand which are eight small bones within the wrist region. Distal radius fractures are the most common fractures of the upper extremity (AAOS, 2009). The radius is the larger of the two forearm bones distally and is concave in shape as it interfaces with the lunate and scaphoid bones. The ulna lies adjacent to the lunate as well as the pisiform carpal bone. The radius, ulna, and the first three bones within the palm of the hand make up the wrist joint. See Figure 2-3 for anatomy of the hand and wrist.

Common conditions affecting the wrist include wrist fractures and conditions such as carpal tunnel syndrome which is a condition of nerve entrapment that results from repetitive motions about the wrist. Wrist fractures can be treated surgically or conservatively. Carpel tunnel syndrome may be treated with conservative bracing or by surgical release of tissues that entrap the nerves.

Beyond the carpal bones are the metacarpals of which there are five. Distal to the metacarpal bones are the bones or

Figure 2-3
Hand/Wrist Anatomy

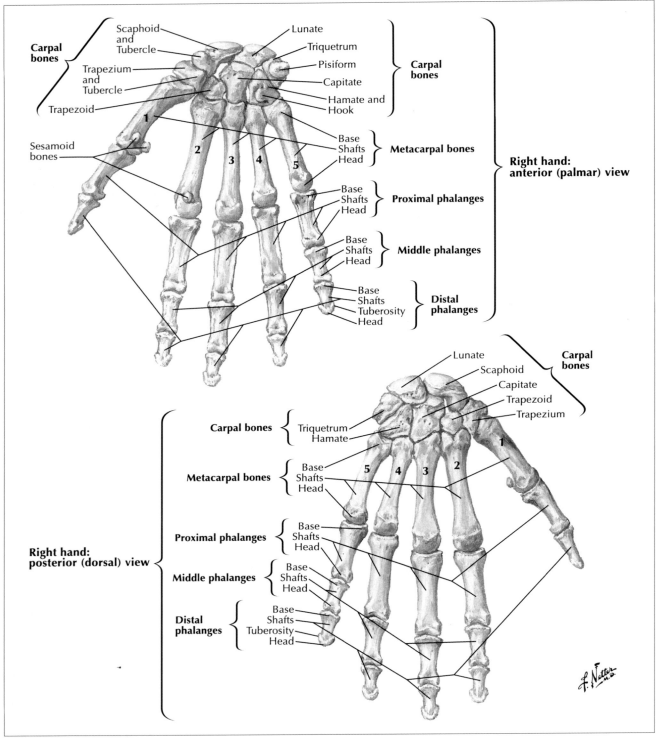

Netter illustration used with permission of Elsevier, Inc. All rights reserved. www.netterimages.com.

fingers, called phalanges. Fractures to any of these structures occur as a result of falls, getting a hand caught in a door, or jamming the hand during a sport activity. Fractures result in pain, swelling, and potential deformity. These bones are routinely splinted until sufficient healing can occur. Anywhere ligaments exist within the wrist and hand, sprains can also arise when the ligaments that connect the bones become stretched or completely torn. Most sprains are cared for using rest, icing, compression, and elevation (RICE).

Lacerations can commonly occur in the hand as a result of work accidents or utilization of knives for cooking. These injuries not only disrupt soft tissues, but they may also sever tendons which can permanently affect hand function if not addressed properly. Animal and human bites are another acute injury seen in orthopaedics. These types of wounds are inspected and cared for with aggressive local wound care and antibiotics. More chronic wrist and hand conditions include arthritis, carpal tunnel syndrome, and contractures of ligaments within the hand.

Physical Assessment

The history is a very important part of any patient assessment. It should be elicited prior to the actual physical exam. Clues to pathology may be conveyed by the patient on this evaluation and lead to the use of additional, adjunctive exam techniques. Alternatively, the medical history may clue the examiner to other causes of shoulder pain or weakness, such as when cervical spine or neurologic pathology exists. Timing the onset of symptoms, precipitating events, and activity modifications used to control symptoms, and the nature of symptoms at rest and with activity will help to understand the causes of pathology and determine interventions to treat the patient's condition. Patients may describe shoulder pain, weakness, popping, catching, stiffness, difficult motion, and feelings of instability. These symptoms should be correlated to the exam. At times, clinicians will employ provocative tests for the shoulder in an effort to provoke sensations of instability and more accurately pinpoint pathology.

Examination of the upper extremity is best accomplished without outer garments to visualize compensation efforts the patient may rely on to perform normal ranges of motion. This is especially true of the shoulder complex where visualization of the anterior, posterior, and lateral chest is important to note weakness and atrophy. The examiner will be able to compare the affected extremity to the unaffected side at rest and then during passive and active motion. Table 2-1 describes and demonstrates normal range of motion for the shoulder. Swelling, contour changes, bruising, and muscle tightness or atrophy should also be noted. Strength assessments of the upper extremity should include all muscle groups of the arm and hand (see Chapter 1, *Musculoskeletal System: Basics of Anatomic Structure and Neurovascular Assessment*, for muscle strength grading). Diminished strength may indicate neurologic or muscle injury, but weakness may also be elicited when painful conditions are present. A neurovascular exam should also be performed for the entire extremity (see Chapter 1).

Impingement signs are maneuvers that "pinch" the rotator cuff and produce pain. They are typically motions that compress the subacromial space and limit the motion of the common tendon within the space. Pain and an inability to produce full motion may indicate a tear, significant inflammation, and/or tendonitis of the rotator cuff. Positive

Table 2-1
Shoulder Range of Motion

Forward Flexion – 180° With arms in full extension and at their side, the patient raises his/her arms straight and above the head, bringing them out in front first, then raising them above and past their head as much as possible.	
Extension – 50° With arms in full extension, the patient stretches their arms behind their back as far as possible. This position is hyperextension.	
Abduction – 180° With arms at their side, the patient lifts his/her arms away from their side and parallel to the shoulders.	
Adduction – 50° With their arms at their side, the patient adducts, crossing the arms at the midline.	
External Rotation – 90° With their elbows flexed and parallel with the shoulders, the patient rotates their palms upward and parallel with their head.	
Internal Rotation – 90° With the elbows flexed and parallel to the shoulders, the patient rotates their palms downward toward the floor and parallel with the body.	

Author creation/photography.

tests, along with reports of ongoing pain in the anterior and lateral shoulder region, especially at night, should raise suspicion of a rotator cuff injury or inflammation. Other pathology such as bicep tendon ruptures or inflammation should also be considered when examining a patient. In any case where an acute event precipitated the painful condition, suspicion of fractures and or sprains should also be foremost. While most shoulder exam techniques are not highly specific to any condition, positive tests are often good indicators of specific injury sites.

In any part of the upper extremity, deformities can be noted in both acute and chronic conditions. In the face of acute events, bruising and immediate swelling often accompany fractures. In more chronic conditions, deformities arise with the destruction of joint spaces as in arthritis, or they can be more obvious as with contractures. Good visual inspection will lead to a more precise diagnosis and appropriate diagnostic testing.

Evaluation of the elbow and wrist joints should include an assessment of strength and a neurovascular exam. Fractures alone or in the face of subsequent swelling can result in progressive nerve injury in the small spaces of the upper extremity. An ability to sense touch over the lateral arm and forearm will indicate an intact axillary nerve. The ability to flex and extend the wrist, pinch and cross the fingers, are strongly supportive of intact radial and ulnar nerves. Any reports of paresthesias or weakness should be reported immediately. When casts are present and the patient reports increasing pain, compartment syndromes are also of concern.

Diagnostics

Once a physical examination has been undertaken, diagnostics are considered. Standard plain radiographs are routinely the first test and the most common procedure performed to identify fractures, dislocations, or other bony pathology such as arthritis. A high riding humerus on x-ray can be helpful in identifying rotator cuff tears, demonstrating that the incompetent cuff is not reinforcing the glenohumeral joint by keeping the humerus on the glenoid. Plain radiographs also easily demonstrate destructive changes within joint spaces whether they are in the shoulder, elbow, wrist, or hand.

Computed axial tomography (CAT) scans, arthrography (intraarticular joint dye injection), and magnetic resonance imaging (MRI) are more sophisticated tests and are indicated for specific conditions. CAT scans can be used to assess fractures, especially when more complex surgical planning is required. MRI may be employed to assess soft tissues in conditions such as RC tears or cartilage tears within the shoulder joint.

Labral (shoulder cartilage) abnormalities such as Bankart lesions and injuries such as superior labral anterior posterior (SLAP) lesions may be diagnosed with MRI. Surgeons will also employ surgical arthroscopy in the face of patient history and physical findings to diagnose specific conditions in the shoulder. Arthroscopic surgery allows immediate surgical intervention to improve the patient's condition,

while allowing direct visualization of the shoulder anatomy. The surgery may be accompanied by an injection of contrast material into the joint to assist visualization of soft tissues.

Electrical testing is employed when carpal tunnel syndrome is suspected. Carpal tunnel syndrome can result from nerve entrapment and swelling of the nerves within the wrist. Electrophysiological testing (EMG) examines the conduction of nerve impulses along the nerve to measure the degree of constriction.

Surgical Anesthesia and Pain Management for the Upper Extremity

Both arthroscopic and open shoulder surgery can be associated with pain significant enough to affect recovery and rehabilitation. Opiates are routinely employed postoperatively, but they are associated with nausea, vomiting, sedation, and somnolence (Neal, McDonald, Larkin, & Polissar, 2003). Adjunctive medications and modalities may also be employed to decrease the need for postoperative opiates. Medications include non-steroidal anti-inflammatory medications (NSAIDs) and non-opiate analgesics such as Acetaminophen (Tylenol®) and Tramadol (Ultram®). Ice is also important for pain control and management of swelling. Pain pumps are frequently employed for postoperative pain management. These devices hold 100 to 150 milliliters of local anesthetic medications that infuse slowly into the incision and or joint space over 24 to 48 hours.

Operative anesthetics can be general, regional, or combined. General anesthetics require intubation and paralytic medications. Regional anesthetics block sensations and motor function to specific regions of the body. Regional anesthetics are performed by anesthesiology and may typically be used to provide pain relief for a period of up to 12 to 24 hours postoperatively. Peripheral or regional blocks help to provide analgesia with fewer side effects, faster functional recovery, and greater patient satisfaction (Liu & Salinas, 2003).

Regional anesthetics for shoulder surgery involve injecting a numbing agent such as lidocaine or bupivacaine around the brachial plexus, which is located within the scalene muscle. The brachial plexus innervates the axilla, rotator cuff, the joint capsule, the subscapularis, and the rest of the arm (Long, Wass, & Burkle, 2002). In some cases, a catheter may be left in place for continuous infusion of the anesthetic medication for longer-term pain relief (Liu & Salinas, 2003; Ekatodramis et al., 2003; Casati et al., 2003). Leakage of solution around the catheter insertion site can occur and should be minimal; reinforcement with gauze and tape may help. Excessive leakage may require removal of the catheter. With outpatient surgery, patients are taught to remove the pain pump once it is empty.

Conscious sedation is a near-anesthetic delivery of medications, used to perform procedures on a patient without loss of consciousness. Patients maintain a degree of consciousness but must be monitored for respiratory depression. Equipment for intubation and medication reversal must be readily available. This type of sedation might be used for relocation of a shoulder dislocation or realignment of a fracture outside of the operating room. Respiratory depression is always a concern when this technique is used. Nursing personnel are typically responsible for administering medications, monitoring vital signs and oxygen saturation, and, often, recovering the patient. Most hospitals have specific policies for the use of conscious sedation.

Common Orthopaedic Shoulder Pathology and Treatment

Shoulder conditions can be acute or chronic, involving the soft tissue and/or the osseous anatomy. Acute shoulder conditions are dislocations or subluxations, muscle ruptures, fractures, and RC tears. RC tears may be both acute and chronic. Other chronic conditions include osteoarthritis, rheumatoid arthritis, secondary or post-traumatic arthritis, and adhesive capsulitis. Arthritis may involve the glenohumeral or the acromioclavicular joints.

Adhesive capsulitis or "frozen shoulder" results from adhesions in the joint capsule that effectively shrink the capsular folds and limit shoulder motion. Patients are often inappropriately labeled as having "frozen shoulder" when presenting with stiffness secondary to pain rather than a documented capsular shrinkage. Adhesive capsulitis tends to occur commonly in diabetes, and it may arise after a soft tissue injury (Wirth, 2001) or spontaneously without any recognized cause.

Shoulder Dislocations/Instability

Shoulder dislocations are defined and described by the direction of displacement of the humeral head. They can be anterior, posterior, inferior, and multidirectional (Wirth, 2001). Injuries to the shoulder architecture include injuries to the bony and soft tissue anatomy. Dislocation may occur traumatically with the motions of abduction, extension, and external rotation, which go beyond what can be controlled by the soft tissue and bony restraints. With dislocation, pain and muscle tensing is common. Other injuries may arise during the dislocation event, such as fractures and cartilage tears. Opiate medications and intra-articular numbing agents facilitate relaxation and pain control during manipulation and reduction. Traction maneuvers to reduce the joint have been employed since Hippocrates (Jobe, 1998). Alternatively, a patient's shoulder may be relocated more slowly with the aid of gravity or weights attached to the affected extremity. With traction or after the application of weights, specific maneuvers are employed to facilitate relocation of the humerus on the glenoid (Swiontkowski, 2001). After relocation, x-rays must be used to confirm proper alignment of the humerus.

Acute dislocations, once reduced, are immobilized to support the shoulder structures and prevent subsequent subluxation, allowing the tissues to heal. The duration of immobilization depends on the type of dislocation, history of previous dislocations, and the patent's age. Nursing care includes neurovascular assessments, pain management, and

patient education about protected motion and activities of daily living. After a first-time dislocation, the shoulder may be immobilized in a sling for up to 6 weeks depending on the patient's age, the expected rate of recurrence, and other associated injuries. Subsequent dislocations are common despite duration or method of immobilization, especially in

Figure 2-4
Pendulum Exercises

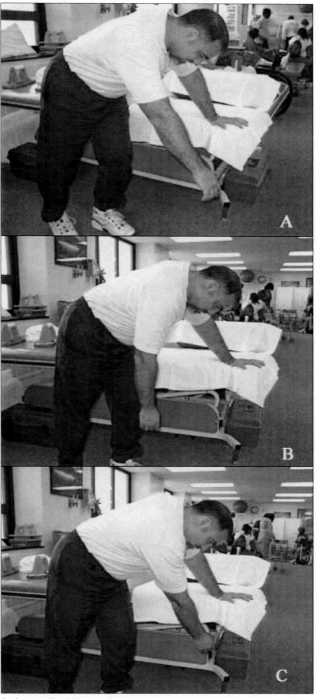

Author creation/photography.

the young (Swiontkowski, 2001; Hovelius et al, 1996). Dislocations in patients younger than 20 years old tend to occur more commonly in association with an avulsion of the labrum, Bankart lesions, and injuries to the glenohumeral ligaments. In contrast, patients older than 50 suffer associated cuff tears and fractures of the humerus (Swiontkowski, 2001). Post-reduction, patients are instructed to move their fingers, elbow, and wrist, and perform pendulum exercises, as seen in Figure 2-4. These exercises help to prevent stiffness and loss of motion (Walch & Boileau, 1997). Pendulum exercises require the patient to lean forward, dangle the affected arm, and create a gentle swinging motion.

Labral pathology such as SLAP lesions can occur with or without dislocation, but they are also common athletic injuries. A traumatic event, such as a fall on an outstretched hand, may result in the humeral head being forced into the labrum and the biceps tendon. The tendon ruptures away from the labrum, or the labrum becomes frayed in the superior anterior or the superior posterior aspect of the joint. Repetitive motion such as pitching baseballs can also force the humeral head beyond the constraints of the joint. SLAP lesions are graded as I through IV, based on the extensiveness of the soft tissue injury and the location of the tear (Kim, Queale, Cosgarea, & McFarland, 2003).

Another soft tissue injury that results during acute dislocation is the Bankart lesion. Bankart lesions involve the anterior glenoid labrum, which is the fibrocartilaginous rim of tissue that deepens the glenohumeral joint. A tear or disruption of the rim results in an alteration of the normal constraints of the joint, contributing to further dislocations and ongoing instability. Surgery may be done to repair the torn labrum, which will help to prevent subsequent dislocations. Bankart lesions and SLAP lesions may be evaluated diagnostically via magnetic resonance imaging (MRI).

Another disorder that is seen due to a traumatic dislocation is a Hill-Sachs lesion. This lesion is an osseous injury (fracture) to the head of the humerus. The lesion is actually an impression fracture of the posterior humeral head that occurs when the dislocated humeral head abuts the anterior glenoid rim. The shoulder abducts, externally rotates too far, and dislocates. Larger lesions are seen with recurrent dislocations (Matsen, Thomas, Rockwood, & Wirth, 1998). A Hill-Sachs lesion is evidence that an anterior dislocation has occurred (Wirth, 2001), although a McLaughlin or Reverse Hill-Sachs lesion (similar to a Hill-Sachs lesion, but in the anterior head) may be seen in posterior dislocations (McMahon & Skinner, 2003). These fractures are actually compression injuries or indentations of the bone. Open reduction or joint reconstruction may be considered if a defect greater than 40 percent exists (Matsen et al., 1998) to prevent eventual arthritic changes within the joint.

Arthroscopic surgery may be employed to surgically treat SLAP lesions, Bankart lesions, and Hill-Sachs lesions. Arthroscopic surgery results in small incisions, each requiring sutures on the front, back, and side of the shoulder joint. The sutures are removed in approximately 5-7 days. The need for immobilization of the patient's arm and physical therapy after surgery is best determined by the surgeon after an evaluation of the shoulder during surgery. This allows for an assessment of tension in the newly repaired soft tissue structures.

Shoulder Separations

A very common shoulder injury is a shoulder separation. This type of injury affects the acromioclavicular (AC) joint. A shoulder separation is different from a dislocation or subluxation of the glenohumeral joint. The AC joint involves the capsular ligaments of the joint itself, as well as the nearby restraining coracoclavicular ligaments that arise from the coracoid. When the AC joint is overstressed, frequently with a direct blow to the shoulder, as when hockey players are checked into the boards, the supporting ligaments become either stretched or disrupted (torn). This causes pain, swelling, bruising, and instability within the shoulder area. Treatment for shoulder separations routinely consists of a sling for comfort, ice, and analgesics, with return to regular activities in approximately 4 to 6 weeks. More severe grades of separations are usually treated surgically (Wirth, 2001).

Biceps Tendon Rupture

A biceps tendon rupture, a common injury, usually occurs in the tendinous portion in the upper arm. Patients often describe sudden pain, swelling, loss of strength, and a visible bulge in their lower arm, with or without an audible snap (Taft, 1996; Wirth, 2001). The injury is usually followed by significant ecchymosis. There is an obvious cosmetic difference in each arm, as the muscle appears to migrate distally. Most patients do not require surgery for this condition, as the rupture is mostly cosmetic and does not routinely limit a patient's function. Usually with conservative care, the pain resolves with rest and the use of a sling. Having the elbow immobilized relaxes the muscle. Distal tendon ruptures, proximal ruptures in younger patients, individuals who perform heavy labor, and/or patients in pain despite conservative treatment, may require surgical intervention. Surgical treatment consists of reattaching the tendon to the humerus bone at the bicipital groove in proximal injures, and to the radial tuberosity in distal tendon ruptures.

Rotator Cuff Tears

Rotator cuff disease or injury is the most common shoulder condition seen in an orthopaedic practice (Cofield et al., 2001). The cuff may wear as a result of repetitive activity, falls, throwing, heavy lifting, or dislocation (Bagwell-Crum, 2001). In general terms, cuff pathology spans simple irritation, abrasion, partial tear, complete tear, capsular tear with muscle disruption and tissue loss, and rotator cuff arthropathy. If surgery is indicated for cuff pathology, the focus includes the bony and ligamentous tissues, as these structures may impinge on the repaired tissue. Older patients tend to have larger tears as a result of fibrosis and degeneration of the tissues, as opposed to younger patients who have healthier tendons. Tears without a traumatic event are not common before the age of 40.

Initially, chronic tears and partial cuff injuries are treated conservatively with physical therapy, pain medications, and steroid injections. Surgery is indicated when conservative treatment fails and the patient has persistent pain, or for more unusual conditions such as large traumatic, acute, or full thickness tears. In the case of chronic tears, most patients also have a component of impingement, whereby the acromion pinches the tendinous complex of the rotator cuff in the subacromial space. In those instances, an acromioplasty is usually performed at the same time as the RC repair to improve the motion of the tendon within the space. Acromioplasty involves debridement or smoothing of the underlying acromion to remove spurs or boney overgrowths. The procedure provides a larger space for the rotator cuff tendon to glide through as the shoulder moves through normal daily motions.

The size of the tear is the most important determinant of outcome after rotator cuff surgery. Postoperatively, the type of therapy and mobilization tends to be driven by the surgeon's visualization of how much tension existed on the RC tendon at the time of repair. Immobilization or slinging after surgery helps to relieve pain, to remind the patient to avoid active use of the arm, and to allow for healing to occur (Cofield et al., 2001). Rehabilitation includes early passive range of motion to avoid stiffness (Yamaguchi et al., 2003). Unfortunately, whether the RC condition is repaired open or arthroscopically, the tissues need to heal prior to being used actively. Healing takes at least 6 weeks and typically longer.

Impingement

Impingement is a condition which arises when the space beneath the acromion and the coracoid ligament narrows. A bursa cushions the cuff beneath the acromion arch, but with narrowing of the space the tissues can become inflamed and frayed, resulting in pain and motion limitations (Bigliani & Levine, 1997). Patients typically complain of pain in the anterior-lateral aspect of the shoulder. With impingement, the supraspinatus is pinched between the humeral head and an opposing structure, either the acromion, AC joint osteophytes, or coracoacromial ligament, leading to inflammation, edema, and bursitis. Osteophytes can overgrow within the space further constraining the ligaments, resulting in degradation of the cuff complex.

The diagnosis of impingement is made by examination. Patients will typically have predictable pain with abduction and internal rotation, or internal rotation and flexion. A small injection of lidocaine or other local anesthetic may be placed into the subacromial space. After the injection, if the subjective symptoms of pain are significantly diminished, the implication is that the symptomatology is due to subacromial impingement. Steroids may also be injected to help reduce the inflammation that is causing the discomfort.

Conservative treatment for impingement is similar to that for a RC tear and consists of physical therapy, non-steroidal-anti-inflammatory medications (NSAIDs), and intraarticular injections. Non-operative care is often successful. Surgical treatment may be required when the patient's symptoms last longer than 6 months despite conservative treatment.

Surgical care involves a decompression of the subacromial space with resection of the coracoacromial ligament, usually an acromioplasty, and possibly a Mumford procedure (Bigliani & Levine, 1997). These procedures are now frequently being performed arthroscopically.

Shoulder Arthritis

Arthritis of the shoulder, like other joints in the body, can result in significant pain. See Chapter 5, *Care of the Patient with Hip, Foot and Ankle Problems*, for a discussion of arthritis. As with other shoulder disorders, patients with arthritis usually present to an orthopaedic surgeon because of pain and/or loss of motion. The patient is examined, and radiographs are routinely taken. Arthritis of the shoulder usually involves one or both of the primary joints, the acromioclavicular joint or the glenohumeral joint. AC joint arthritis is common, but patients are not as routinely symptomatic as they are with glenohumeral joint arthritis. Patients with AC arthritis more commonly report pain that is due to cuff impingement and demonstrate tenderness over the AC joint. With AC joint pathology patients have pain with flexion, cross-body motions, and complain of pain during sleep. Treatment for AC arthritis may involve NSAIDs, narcotic medications, physical therapy, intra-articular steroid injections, and/or surgery (Swiontkowski, 2001). The Mumford procedure is a surgical technique used to remove the distal clavicle. It can be done arthroscopically or through an open incision.

Glenohumeral joint arthritis behaves more like the other large joint arthritides. The cause of the arthritis may be osteoarthritis (OA), rheumatoid arthritis (RA), or post-traumatic, secondary arthritis. Pain management in arthritic conditions may include NSAIDs and narcotics, heat, and activity modifications. Intra-articular steroid injections may also be employed to treat the associated acute and subacute synovitis. Most doctors recommend limiting injections to

Figure 2-5
Hemiarthroplasty

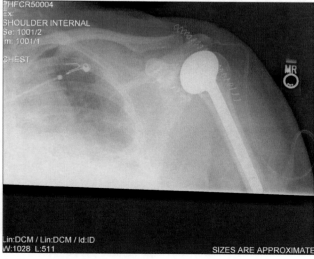

Author creation/photography.

Figure 2-6
Reverse Total Shoulder

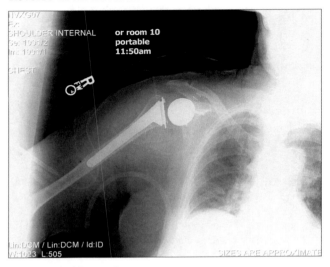

Author creation/photography.

3 per year if they prove to be effective, because steroids may adversely affect the cartilage and tendons of the rotator cuff (Chen, Joseph, & Zuckerman, 2003). Yet, when compared to physical therapy alone, patients receiving injections along with therapy demonstrated better outcomes related to pain and disability (van der Windt et al., 1998).

Shoulder arthroplasty is a surgical intervention for arthritis in patients who have failed conservative treatment. Other indications for arthroplasty include avascular necrosis, osteonecrosis, complicated proximal humerus fractures, malunion of a previous fracture, and pathology. Goals of joint replacement include better motion, function, and pain relief. Strength is rarely restored. Shoulder hemiarthroplasty (Figure 2-5) involves replacement of the humeral head with an endoprosthesis. The prosthesis articulates with the native glenoid. Two additional procedures exist to resurface the glenoid and the humeral head. In total shoulder arthroplasty, the humeral head is replaced with a hemispheric head much like that of a hip replacement. The glenoid is resurfaced as well. Candidates for this procedure have an intact rotator cuff. A reverse total shoulder arthroplasty is a more recent procedure (FDA approved in 2004) for those with a completely torn rotator cuff or a previous total shoulder arthroplasty (AAOS, 2007). For this procedure, the glenoid is resurfaced with a hemispheric component, much like the head of the humerus. The humerus is replaced with a socket-like prosthesis, thus "reversing" the typical placement of the components (Figure 2-6).

The decision to perform total shoulder arthroplasty versus hemiarthroplasty depends upon the patient's history, wear of the joint, bony pathology, condition of the soft tissues (especially the RC), and surgical philosophy. Both procedures provide pain reduction and usually improved motion and function (Sperling, Cofield, & Rowland, 1998). As with any arthroplasty, life of the implant will vary, but appropriate patient selection is important when predicting

success. The integrity of the RC is one of the most important determinants of outcome. If a patient has a non-repairable cuff tear, outcome of total shoulder arthroplasty is often poor due to glenoid loosening (Cofield et al., 2001). In these cases, hemiarthroplasty or reverse shoulder arthroplasty may be recommended (Smith & Matsen, 1998) as these designs help to compensate for compromised cuff integrity. Reverse shoulder arthroplasty patients achieve greater than ninety degrees of abduction and no adduction deficits (Gutierrez, Comiskey, Luo, Pupello, & Frankle, 2008). Complications of arthroplasty include problems with balancing of the humerus on the glenoid (instability), loosening, fractures, rotator cuff tears, heterotropic ossification, nerve injury, and infection (Cuomo & Checroun, 1998).

On the day of surgery, the patient is seen in the preoperative suite by an anesthesiologist and his/her surgeon. The surgical site should be confirmed by the surgeon at that time and initialed or signed. Preoperative antibiotics are administered and usually continued for twenty four hours after the procedure. For upper extremity surgeries, patients are given an operative anesthetic: general, regional, or both. Surgery is often performed with the patient in a beach chair position, which is a slightly reclined, sitting position.

The surgery is usually accomplished through a classic deltopectoral approach, in which the interval between the deltoid and the pectoralis major is dissected with an attempt to preserve the cephalic vein. The subscapularis tendon and the underlying joint capsule are divided, exposing the joint. The humeral head is dislocated and then resected. If a total shoulder arthroplasty is to be performed, the glenoid is resurfaced and a plastic component is implanted. For a total shoulder arthroplasty and a hemiarthroplasty, a metallic stem is usually implanted with a modular head component. The stem is either press-fit or cemented into the humeral canal after reaming. Sizing of the head is important to balance the joint. Overstuffing the joint is not desired, and proper rotation is required to prevent dislocation. The rotator cuff is inspected, and the soft tissue structures are balanced (Chen et al., 2003). With a reverse total shoulder arthroplasty, the components are different in that the stem side which is implanted into the humerus is concave and has the appearance of a cup. The glenoid is resurfaced and a rounded or hemispheric component is put in place.

Immediately after surgery, the patient's arm is supported in a sling or immobilizer. A sling is used for approximately 2 to 6 weeks, especially when sleeping, to protect the shoulder. The sling is essential to protect the repair of the subscapularis tendon and the capsule, which are at risk for disruption especially with external rotation. Dressings are placed over the incision. Drains are not routinely used. Pain management can be accomplished several ways, using opioids, ice, NSAIDs, long acting regional blocks, and/or pain pumps. Patients are at a very small risk for venous thromboembolism, compared to patients having hip or knee replacement. Thrombolytic prevention is at the discretion of the surgeon. Anti-embolic hose and foot pumps or venous sequential pumps are often employed until the patient is ambulatory. Lower extremity mobility should resume quickly, although patients may require assistance initially for balance and ADLs. Patients are frequently discharged home as early as the first postoperative day.

Rehabilitation begins immediately for patients after a total shoulder arthroplasty. For patients undergoing reverse arthroplasties, therapy doesn't begin until the sling is removed at about 6 weeks. All patients are initially instructed on passive range of motion of the shoulder for the first 4 to 6 weeks (Chen et al., 2003). These patients should not push, pull, or lift with the surgical extremity until instructed by their physician. Weight-bearing restrictions preclude lifting objects and forcing weight through the hand of the affected extremity.

Total shoulder arthroplasty reconstructs the joint to be more like the original, native anatomic structures. Reverse total shoulder arthroplasty surgery is performed for an incompetent rotator cuff as well as arthritis within the glenohumeral joint. Therefore, functional outcomes after surgery may be better for total shoulder arthroplasty patients than reverse total shoulder patients.

Isometric exercises and active assisted range of motion exercises are initiated approximately 4 to 6 weeks after surgery for total shoulder arthroplasty. Resistive strengthening exercises begin 10 to 12 weeks later. The primary goal of surgery is pain relief and improved range of motion which may require 6 to 12 months to maximize. Abduction will be the first motion a patient loses with arthritis and the last motion to recover after surgery. Internal rotation is often a problem as well. Internal rotation of the shoulder is required for routine hygiene during toileting, reaching into a back pocket, and hooking a bra.

The nature of the implant for a reverse total shoulder arthroplasty restricts internal rotation and elevation of the arm. Therefore, to prevent disruption of the implant during rehabilitation, the shoulder must not be internally rotated or raised higher than the top of the head. These restrictions may interfere with normal daily routines such as hygiene and dressing. Rehabilitation begins 6 weeks postoperatively and focuses primarily on strengthening the deltoid to compensate for the position restrictions. Even with motion restrictions, rehabilitation for the patient with reverse total shoulder arthroplasty typically takes less time than that for total shoulder arthroplasty.

As with any total joint arthroplasty procedure, antibiotic prophylaxis prior to dental procedures must be considered for patients who have undergone total shoulder or reverse total shoulder arthroplasty. The American Dental Association and the Academy of Orthopaedic Surgeons (AAOS) issued an advisory statement in 2003 regarding antibiotic prophylaxis for dental procedures. Prophylactic antibiotics are recommended for total joint arthroplasty patients who are undergoing high risk dental procedures within two years of their surgery. High risk procedures include dental extractions, dental implants, root canals beyond the apex, and prophylactic cleaning of teeth or implants where bleeding is anticipated. See Chapter 4, *Care of the Patient with Knee Problems*, for further discussion of prophylactic use of antibiotics prior to dental procedures for total joint arthroplasty procedures.

Common Orthopaedic Elbow, Wrist, and Hand Conditions

Chronic conditions of the elbow include arthritis and tendonitis. Total elbow arthroplasty may be used to treat patients with disability and pain related to arthritis when conservative measures have failed. Elbow arthroplasty provides good clinical results, even in younger patients, with studies demonstrating acceptable survival rates of the implants (Celli & Morrey, 2009). Nursing care will focus on pain management, swelling, and elevation with hand motion to promote circulation and reduction of swelling.

Another common condition affecting the elbow is tendonitis or "tennis elbow". This condition arises when repetitive motion of the elbow results in inflammation of the tendons around the elbow. Bursitis can also arise in these tissues. NSAIDs, non-opioid analgesics, splinting, rest from aggravating activities, and icing in the acute phase are most beneficial.

Within the wrist structures, carpal tunnel is one of the most common conditions. The nerves become entrapped within the soft tissues resulting in pain and numbness within the palm of the hand. Pain can be especially pronounced at night. Carpal tunnel syndrome can be diagnosed accurately using clinical criteria (Graham, 2008). The Tinel sign can be used to distinguish carpal tunnel syndrome by lightly tapping over the inside of the wrist. A positive sign elicits pain and paresthesias over the hand, ring, and little fingers. Electro-diagnostic testing (EMG) as previously described may also be used as a diagnostic tool. Initial conservative care may include wrist splints to alleviate discomfort, steroid injections, and elimination or reduction of aggravating activities. Patients may require surgical release of soft tissues in an effort to relieve the nerve entrapment.

A common entrapment condition within the hand is "trigger finger". The condition is treated in the early stages with cortisone injections (Rozental, Zurakowski, & Blazer, 2008). When conservative measures fail, surgical release can be used. The surgical procedure is performed in an outpatient setting using a small bevel needle to release the tissues. Post procedure, the patient will require icing and minimal local wound care.

Not unlike the elbow and the shoulder, the hand can be afflicted with arthritis significant enough to warrant resection arthroplasty. Initial treatment for arthritis of the hand includes splinting and steroid injections. Surgery is indicated for pain relief and restoration of function. Any arthritic joint in the hand can undergo arthroplasty, although thumb arthroplasty is the most common replacement surgery performed. Hand arthroplasties are typically performed in an outpatient setting. Post-thumb arthroplasty, patients are typically placed in a thumb-spica cast. Physical therapy is started one month postoperatively. Grip and pinching exercises are delayed for approximately 6-8 weeks (Tomaino, 2008).

Fractures of the upper extremity

Fractures of the upper extremity may involve any of the bony structures of the shoulder. The clavicle, scapula

Figure 2-7
Open Reduction Internal Fixation:
   A. Proximal humerus fracture with screw fixation
   **B. Proximal humerus fracture with plate
      and screws**

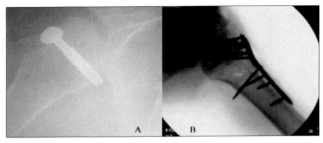

Author creation/photography.

(acromion, coracoid, or glenoid), or the humerus may be affected. Fractures also arise in the distal humerus, the radius and ulna, and within the bones of the hand. Fractures may result because of a fall on an outstretched hand, a blow to the upper extremity, or complex twisting or stretching beyond the normal constraints. Open fractures to any of these areas are considered a surgical emergency; patients should be taken to the operating room for immediate irrigation and drainage to prevent infection.

Clavicle fractures are extremely common, especially in children (Schoen, 2000). They are described based on the location of the fracture and degree of bony displacement. Patients are usually treated with a figure-of-eight strap, which wraps over the anterior aspect of each shoulder to keep the shoulders back and the clavicle in good alignment, or an arm sling (Wirth, 2001). Immobilization is primarily for pain control rather than fracture reduction. Mid-clavicle fractures comprise 80 percent of clavicle fractures. These fractures heal quite readily in a hanging-arm-cloth sling alone or a figure-of-eight sling (Schmitt, 1999). Displaced fractures, especially those that disrupt the acromioclavicular joint dynamics, may require an open reduction internal fixation (ORIF).

Fractures affecting the glenoid of the scapula are intra-articular fractures. Fractures involving more than 25 percent of the glenoid fossa or resulting in shoulder instability require an ORIF. The repair of soft tissue structures such as the capsule, labrum, or ligaments may also be required, depending upon the amount of disruption or injury at the time of fracture (Butters, 2001). Surgical incisions are routinely on the anterior aspect of the shoulder, with an ORIF requiring the use of screws. Fractures of the scapula, acromion, glenoid, or coracoid are less common and are associated with much higher traumatic forces such as seen with motor vehicle accidents. These fractures are often treated effectively with a sling and pain medications, unless significant displacement exists.

Fractures of the humerus are described as humeral shaft fractures and classified as either proximal, mid, or distal. Fractures to the distal shaft of the humerus may include fractures within, through, and above the elbow joint. Non-articular involvement and satisfactory reduction are indications for conservative care, while surgery may be indicated for patients suffering from neurovascular deficits, poor reductions, severe comminution, and fractures disrupting the articular surface (Altizer, 2003).

Mid-shaft humerus fractures are routinely treated with a sling, a hanging arm cast, or a fracture splint. They may also be treated with a combination U-shaped splint and sling. Union for most fractures is typically seen at 6-8 weeks. Surgical intervention may be required when good alignment is not possible because of the patient's physical characteristics. A large abdomen or pendulous breasts may result in unacceptable angulation of the fracture fragments. Fixation is therefore necessary to ensure optimal alignment and later functional ability. Fractures resulting in vascular or nerve injury, pathologic fractures, or those requiring fixation to facilitate early mobilization may require surgical care (Altizer, 2003). Humerus fractures may be surgically treated with compression plating, interlocking nails, or flexible nails. These may be inserted either proximally or distally to the fracture site (Gregory, 2001).

Proximal humerus fractures include fractures to the head and neck. Fractures of the proximal humerus are often classified as 1-, 2-, 3-, and 4-part fractures. Other descriptions may include compressed, displaced, or non-displaced fractures. Fractures can also be described according to their anatomic location such as the greater or lesser tuberosity, the proximal shaft, and the humeral head. Patients typically experience swelling, pain, and bruising in the shoulder or around the upper arm (Wirth, 2001).

Many proximal humerus fractures are minimally or non-displaced, so there is no need for surgery. These fractures are treated with a sling for a period of 3 weeks, or until callus formation is seen on x-ray. If the fracture is reduced but unstable because alignment is not consistent, then percutaneous pinning may be done (Flatow, 2001), or an ORIF may be performed as seen in Figure 2-7. Other surgical care involves plating, hemiarthroplasty, total shoulder arthroplasty, or reverse shoulder arthroplasty, depending on the fracture location, degree of comminution, the integrity of the rotator cuff, and the extent of displacement. Open reduction or shoulder arthroplasty is indicated for 3- and 4-part fractures, significant displacement, and shoulder instability. With ORIF, patients are started initially on passive range of motion, and then progressed to active assisted motion at approximately 6 weeks when callus is evident on follow-up radiographs.

Pathologic fractures occur secondary to osteoporosis, metabolic bone diseases, and cancer. Common cancers that spread to the bone are prostate, lung, breast, kidney, and thyroid. Fracture care in the case of metastatic disease involves immediate stabilization of the bony architecture to provide pain relief and improve the patient's remaining quality of life.

Prophylactic fixation of an impending pathologic fracture is indicated when there is a risk of progression to a complete fracture. Fixation is indicated for increasing pain or when the size of the fracture reaches critical levels, usually 50% of the diameter of the bone as seen on x-rays. Fixation is usually accomplished with an intramedullary fixation device in a closed fashion, without opening the fracture site. This allows for radiation early in the postoperative period.

If an open surgical approach is necessary, an intramedullary nail may be used. Intramedullary nails are inserted after the canal of the bone is reamed. The intramedullary nail is passed through the cortex of the bone and screws are inserted at the proximal and distal end of the nail (Swiontkowski, 2001). Patients who have intramedullary fixation are able to immediately bear weight on the extremity due to the support of the nail. Weight bearing may be limited in the patient with complex or unstable fractures, with osteoporotic bone, and after a difficult fixation. If radiation and/or chemotherapy are planned, surgical wounds should be allowed to heal and mature to prevent tissue breakdown or infection.

Elbow, forearm (radius & ulna), and hand fractures can arise due to a fall on an outstretched hand or after a traumatic blow to the upper extremity as seen with motor vehicle accidents. As with other bones and joints, care is guided by fracture care principles. If there is acceptable alignment of the osseous structures, the initial goal is to splint and or cast the extremity for approximately 6 weeks, followed by therapy to regain range of motion. Malalignment, fractures involving the joint surface, inability to achieve and sustain alignment, and open fractures often require surgical care. The patient age, co-morbidities, and condition of the osseous structures help to determine the need and potential success of surgical intervention.

Elbow fractures are technically complex injuries to manage. Most elbow fractures with associated dislocations require surgical care (Wolf, Athwal, Shin, & Dennison, 2009). Wrist fractures commonly involve the distal radius and are often seen with osteoporosis, and are therefore considered fragility fractures. These injuries respond well to casting unless reduction is difficult to maintain. With difficult reductions, surgery may be employed. Phalanges are often common fracture sites and heal well with splinting.

Generalized Nursing Care

Common themes emerge when caring for patients with upper extremity orthopaedic conditions. Orthopaedic injuries and/or conditions can result in considerable pain. Patients need to understand proper use of medications, signs and symptoms of infection, potential for neurovascular complications, maintenance of skin integrity, cast and splint care, activity restrictions, and adaptive strategies for managing ADLs. See Table 2-2 for a list of nursing diagnoses for the patient with upper extremity conditions.

Physical therapy and occupational therapy are critical to identifying home equipment and ways to compensate for deficits in mobility and function. With shorter hospital stays, the promotion and reinforcement of self-care are essential. Pendulum exercises are often taught to patients to keep the

Table 2-2

Nursing diagnoses for the patient with upper extremity conditions

Acute pain related to shoulder injury
Self-care deficit
Skin integrity, potentially impaired
Physical mobility, impaired
Knowledge deficit

elbow and shoulder mobile, prevent stiffness, and promote circulation in the extremity.

Patient education should focus on teaching patients how to identify problems with circulation and skin integrity. Older patients often have frail, thin skin at increased risk for breakdown. Casts and splints should be well-padded to prevent skin tears and irritation. They should be adequately covered during bathing, and patients should be instructed to never insert anything down into the cast or splint. A hair dryer set on a cool setting can be aimed into the sides of the cast to relieve itching if needed.

Patients should understand principals of elevation and icing during the acute injury phase to reduce swelling and promote comfort. Patients and their support persons should understand monitoring for neurovascular compromise and techniques for reducing swelling when cylindrical casts have been applied. Casts may be split and then over-wrapped with an ace wrap to accommodate swelling after surgery. Casts are routinely removed at the follow-up visit to facilitate wound inspection and staple or suture removal. Fresh casts are often reapplied if needed. For those patients treated in a sling or splint, application should be taught to support the upper extremity and keep swelling to a minimum. Sleeping can be problematic for patients. Sleeping in a recliner may promote rest until the patient is more comfortable. Clothing application can be difficult with upper extremity conditions. Clothes that button down the front will make dressing easier.

Bathing becomes an important concern with any upper extremity injury or surgery. Patients need to be counseled regarding steadiness on wet surfaces while navigating a shower or tub, especially without the use of two hands. Generally, 48 hours after surgery, incisions may be exposed to water while showering and should be patted dry. Some physicians may prefer to keep the incision dry until staples or sutures are removed. In this case, the incision can be covered by an impermeable material such as saran wrap while bathing. The armpit must be kept dry without the use of powder or deodorants until the incision is healed. If shoulder movement is restricted, patients are encouraged to dry the armpit well by slipping a towel between the arm and chest and moving it gently back and forth. Feminine pads can be tucked between the arm and chest to absorb excess moisture and avoid maceration.

Patients should be counseled that postoperative activity and range of motion is determined by the physician and based on the assessment of tissue structures at the time of surgery. Therapy is tailored to the patient's needs and capabilities over several months. Patients may be encouraged to perform therapy in several short sessions a day to prevent fatigue and achieve optimal results (Chen et al., 2003). Patients are instructed that pendulum exercises, elbow range of motion, and isometric hand exercises will prevent muscle atrophy and stiffness. Patients should be thoroughly educated about the signs and symptoms of infection, and understand when to notify the surgeon.

Summary

The upper extremity is a complicated structure that is versatile yet vulnerable to an assortment of injuries and chronic conditions. Patients with upper extremity disorders require information about their conditions, but, more importantly, they need guidance and instruction regarding self-care. They should be taught strategies to allow them to adapt to limitations imposed by their conditions. Patients with upper extremity disorders need the expertise of orthopaedic nurses who understand their condition, needs, and limitations. Knowledgeable patients are empowered to care for themselves and will thrive despite their disabilities.

References

Altizer, L. (2003). Forearm and humeral fractures. *Orthopaedic Nursing, 22*(4), 266-273.

American Academy of Orthopaedic Surgeons (2007). *Reverse total shoulder arthroplasty.* Retrieved on January 26, 2010 from http://orthoinfo.aaos.org/topic.cfm?topic=A00094

American Academy of Orthopaedic Surgeons (2009). *Wrist fractures.* Retrieved on January 26, 2010 from http://www.aaos.org

American Dental Association and American Academy of Orthopaedic Surgeons (2003). Antibiotic prophylaxis for dental patients with total joint replacements. *The Journal of the American Dental Association, 134,* 895-899.

Bagwell-Crum, C. (2001). The shoulder. In D. Schoen (Ed.), *Core curriculum for orthopaedic nursing* (4th ed., pp. 419-437). New Jersey: NAON.

Bigliani, L., & Levine, W. (1997). Current concepts review—Subacromial impingement syndrome. *Journal of Bone and Joint Surgery, 79*(12), 1854-1868.

Butters, K. (2001). Fractures of the scapula. In R. Bucholz, & J. Heckman (Eds.), *Rockwood and Green's fractures in adults* (5th ed., pp.1079-1107). Philadelphia: Lippincott.

Casati, A., Borghi, B., Fanelli, G., Montone, N., Rotini, R., Fraschini, G., ...Chelly, J. (2003). Interscalene brachial plexus anesthesia and analgesia for open shoulder surgery: A randomized, double-blinded comparison between Levobupivacaine and Ropivacaine. *Anesthesia Analgesia, 96,* 253-259.

Celli, A., & Morrey, B (2009). Total elbow arthroplasty in patients forty years of age or less. *Journal of Bone and Joint Surgery, 91,* 1414-1418.

Chen, A., Joseph, T., & Zuckerman, J. (2003). Rheumatoid arthritis of the shoulder. *Journal of the American Academy of Orthopaedic Surgeons, 11*(1), 12-24.

Cofield, R., Parvizi, J., Hoffmeyer, P., Lanzer, W., Ilstrup, D., & Rowland, C. (2001). Surgical repair of chronic rotator cuff tears. *Journal of Bone and Joint Surgery, 83*(1), 71.

Cuomo, F., & Checroun, A. (1998). Avoiding pitfalls and complications in total shoulder arthroplasty. *Orthopedic Clinics of North America, 29*(3), 507-517.

Ekatodramis, G., Borgeat, A., Huledal, G., Jeppsson, L, Westram, L., & Sjovall, J. (2003). Continuous interscalene analgesia with Ropivacaine 2mg/ml after major shoulder surgery. *Anesthesiology, 98*(1), 143-150.

Flatow E. (2001). Fractures of the proximal humerus. In R. Bucholz, & J. Heckman (Eds.). *Rockwood and Green's fractures in adults* (5th ed., pp. 997-1040). Philadelphia: Lippincott.

Graham, B. (2008). The value added by electrodiagnostic testing in the diagnosis of carpal tunnel syndrome. *Journal of Bone and Joint Surgery, 90,* 2587-2593.

Gregory, P. (2001). Fractures of the shaft of the humerus. In R. Bucholz, & J. Heckman (Eds.), *Rockwood and Green's fractures in adults* (5th ed., pp. 973-996). Philadelphia: Lippincott.

Gutierrez, S., Comiskey IV, C., Luo, Z., Pupello, D., & Frankle, M. (2008). Range of impingement-free abduction and adduction deficit after reverse shoulder arthroplasty. *Journal of Bone and Joint Surgery, 90,* 2606-2615.

Hovelius, L., Augustini, B., Fredin, H., Johansson, O., Norlin, R., & Thorling, J. (1996). Primary anterior dislocation of the shoulder in young patients: A ten-year prospective study. *The Journal of Bone and Joint Surgery, 78,* 1677-1684.

Jobe, C. (1998). Gross anatomy of the shoulder. In C. Rockwood, & F. Matsen (Eds.), *The shoulder* (2nd ed., pp. 34-63). Philadelphia: W.B. Saunders.

Kim, T., Queale, W., Cosgarea, A., & McFarland, E. (2003). Clinical features of the different types of SLAP lesions. *Journal of Bone and Joint Surgery, 85-A*(1), 66-71.

Lindenhovius, A., Buijze, G., Kloen, P., & Ring, D. (2008). Correspondence between perceived disability and objective physical impairment after elbow trauma. *The Journal of Bone and Joint Surgery, 90,* 2090-2097.

Long, T., Wass, C., & Burkle, C. (2002). Perioperative interscalene blockade: An overview of its history and current clinical use. *Journal of Clinical Anesthesia, 14*(7), 546-556.

Liu, S., & Salinas, F. (2003). Continuous plexus and peripheral nerve blocks for postoperative analgesia. *Anesthesia Analgesia, 96,* 263-272.

Matsen, F., Thomas, S., Rockwood, C., & Wirth, M. (1998). Glenohumeral instability. In C. Rockwood, & F. Matsen, (Eds.), *The shoulder* (2nd ed., pp. 611-754). Philadelphia: W.B. Saunders.

McMahon, P., & Skinner, H. (2003). Sports medicine. In H. Skinner (Ed.), *Current diagnosis and treatment in orthopedics* (3rd ed., pp. 155-204). New York: McGraw-Hill.

Musgrave, D., & Rodosky, M. (2001). SLAP lesions: Current concepts. *The American Journal of Orthopedics, 30*(1), 29-38.

Neal, J., McDonald, S., Larkin, K., & Polissar, N. (2003). Suprascapular nerve block prolongs analgesia after nonarthroscopic shoulder surgery but does not improve outcome. *Anesthesia Analgesia, 96,* 982-986.

Orfaly, R. (2001). Elbow and forearm. In W. Greene (Ed.), *Essentials of musculoskeletal care,* (2nd Edition, pp. 163-169). Rosemont: American Academy of Orthopaedic Surgeons.

Rozental, T., Zurakowski, D., & Blazar, P. (2008). Trigger finger: Prognostic indicators of recurrence following corticosteroid injection. *Journal of Bone and Joint Surgery, 90,* 1665-1672.

Schmitt, M. (1999). *Evaluating the Shoulder. Patient Care for the Nurse Practitioner, 2*(3), 42-53.

Schoen, D. (2000). Care of a patient with shoulder and elbow injury. In *Adult orthopaedic nursing* (pp. 403-444). Philadelphia: Lippincott.

Smith, K., & Matsen, F. (1998). Total shoulder arthroplasty versus hemiarthroplasty. *Orthopedic Clinics of North America, 29*(3), 491-503.

Sperling, J., Cofield, R., & Rowland, C. (1998). Neer hemiarthroplasty and Neer total shoulder arthroplasty in patients fifty years old or less. *The Journal of Bone and Joint Surgery, 90,* 464-473.

Swiontkowski, M. (2001). In *Manual of orthopaedics* (5th ed., pp. 185-213). Philadelphia: Lippincott.

Taft, T. (1996). Shoulder injuries in sports. In J. Richmond, & E. Shahady (Eds.), *Sports medicine for primary care* (pp. 211-283). Cambridge: Blackwell Science.

Tomaino, M. (2008). Resection arthroplasty of the thumb basilar joint. In K. Chung (Ed.), *Hand and wrist surgery: Operative technique, 2* (pp. 589-598). Philadelphia: Elsevier.

Walch, G., & Boileau, P. (1997). Rotator cuff tears associated with anterior instability. In J. Warner, J. Iannotti, & C. Gerber (Eds.), *Complex and revision problems in shoulder surgery* (pp. 65-97). Philadelphia: Lippincott.

Wirth, M. (2001). Shoulder. In W. Green (Ed.), *Essentials of musculoskeletal care* (2nd ed., pp. 105-160). Rosemont: American Academy of Orthopaedic Surgeons.

Wolf, J., Athwal, G., Shin, A., & Dennison, D. (2009). Acute trauma to the upper extremity: What to do and when to do it. *Journal of Bone and Joint Surgery, 91,* 1240-1252.

Van der Windt, D., Koes, B., Deville, W., Boeke, A., Jong, B., & Bouter, L. (1998). Effectiveness of corticosteroid injections versus physiotherapy for treatment of painful stiff shoulder in primary care: Randomized trial. *British Medical Journal, 317*(7), 1292-1296.

Yamaguchi, K., Levine, W., Marra, G., Galatz, L., Klepps, S., & Flatow, E. (2003). Transitioning to arthroscopic rotator cuff repair: The pros and cons. *The Journal of Bone & Joint Surgery, 85-A*(1), 144-154.

Chapter 3

Care of the Patient with Spine Problems

Lisa A. Olds, BSN, RN, ONC®

Objectives

- Identify common anatomical structures and functions of the spine.

- Outline common treatment options for cervical and lumbar spine disorders.

- Detect pertinent signs and symptoms of serious postoperative complications related to cervical and lumbar spine surgeries.

- Describe nursing interventions in caring for patients with cervical and lumbar spine disorders.

Key Terms

Allograft bone: sterilized bone from a bone bank.

Annulus fibrosus: the outer ring of the disc that is made of numerous concentric layers of thick, fibrous tissue.

Autogenous bone graft: live bone harvested from the patient.

Bone spurs: degenerative overgrowth of bone in and around the vertebral and neural foramina causing spinal cord or nerve root compression; also called osteophytes.

Corpectomy: removal of the center portion of the vertebral body; similar to a vertebrectomy.

Dural tear: unintentional opening of the dura mater during a spinal procedure, allowing cerebral spinal fluid to escape; is usually repaired immediately.

Epidural steroid injection: the placement of solution, typically containing an anesthetic and a corticosteroid, by insertion of a needle into the epidural space to help relieve pain and decrease inflammation of the nerve.

Foramen: an opening or passageway in bone.

Herniated disc: nucleus pulposus escapes through a tear in the annulus fibrosus.

Instrumentation: implantable, metal, bone fixation devices such as plates, rods, screws, or wires.

Kyphoplasty: percutaneous procedure performed by inserting a small instrument into a fractured vertebra that allows a small balloon to be inserted and inflated to create a cavity into which bone cement is injected; restores vertebral body height and stabilizes the compression fracture.

Kyphosis: posterior curvature of the spine as seen in the thoracic and sacral regions; if curvature is exaggerated, it is considered a spinal deformity.

Lordosis: anterior curvature of the spine as seen in the cervical and lumbar regions; if curvature is exaggerated, it is considered a spinal deformity.

Myelopathy: spinal cord dysfunction caused by compression of the spinal cord resulting in problems such as gait disturbances, bowel and bladder dysfunction, and changes in sensory, motor, and reflex function.

Nucleus pulposus: the center of the disc that is made of a soft, gelatinous material.

Pseudarthrosis: failure of bone to heal in the location of an attempted spinal fusion within one year after initial surgery.

Radiculopathy: nerve root compression resulting in nerve dysfunction evidenced by changes in sensory, motor, and reflex function.

Scoliosis: an abnormal lateral curvature of the spine with possible abnormal rotation of the vertebrae.

Spondylolisthesis: described as the "slipping" of a vertebra from its normal position.

Stenosis: narrowing of a passageway.

Vertebrectomy: removal of the center portion of the vertebral body; similar to a corpectomy.

Vertebroplasty: percutaneous procedure done by inserting a large needle into a fractured vertebra in order to inject bone cement to stabilize the compression fracture; does not restore normal vertebral body height.

The spine is the center of the body. It protects essential neural structures from injury. The spine serves as an anchor for forceful muscles that perpetually pull on the small bones. While supporting the weight of the body, the spine must withstand additional mechanical forces as the body performs various activities. The pieces of the spine fit together like an intricate puzzle. When the many components of spinal anatomy are not working in harmony, problems can arise.

Neck and back pain plague millions of people on a daily basis. Pain and dysfunction may begin to interfere with everyday activities. Whether pain persists over weeks or years, when a patient's quality of life is in jeopardy, the search for relief begins.

This chapter provides a review of spinal anatomy for better understanding of cervical and lumbar diagnoses, in addition to various treatment options. A fundamental knowledge of spinal disorders is the key element to understanding how to care for patients with spine problems.

Anatomy of the Spine

The human spine is composed of 33 vertebrae that are separated into five regions. Each region consists of a group of vertebrae that is unique in size, shape, and number. The vertebral column (see Figure 3-1) begins with the cervical region that is composed of seven vertebrae and is generally known as the neck area of the body. Next, the thoracic region includes 12 vertebrae and refers to the body's chest area. The lumbar region, commonly recognized as the low back area, consists of five vertebrae. The sacral region consists of five fused vertebrae that form a solid piece of bone called the sacrum and refers to the back of the pelvis area. Lastly, the coccygeal region is composed of four small vertebrae that are fused to form the coccyx, also known as the tailbone area.

Although each region's vertebrae have very distinct characteristics, most vertebrae possess several common structures (see Figure 3-2). A typical vertebra has a large, thick body that is positioned at the front or anterior portion of the vertebral column. Protruding off the back of the body, there are two bridges of bone called pedicles; one is positioned to the right back edge of the body, and the other is positioned to the left back edge. The pedicles join the vertebral body to a bony arch that forms the posterior or back aspect of the vertebral column. This arch is composed

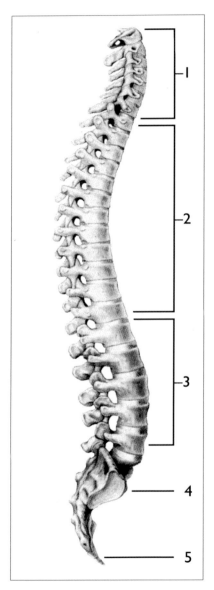

**Figure 3-1
Lateral view
of spine:**

1. Cervical Region;
2. Thoracic Region;
3. Lumbar Region;
4. Sacral Region;
5. Coccygeal Region.

Reproduced with permission from DePuy AcroMed™.

of two laminae with one reaching from the left side and the other from the right side. The laminae meet in the center and elongate to form the spinous process. With gentle palpation, the spinous processes can usually be felt under

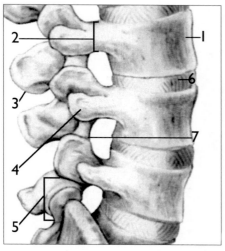

**Figure 3-2
Spinal anatomy:**

1. Vertebral Body;
2. Pedicle;
3. Posterior Spinous Process;
4. Transverse Process;
5. Facet Joint;
6. Disc;
7. Neural Foramen.

Reproduced with permission from DePuy AcroMed™.

the skin, running down the midline of the back. To the outer side of each lamina, there is a transverse process that extends laterally. The spinous and transverse processes function as levers for the many muscles that attach to them. The major muscle groups that support the vertebral column are the erector spinae, multifidi, interspinalis, quadratus lumborum, and psoas muscles. The abdominal and the gluteal muscles also play an important role in assisting the spinal muscles (Mayer, 1999).

Between the transverse processes and the laminae, there are the superior and inferior articular processes called facets. The two inferior facets of a vertebra interact with the two superior facets of the vertebra below, forming two individual facet joints. These joints are synovial joints that allow for flexion, extension, and rotation in the cervical, thoracic, and lumbar regions of the spine. The primary function of the facet joints is to allow for very simple gliding movements to occur between the vertebrae.

There are numerous ligaments that work to stabilize the spine (see Figure 3-3). Interspinous ligaments connect adjacent spinous processes (Kirschblum & Benevento, 2009). They are found in-between the spinous processes from C2-C3 through L5-S1. The supraspinous ligament begins at the tip of the C7 spinous process. It connects to the tip of each spinous process as it continues into the lumbosacral region (Yoganandan, Halliday, Dickman, & Benzel, 2005). The ligamentum flavum aids the facet joints by stretching during flexion and staying taut during extension. These movements help to control the motion of the vertebrae. The ligamentum flavum can be found within the spinal canal, under the laminae. It connects the anterior surface of one lamina to the posterior surface of the lamina below.

Another type of joint found in the spine is a symphysis or flexible joint where fibrous cartilage connects bone. Here, an intervertebral disc connects the bodies of two vertebrae. Two main ligaments assist these joints (see Figure 3-3). The first is the anterior longitudinal ligament that can be found along the front, smooth portion of the vertebral bodies. This

strong band begins at the occipital bone of the skull and extends down to the sacrum. The second ligament is the posterior longitudinal ligament that is adhered to the back of the vertebral bodies, inside the spinal canal. These ligaments lend support to the vertebral column by connecting all the vertebral bodies and discs.

The primary functions of the disc are to absorb stresses and shocks transferred along the spine and to allow mobility. The disc is comprised of two parts. The outer ring, or annulus fibrosus, consists mostly of collagen fibers that are organized into concentric layers. These layers provide elasticity and strength. They also provide support to the inner portion of the disc, known as the nucleus pulposus. The nucleus pulposus is soft and gelatinous. It is made mostly of water. The disc tissue is avascular in adults. Nutrients for the disc cross through superior and inferior cartilaginous end plates. This cartilage serves as the interface between the disc and the vertebral body (Rao & Bagaria, 2006).

Within the confines of the posterior side of the vertebral body, the two pedicles and the laminae, there is a small amount of open space called the vertebral foramen or spinal canal. All vertebrae in the cervical, thoracic, and lumbar regions have this foramen. It allows the spinal cord to descend from the brain through the base of the skull, into the cervical region, and down to the lumbar region. There are 31 pairs of spinal nerve roots that extend from the spinal

**Figure 3-3
Spinal Ligaments**

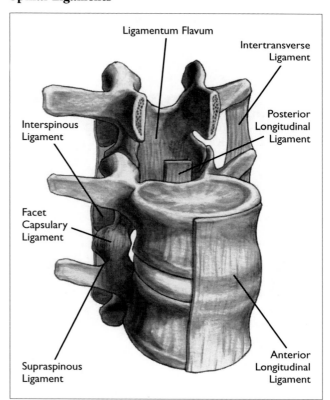

Courtesy of www.Spinecme.org.

cord. They are divided by regions into: eight cervical, twelve thoracic, five lumbar, five sacral, and one coccygeal. To innervate the appropriate area of the body, each pair of nerve roots must leave the vertebral foramen. There is an opening just under each pedicle, moving laterally, where the nerve root exits the vertebral foramen. This opening is called an intervertebral or neural foramen (see Figure 3-2).

Although the spinal cord tapers to an end between the first and second lumbar vertebrae, there are some nerve roots that have to travel down toward the bottom of the vertebral column before exiting. This collection of lumbar, sacral, and coccygeal nerve roots is called the cauda equina. Three layers of connective tissue, called the meninges, protect the brain, spinal cord, and nerve roots. The outer layer, the dura mater, is the thickest and toughest. The dura encapsulates the brain, spinal cord, and spinal nerves until they exit the spinal canal. Inside the dura, cerebral spinal fluid bathes the brain, spinal cord, and nerves, and helps to cushion these delicate structures.

Of all the spinal nerves, the sciatic nerve is most notable. The largest nerve in the body, the sciatic nerve is a conglomeration of portions of the fourth and fifth lumbar nerves, joined with portions of the first four sacral nerves (Jenkins, 2009). It runs down the posterior aspect of the thigh and then splits into two main branches just above the knee. These branches continue down either side of the lower leg into the foot.

Natural curvatures of the spinal regions develop in early childhood as an adaptation to upright posture. There are four spinal curves that alternate between lordosis and kyphosis. The curves in the cervical and lumbar regions are described as lordotic, whereas the curves in the thoracic and sacral regions are kyphotic. These curves give the spine a distinct S-shaped appearance. This is best observed from a lateral or side view of the spine.

The functional or moveable portion of the spine is called a motion segment. It consists of two vertebrae, the disc in-between, and the associated soft tissue. These motion segments allow the spine the capability of flexion, extension, lateral flexion, and rotation. The normal neck moves as much as 130 degrees in flexion and extension, 75 degrees in lateral bending, and 160 degrees in rotation (Johnson, Murphy, & Southwick, 1999). In the lumbar spine itself, normal range of motion is approximately 40-60 degrees of flexion, 20-35 degrees of extension, 15-20 degrees of lateral flexion, and 3-18 degrees of rotation (Rauscher, 2001).

Although numerous similarities in the spine have been discussed, there are also important differences that should be mentioned. Vertebrae in the cervical region are small in comparison to those in the thoracic and lumbar regions. As the vertebrae cascade from top to bottom, they grow progressively larger. The lumbar vertebrae are the largest. Intervertebral disc size follows the same progressive increase. In addition to size, there is a significant difference in the shape and function of the first two cervical vertebrae. The first cervical vertebra, or atlas, does not have a vertebral body or a spinous process. The shape of the atlas is similar to a ring. It has a much larger vertebral foramina because it must accommodate a bony projection rising from the vertebral body of the second cervical vertebra, or axis. This projection, referred to as the dens or the odontoid process, serves as a pivot between the first two cervical vertebrae, allowing for rotation of the head.

When referring to a specific vertebra, it is customary to name it by the first letter of the region it is located in and by the number representing its place within the region. For example, the fourth cervical vertebra would be identified as C4. The second lumbar vertebra would be identified as L2. The discs are named by the vertebra above and the vertebra below. The disc between the third and fourth lumbar vertebrae is referred to as the L3-L4 disc.

Diagnostics

There are several common types of diagnostic imaging that can be performed in order to evaluate the spine. The most common type of imaging is a plain radiograph or x-ray. Radiographs show bony structures well but are unable to show soft tissue structures such as nerves or discs; therefore, radiographs of the spine only give partial information and are best paired with more sensitive imaging studies.

Magnetic resonance imaging (MRI) is considered to be the study of choice for imaging the spine. It is noninvasive, and can visualize the neural elements, intervertebral discs, and spinal ligaments with remarkable clarity. It also offers the ability to image the spine in both axial and sagittal planes. MRI can be enhanced with the addition of gadolinium, injected intravascularly, which helps to improve the visualization of scar tissue. Gadolinium-enhanced MRI is currently the most accurate imaging test to distinguish recurrent disc herniation from postoperative scarring, with a reported accuracy as high as 100% (Bell & Ross, 1997).

Computed tomography (CT) is a noninvasive study that is able to directly visualize the spine and can be done on an outpatient basis. A CT scan is able to distinguish the difference between soft tissue and bone as the cause of the neural compression. Advances in CT technology can now provide coronal, sagittal, and three-dimensional images that can provide more complete information. Because the CT can provide exceptional bony detail, it is helpful in more clearly defining fractures, tumors and infections in the spine (Yu & Williams, 2006).

A myelogram is an invasive procedure that is able to show changes in soft tissue. The test is performed by injecting a contrast dye into the subarachnoid space just inside the dura where the dye mixes with the cerebral spinal fluid. If the injection is done in the lumbar region, the dye will circulate upward toward the brain. If the injection is done in the cervical region, the dye will circulate downward. The dye highlights the neural structures of the spinal canal. If there is compression of the neural structures, the contrast dye cannot flow freely. Thus, the myelogram images will show a brightened area that continues to the vertebral level where the dye is trapped. The rest of the spinal canal will remain dark because the dye is unable to pass the compressed area.

This kind of information is considered indirect evidence of a problem because the myelogram itself does not show what is causing the compression. It only indicates that there is a compression and at what level it has occurred.

Because of the invasive nature of the myelogram, the patient is usually kept for observation for several hours. During this time, the patient rests in bed with their head elevated. This position helps the dye to settle toward the base of the spinal canal. The dye is usually water-soluble, which helps to decrease side effects including nausea, vomiting, or headaches. The patient is encouraged to drink plenty of fluids to help eliminate the dye. Occasionally, this typical outpatient procedure may require overnight hospitalization if side effects are persistent. Complications of a myelogram may include a dural tear, reaction to the contrast dye, or infection. It is important to instruct the patient to report persistent nausea, vomiting, headaches, or fevers to the physician.

Despite the individual limitations of the myelogram and CT, the two tests combined provide a wealth of information. The contrast dye introduced through the myelogram helps to enhance the accuracy of the CT. Because of the quality of information these combined tests can offer, it is quite common for them to be ordered together. The combined test is usually referred to as contrast enhanced computed tomography (myelo-CT).

Nerve function tests are performed to substantiate abnormalities found on a clinical exam, as well as to help differentiate between radiculopathy and myelopathy. Electromyography (EMG) is done by sending electrical impulses through nerves and recording the muscles' response. Nerve Conduction Velocity (NCV) measures how well a nerve is able to transmit an electrical impulse.

Discography is an invasive test used to diagnose and treat back pain. This controversial test is performed by injecting contrast into the suspected troublesome disc to see if the patient's typical pain pattern can be reproduced (Williams & Park, 2003). This test is indicated when a patient's pain symptoms have not improved after surgery, and other tests, such as CT, MRI, or myelogram, have failed to identify any source of unrelenting spinal pain (Charuk, 2006).

A bone scan is another useful tool for evaluation of the spine. This test assists to confirm the presence of tumors, traumatic injuries, infections, fractures, and arthritic problems. A radioisotope is administered intravenously, which circulates through the body. The radioisotope is present in areas of increased bone activity and will show as a highlighted area on the images. Bone scans have a low sensitivity and therefore are best utilized in conjunction with higher-sensitivity tests such a MRI.

Degenerative Changes in the Spine

Degenerative disc disease is the same no matter where it occurs in the spine. Progressive degenerative changes begin in the spine from the third through the fifth decades of life (Wiesel, 1997). The intervertebral disc is the first structure to show signs of aging (see Figure 3-4). The disc is made

Figure 3-4
Examples of Degenerative Changes in the Spine

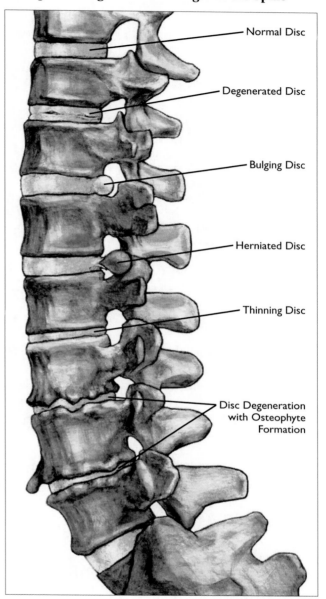

Normal Disc

Degenerated Disc

Bulging Disc

Herniated Disc

Thinning Disc

Disc Degeneration with Osteophyte Formation

Courtesy of www.Spinecme.org.

mostly of water; as aging occurs, the water content decreases. There are biochemical changes that occur in the disc that alter the molecular meshwork. The disc slowly loses the ability to distribute stress evenly, which can lead to a disc herniation. There is a loss of disc height that brings the vertebral bodies closer together. Over time, this can lead to degenerative changes in the bony structures of the spine. The facet joints and the vertebral bodies begin to endure more mechanical stress, which may eventually lead to the formation of osteophytes or bone spurs. The ligaments also thicken and lose elasticity which may lead to spinal instability. Soft tissue pain may also develop. In time, all of these degenerative changes can contribute to the narrowing of the spinal canal and the neural foramina, a condition better known as stenosis. At this point, the nerve roots and potentially the spinal cord may be in jeopardy of being compressed.

Common Problems and Treatments of the Cervical Spine

The most common symptoms described by patients with cervical spine conditions may include pain in the neck or upper extremities, numbness or tingling in the upper extremities, and muscle weakness. These symptoms can progress slowly over time and may be caused by degenerative disc disease or stenosis. Acute injuries such as a fracture, dislocation, or herniated disc may trigger these symptoms to occur very abruptly. Depending on the cause, severity, and duration of the symptoms, there are operative and nonoperative methods to treat cervical diagnoses.

Cervical Degenerative Disc Disease

Cervical degenerative disc disease is usually best evaluated by MRI. For the evaluation of neck, arm, and shoulder symptoms, MRI of the cervical spine has quickly become the main diagnostic test (Williams & Park, 2003). Standard radiographic

Figure 3-5
Lateral Cross Section View of an Anterior Cervical Discectomy and Fusion Procedure

The disc has been removed and the bone graft is inserted.

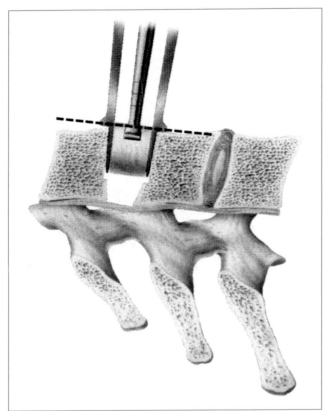

Reproduced with permission from DePuy AcroMed™.

Figure 3-6
Anterior View of an Anterior Cervical Discectomy and Fusion Procedure

The disc has been removed and the bone graft is inserted.

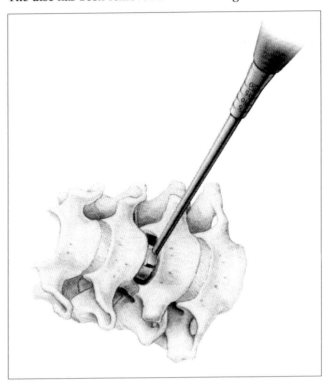

Reproduced with permission from DePuy AcroMed™.

films, used in conjunction with the MRI, show disc space height and often reveal a loss of normal cervical lordosis. When treatment options are considered, it is important to know that most patients respond well to nonoperative or conservative treatment. This treatment usually includes short periods of rest, massage, ice or heat, and anti-inflammatory agents with active mobilization as quickly as possible (Williams & Park, 2003). Occasionally, cervical traction and cervical collars may be used. Once the acute pain subsides, neck and shoulder exercises can be helpful.

Surgical intervention is indicated when persistent or recurrent upper extremity pain is not responsive to conservative treatment, neurologic deficits progress, significant radicular pain is present with an unchanged neurologic deficit, and confirmatory imaging studies are consistent with clinical assessment (Fischgrund & Herkowitz, 1997). The most common cervical procedure is the anterior cervical discectomy and fusion. The surgical incision is routinely made on the front, left side of the neck to minimize the chance of injuring the recurrent laryngeal nerve. The nerve is protected anatomically on the left side of the neck. A cut is made into the anterior longitudinal ligament and the degenerated disc is removed through the opening. If there is additional pressure on the nerves from a herniated disc or stenosis, the nerves will be decompressed or freed.

Between the vertebral bodies, a bone graft is then inserted in place of the disc (see Figures 3-5 and 3-6). Over several months, bone cells will grow into the bone graft and form a fusion that joins one vertebral body to the other. The use of allograft bone verses an autogenous bone graft is a decision made by the physician and the patient. It is common practice to use allograft bone for cervical procedures. Recovery from surgery is thought to be quicker and easier since the autogenous bone graft donor site, typically the anterior iliac crest, can be very painful and may inhibit mobility.

The use of anterior cervical instrumentation has become more widespread. The cervical plate (see Figure 3-7) provides stability and helps to prevent the bone graft from dislodging. A similar surgical procedure is done for the treatment of cervical myelopathy. When multiple levels need to be decompressed and fused, an anterior cervical corpectomy (also may be referred to as a vertebrectomy), fusion, and instrumentation may be performed (see Figure 3-8). When a corpectomy is performed, the center portion of the vertebral bodies as well as the discs are removed and replaced by a bone graft (see Figures 3-9, 3-10, and 3-11).

There are also several posterior cervical procedures that are used to treat herniated discs and stenosis. A posterior decompressive cervical laminectomy is done through an incision on the back of the neck, sometimes extending to the occiput. The posterior laminectomy consists of removing the laminae, and potentially a portion of the facets, in order to open the spinal canal and allow more room for the neural structures. Instability may occur, causing the vertebrae to fall forward, producing kyphosis. The development of postlaminectomy kyphosis after a multilevel posterior cervical decompressive laminectomy with partial facet

Figure 3-7
Anterior View of an Anterior Cervical Discectomy and Fusion Procedure with Instrumentation

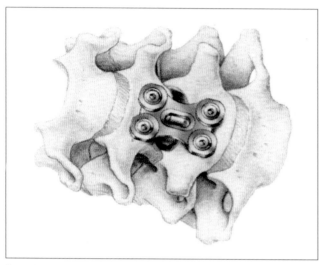

Reproduced with permission from DePuy AcroMed™.

Figure 3-8
Anterior View of an Anterior Cervical Corpectomy Being Performed

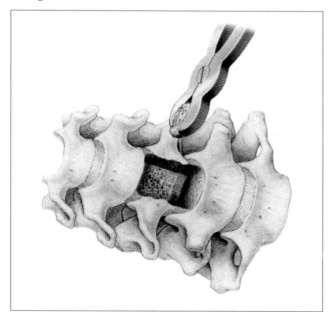

Reproduced with permission from DePuy AcroMed™.

Figure 3-9
Lateral Cross Section View of a Completed Anterior Cervical Corpectomy

The discs and vertebral bodies have been removed and the bone graft sized.

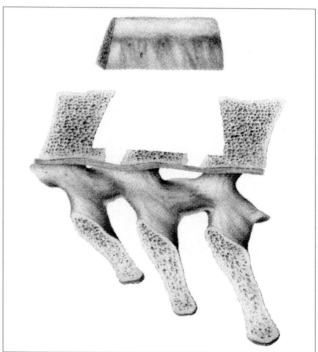

Reproduced with permission from DePuy AcroMed™.

Figure 3-10
Anterior View of an Anterior Cervical Corpectomy and Fusion Procedure

The bone graft is inserted.

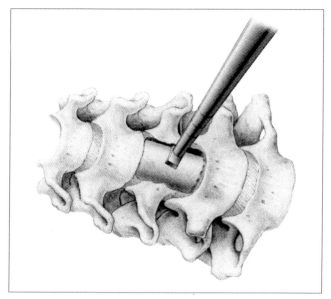

Reproduced with permission from DePuy AcroMed™.

removal is a noteworthy concern. Performing a posterior fusion with the decompressive laminectomy can provide strength and stability to the cervical spine over time. With the addition of instrumentation, such as screws and rods, this procedure can be used to give immediate supplemental support to multilevel anterior cervical procedures and to a posterior decompressive cervical laminectomy. This combined technique can improve stability, promote fusion healing, and can prevent the development of kyphotic deformity (Kim & Vaccaro, 2008). Posterior cervical laminoplasty is another surgical option used to achieve decompression. Instead of totally removing the laminae, they are hinged with sutures on one side, like a door. The open side is kept open with a small amount of fat so that the "door" does not close completely.

More recently, total cervical disc replacement implants have been developed for the treatment of cervical degenerative disc disease with the FDA approving the first cervical disc implant in the United States in July, 2007. The cervical disc arthroplasty is performed similarly to an anterior cervical discectomy and fusion procedure.

After most cervical surgeries, the patient is usually placed in a rigid, cervical collar. If instrumentation is used, the amount of time spent in the cervical collar is greatly reduced. Most patients are required to wear the collar for at least 6 weeks if a plate is not used. If instrumentation is used, the amount of time spent in the cervical collar is greatly reduced and varies by surgeon. Patients are instructed to avoid lifting more than 10 pounds, limit repetitive upper extremity activities, and avoid pushing and pulling during the recovery period.

Depending on the physical demands of the job and an employer's ability to accommodate activity restrictions, the patient may return to work within a few weeks to several months following surgery.

Fractures and Dislocations of the Cervical Spine

There are numerous types of fractures and dislocations that can occur in the cervical spine depending on the specific mechanism of injury. Cautious body positioning and frequent respiratory and neurological assessments should be performed until spine injury is either confirmed or ruled out for all patients for whom the mechanism of injury suggests fracture. A fracture of the dens or odontoid process can occur when a patient sustains a blow to the head, forcing the head abruptly forward. An example of this is falling down a set of stairs and hitting the back of the head on a step. These fractures are classified into three types depending on the exact location of the break in the bone. The degree of displacement of the fracture can greatly affect treatment. Facet dislocations, one of the most common cervical spine injuries, are often associated with motor vehicle accidents or falls from heights and usually occur at C5-C6 or C6-C7 (Connolly, Abitbol, Martin, & Yaun, 1997). Cervical traction may be indicated to help restore normal alignment in both fractures and dislocations. The patient may require surgical intervention in order to stabilize the spine, particularly after a dislocation. After surgery, the patient will typically wear a rigid cervical collar for several weeks while the injury heals.

If there has been minimal or no displacement of a fracture or if, after surgery, the surgeon wants to insure the head and

Figure 3-11
Anterior View of an Anterior Cervical Corpectomy and Fusion Procedure with Instrumentation

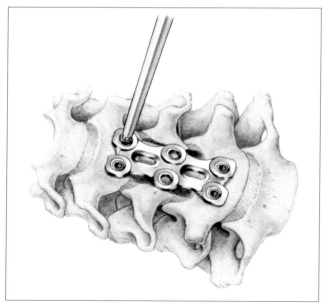

Reproduced with permission from DePuy AcroMed™.

Figure 3-12
Halo Brace Provides Ridged Stability for the Cervical Spine

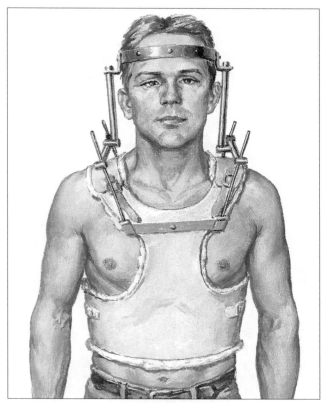

neck remain immobile, the patient may be placed in a halo brace (see Figure 3-12). The advantage of this type of brace is good stabilization with immediate mobility (Hickey, 1997). The halo brace consists of a cranial ring, four metal pins that attach the ring to the patient's skull, vertical bars, and a vest worn on the torso. The cranial ring, made of lightweight metal or composite materials, may be a continuous ring or open posteriorly. Prior to pin placement, local anesthetic is typically injected at the proposed insertion points on the head. The pins are pushed through the skin and rest up against the skull. Proper tightening of the pins ensures that they do not puncture the skull. Once secured to the head, the ring is then secured to the vest by lightweight rods. Traction is provided by the vest and maintained by the vertical rods. The vest is adjusted for stabilization and comfort. Typically, positioning of the cervical spine is checked by x-ray. After proper alignment is confirmed, the patient can ordinarily be mobilized. The patient may need to wear the halo brace for approximately 3 months, depending on the type of fracture.

If the patient is conscious and awake during the application of the halo brace, they may be fearful and anxious. It is important to assess the patient's understanding of the procedure and answer any questions, hopefully easing the patient's apprehension. Offering emotional support during the procedure can also be very comforting. If possible, pain medication or a mild sedative should be offered to the patient.

When caring for a patient in a halo vest, there are several nursing considerations. Skin under the vest must be assessed for breakdown, especially at pressure points. Skin should be cleansed at least daily with light soap and water, then dried thoroughly. Avoid creams or lotions under the vest. Hair washing can be performed by padding the vest with plastic to keep it dry and cleansing the pins immediately following the process. Hairdryers must be avoided as the halo pins can become heated, causing loosening. The vest liner should be replaced if it becomes wet or soiled.

Pin site care must be provided to the insertion points on the head. Care must be taken to keep the pin sites clean and free of infection. Pin sites are usually cleansed one to two times a day with a solution made from equal parts of hydrogen peroxide and saline. The halo bars or vest should never be used to move the patient as this may loosen the system. It is imperative to patient safety that an emergency wrench is kept on the vest at all times. In the event of an emergent situation such as cardiac arrest, the nurse must be familiar with how to release the screws and remove the front half of the vest to perform CPR.

The physician will determine what specific activity restrictions are necessary for the patient. Generally, patients are instructed to avoid lifting more than 5-10 pounds, limit repetitive upper extremity activities, and avoid pushing and pulling during the recovery period.

Nursing Considerations for the Cervical Spine

Nursing considerations when caring for patients with cervical spine conditions include, but are not limited to, the following considerations (see Table 3-1). Skin under the cervical collar must be assessed for breakdown, especially at pressure points such as the chin and the occiput. Extra attention must be given to patients who have altered mobility or who are bedridden. These patients are at high risk for developing skin breakdown on the occiput due to extended periods of pressure exerted by the edge of the collar. Cervical collar application and removal techniques may vary somewhat by the specific collar type. However, when opening any collar to provide skin care, be sure to maintain the patient's head and neck in a neutral position. Do not allow the head to turn from side to side or move up and down. When reapplying the collar, be sure to assess the positioning of the head and the placement of the collar for proper alignment. The collar straps should be fastened just enough to keep the head and collar securely in place.

It is common for patients to have some degree of difficulty swallowing due to tissue swelling in and around the esophagus caused by intubation and manipulation of the neck tissue during the surgery. Most patients report feeling like there is a lump in their throat when they swallow. They may also report that it feels as though food or medication catches in that area. This feeling may take several days to

Table 3-1
Nursing Diagnoses, Outcomes, and Interventions for the Cervical Spine

Diagnoses	Outcomes	Interventions

A. Skin integrity, potentially impaired
  1. Pressure points
    a. cervical collar
    b. halo vest
	• Patient verbalizes adequate comfort in cervical collar or halo vest
	• Skin integrity is maintained.
		• Evaluate cervical collar or halo vest for proper fit and application
		• Assess skin frequently for signs of redness, blisters, tenderness

B. Swallowing, altered post-operative	• Patient able to swallow with minimal difficulty	• Assess patient's ability to swallow liquids and solids
C. Physical mobility, impaired	• Patient verbalizes understanding of activity requirements and restrictions • Patient complies with activity requirements and restrictions	• Instruct patient to avoid tasks that require repetitive upper extremity movements, pushing and pulling, prolonged overhead tasks, or lifting greater than 10 pounds • Instruct patient to walk a comfortable distance several times a day • Instruct patient to limit daily tasks to light duty activities
D. Neurologic status, altered postoperative	• Patient's neurologic status remains unaltered	• Assess patient's neurological status as ordered • Notify physician about deviations from the patient's norm immediately
E. Knowledge, deficient	• Patient verbalizes understanding of healing process	• Assess patient's knowledge of healing process related to cervical spine surgery • Provide additional information as necessary
F. Coping, ineffective	• Patient verbalizes decreased anxiety related to healing process	• Provide encouragement to patient

several weeks to resolve. The patient's nutritional status may be affected by prolonged difficulty swallowing. The patient might also be at risk for aspiration, as the muscles of the esophagus are not able to control food and liquid well. Generally, patients should start with a liquid diet. Based on the patient's toleration, their diet will progress to soft foods. Patients should be instructed to eat slowly, taking small bites and chewing thoroughly. Patients often report difficulty swallowing oral secretions when resting in bed. Elevating the patient's head and shoulders by using a wedge pillow or by raising the head of the bed 30 degrees, can aid swallowing and increase patient comfort.

One of the most serious postoperative complications of cervical spine surgery is an upper airway obstruction. The obstruction may be caused by a hematoma, pharyngeal edema, or a dislodged plate or bone graft. Pressure is applied to the trachea and esophagus by any one of these causes, creating an emergent situation. If the patient is conscious, they might begin to feel they are having difficulty breathing, swallowing, or talking. They may also appear restless, cyanotic, tachycardic, and tachypnic (Guyer, Delmarter, Fulp, & Small, 1999). Intubation may be necessary to maintain the airway. The patient may be taken to the operating room so that the surgeon can explore the surgical site and minimize the obstruction.

Additional surgical complications may include, but are not limited to, perforation of the trachea, esophagus, or vascular vessels, dural tear, and permanent spinal cord or nerve injury. Other postoperative complications that may develop during the extended period of postoperative healing may include infection of the surgical or graft site, loosening of the plate or screws, pseudarthrosis, sore throat, and hoarseness.

Spinal Cord Injury

More than 1 million people in the United States are affected by spinal trauma each year. The incidence of traumatic spinal cord injury (SCI) is approximately 11,000 new cases each year in the United States (Inamasu & Guiot, 2006). The primary cause of SCI is motor vehicle accidents. The second most common cause of SCI is falling, especially in older adults. Violence-related injuries rank third, particularly in younger men (Kirschblum & Benevento, 2009).

Approximately one half of traumatic SCI's occur in the cervical spine, with C5 being the most common neurological level of injury. Injuries to the cervical segments of the spinal cord, resulting in loss of motor or sensory function is called tetraplegia, which is considered the preferred term instead of quadriplegia (Kirschblum & Benevento, 2009). People with tetraplegia experience impairment in the use of their upper and lower extremities, trunk, and pelvic organs. They may also be unable to breathe independently and may require ventilator assistance, especially in the acute phase of hospitalization (Vocaturo, 2009). Paraplegia is the loss of motor or sensory function due to injuries to the thoracic, lumbar, or sacral segments of the spinal cord. These people typically maintain use of their upper extremities. Impairment of the trunk, pelvic organs, and lower extremities depends on the level of injury. The most common level for paraplegia is T12 (Kirschblum & Benevento, 2009).

SCI's are further divided into complete or incomplete injuries. A complete spinal cord injury is described as no motor or sensory function from the level of the injured spinal cord segment down through the lowest sacral spinal cord segment. An incomplete spinal cord injury is described as the presence of motor or sensory function below the injured spinal cord segment through the lowest sacral spinal cord segment.

Meticulous physical and neurological examinations are essential for successfully treating patients with SCI. Due to the traumatic nature of the event that led to the SCI, these patients may have other injuries that need to be identified. There is also a high risk for developing respiratory, cardiac, pulmonary, and hemodynamic complications as a result of the SCI.

Common Problems and Treatments of the Lumbar Spine

Patients with lumbar spine conditions describe symptoms including back pain and lower extremity numbness, tingling, weakness, and pain. Just as with the cervical spine, over time, these symptoms can progress slowly and be exacerbated by degenerative changes. Acute injuries can cause symptoms to rapidly materialize. Numerous operative and nonoperative treatments are available to treat these lumbar diagnoses.

Degenerative Lumbar Disc Disease and Disc Herniations

Lumbar disc herniations related to degenerative lumbar disc disease are most likely to occur in the third and fourth decades of life. The pairing of the progressive degenerative changes and vigorous lifestyles maintained by people in this age group contribute to an increased incidence of disc herniations. The most commonly affected discs are L4-L5 and L5-S1. The patient may present with one or more symptoms including back pain, lower extremity radiculopathy, which may include pain, numbness, or tingling, limited motion of the back, or difficulty walking. Radicular pain is described as sharp, shooting pain that travels from the back, through the buttock, and down the leg (Mignucci & Bell, 1999). If the pain extends below the knee, it is often referred to as sciatica, caused by compression of the sciatic nerve. Disc herniation is a frequent cause of sciatica; however, there are many other potential causes. Not only does the herniated disc cause compression of the nerve root, it is also thought that chemicals leaking from the damaged disc may also cause irritation (Mignucci & Bell, 1999). Symptoms vary based on rest and activity patterns. Rest usually helps to relieve symptoms, whereas walking, standing, and sitting usually exacerbates symptoms.

Nonoperative treatments may include a short period of bedrest, anti-inflammatory agents, muscle relaxants, oral steroids, antidepressants, epidural steroid injections, physical therapy, and traction (Wisneski, Garfin, Rothman, & Lutz, 1999). Ordinarily, failure of nonoperative treatments after a 6- to 12-week trial period, persistence of incapacitating symptoms in the lower extremities, and confirmatory imaging studies coinciding with clinical assessment will lead to an evaluation for surgical intervention. The MRI is the diagnostic test of choice in preparing for surgery.

The most common surgical procedure performed is a laminotomy and disc excision. A small incision is typically made on the midline of the back, over the involved disc level. Laminotomy refers to the removal of a small portion of the lamina for better visualization of the nerve root. Disc excision is the removal of the portion of the disc that has herniated and is causing nerve root compression. This procedure is also referred to as a lumbar discectomy. The purpose of this surgery is to relieve leg pain; it may or may not relieve back pain. A one-night stay in the hospital may be necessary. Once the patient is tolerating oral intake, urinating sufficiently, able to ambulate safely, and pain is controlled by oral medication, the patient is usually ready for discharge.

Lumbar Stenosis

Lumbar spinal stenosis is a term used to describe a complex set of symptoms, physical findings, and radiographic abnormalities caused by narrowing of the spinal canal or neural foramina (Mirkovic et al., 1999). Narrowing of these openings can be caused by bony or soft tissue structures (see Figure 3-13). Although there are multiple classifications for spinal stenosis, degenerative stenosis of the lumbar spine is the most common type. It is ordinarily the result of arthritic changes that develop as part of the natural aging process. Symptomatic lumbar stenosis occurs most often in the fifth to seventh decades of life (Hai, 2004).

Initial symptoms of spinal stenosis may be vague, but include a lengthy history of low back discomfort and stiffness that is usually irritated by activity and relieved by rest. Advancing degenerative changes, such as thickening of the ligamentum flavum, herniated discs, hypertrophied facet joints, or osteophytes, continue to cause narrowing in the lumbar spinal canal. This deterioration can lead to numbness, tingling, weakness, cramping, aching, and burning pain in one or both legs. These symptoms start in the low back and buttocks, proliferating to the thighs, knees, calves, and feet. These symptoms exemplify neurogenic

Figure 3-13

Common Degenerative Changes that result in Spinal Stenosis which can Lead to Nerve Compression

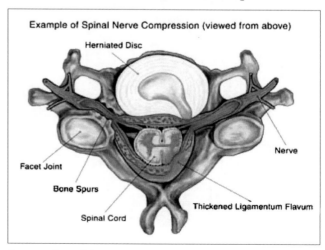

Example of Spinal Nerve Compression (viewed from above)

Herniated Disc
Facet Joint
Bone Spurs
Spinal Cord
Nerve
Thickened Ligamentum Flavum

Courtesy of www.Spinecme.org.

Figure 3-14
Posterior View of Autogenous Bone Graft Harvesting and Placement

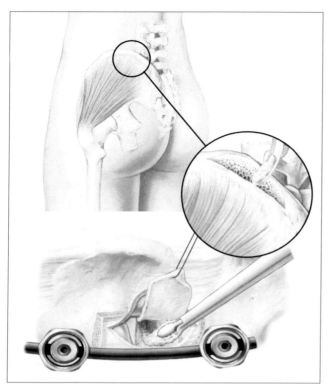

Reproduced with permission from DePuy AcroMed™.

Figure 3-15
Lateral Cross Section View of Lumbar Spine with Pedicle Screw Implants

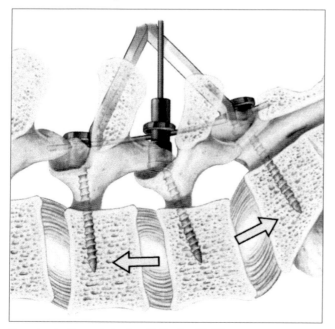

Reproduced with permission from DePuy AcroMed™.

claudication and are defined by the onset of lower extremity pain, parathesias, or motor symptoms when walking (Mirkovic et al., 1999).

As the condition worsens, the distance a patient can comfortably walk becomes shorter. Often, there is limited ability to stand for a prolonged period of time. Walking and standing increase lumbar lordosis, accentuating canal and foraminal narrowing, thus causing nerve compression. The patient may be able to temporarily relieve the symptoms by sitting or leaning forward on a shopping cart or counter. These activities reduce the lordosis by separating the vertebrae just enough to relieve the nerve compression.

Most patients do not seek treatment until the symptoms worsen and disrupt activities of daily living. Nonoperative treatment is typically initiated. Treatment for lumbar spinal stenosis includes very similar options to those discussed for disc herniations. Most patients with mild stenosis improve with nonoperative treatment. Those patients who experience failure of nonoperative treatments after a 6- to 12-week trial period, persistence of incapacitating symptoms in the lower extremities, and have confirmatory imaging studies coinciding with clinical assessment will pursue an evaluation for surgical intervention. Standard diagnostic imaging for spinal stenosis includes radiographic films as well as MRI or myelo-CT.

The goal of surgery is to relieve neural compression. The standard surgical procedure is a decompressive lumbar laminectomy (Russell & Hanley, 1999), in which a midline incision is made over the spinous processes of the involved vertebrae. The muscles and ligaments are separated from the spinous processes and the laminae. Total extraction of the spinous processes and the laminae (laminectomy) is completed. If bone spurs are present, they are trimmed away from the facet joints (facetectomy) and the neural foraminae (foraminotomy). In addition to the bone, some of the hypertrophied ligamentum flavum may be removed, accomplishing the decompression of the neural structures. Great care must be taken when removing the ligamentum flavum in order to guard against tearing the delicate dura positioned right beneath. Occasionally, a disc herniation is present along with the spinal stenosis. The herniated portion of the disc is excised as part of the procedure.

Spinal stenosis may recur as a result of spine surgery and further degenerative changes. After a laminectomy, instability occasionally evolves, resulting in the development of spondylolisthesis and recurrent stenosis. The length of stay in the hospital and the discharge plan after this type of surgery vary based on the patient's age, overall health, support systems, living arrangements, mobility, and number of spinal levels involved.

Degenerative Spondylolisthesis

The word spondylolisthesis is derived from the Greek root spondylos, which means vertebra, and olisthesis, which means to slip or slide down a slippery incline (Balderston, 1997). Like spinal stenosis, there are numerous classifications of spondylolisthesis. Symptoms produced by degenerative spondylolisthesis usually present after the

Figure 3-16

Posterior view of lumbar spine with pedicle screw implants and rods. The top of each screw is locked down to secure the rod.

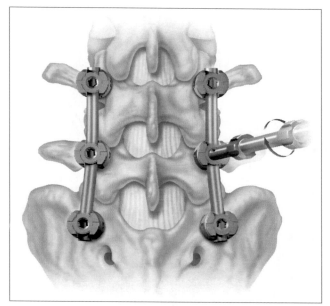

Picture from Depuy AcroMed™ Expedium Surgical Technique Brochure, p. 15.

fourth or fifth decade of life. This condition occurs more frequently in females and is more common in people with diabetes mellitus (Floman, 2008). Degeneration of the disc coupled with severe degenerative changes of the facet joints allows forward vertebral slippage (Amundson, Edwards, & Garfin, 1999). The slip typically does not exceed one-third of the vertebral body width. The L4 - L5 segment is most commonly affected.

Symptoms may be similar to those described for spinal stenosis, since they follow the pattern of neurogenic claudication or typical sciatica. The onset of pain is usually slow and progressive, with long periods of remission. Nonoperative treatments are the same as those detailed for degenerative disc disease.

The goal of surgery is to relieve back and leg pain and to maintain the stability of the spine. The most successful clinical outcomes for patients with degenerative spondylolisthesis occur as a result of a decompressive laminectomy combined with a posterolateral intertransverse process arthrodesis (Amundson et al.,1999). The decompressive laminectomy is completed as explained for treatment of spinal stenosis. Posterolateral intertransverse process arthrodesis translates to placing autogenous bone onto the transverse processes in order for a fusion to form. After exposing the transverse processes on both sides of the vertebra, cortical bone is scraped off to reveal cancellous bone. The autogenous bone may be harvested from the posterior aspect of the iliac crest (see Figure 3-14). The bone harvesting is typically done through the same spine incision. Autogenous bone may also be harvested from the removed laminae. This bone is usually

ground up using a bone mill. The autogenous bone is then placed on top of the exposed cancellous surface of the transverse processes. Pedicle screw implants (see Figures 3-15 and 3-16) are typically used to enhance the arthrodesis. A drain is usually placed near the incision to help control and monitor postoperative drainage. Over the course of approximately 3 months, the fusion begins to solidify. During this time, patients may be able to return to light duty work. Heavy physical labor should be avoided for at least 6 months or longer. It can take up to a year for a successful fusion to take place.

The use of instrumentation in lumbar fusion procedures is continuously evolving. Most studies report that fusion rates are better with instrumentation, but clinical results are not different from those after noninstrumented fusions (Linville, 2003). There are many different types of instrumentation systems, each with their own purpose. The advantages of using instrumentation are to reduce spinal deformities, provide stability to the spine, and increase chances for successful fusion (Zdeblick, 1997). Pedicle screws, intervertebral fusion cages, rods, plates, and wires are general examples of different types of spine fixation devices.

Other fusion procedures include posterior lumbar interbody fusion (PLIF), anterior lumbar interbody fusion (ALIF), and transforaminal lumbar interbody fusion (TLIF). Intervertebral fusion cages are filled with cancellous bone and then inserted in the disc space between two vertebrae (see Figures 3-17 and 3-18). Disc material is removed prior to cage insertion. These procedures can be effective in the treatment of discogenic lumbar pain. When used in combination with

Figure 3-17

Sagittal View of Lumbar Spine with Fusion Cages that are Packed with Bone Graft

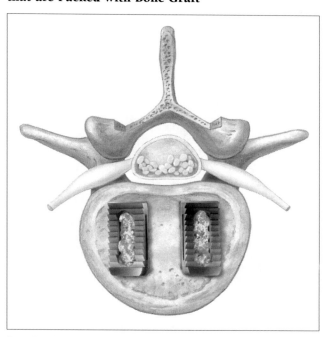

Reproduced with permission from DePuy AcroMed™.

Figure 3-18

Lateral Cross Section View of Lumbar Spine with Pedicle Screw Implants, Interbody Fusion Cages, and Bone Graft

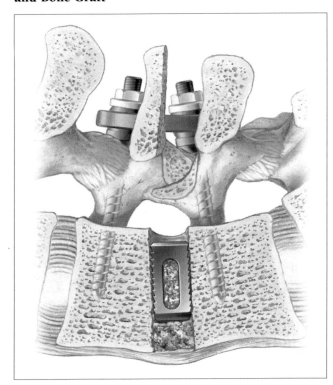

Reproduced with permission from DePuy AcroMed™.

other standard fusion procedures, the rate of fusion is even more successful (Perry, Kim, & Garfin, 2008).

Bone morphogenic proteins (BMPs) may provide a potential alternative to standard bone graft materials. BMPs have been proven to stimulate bone production. The specific use of rhBMP-2 with an intervertebral fusion cage for anterior spinal fusion has been approved by the FDA. Wider use of BMPs to promote bone growth in spinal fusion is currently being studied (Perry, Kim, & Garfin, 2008).

Another treatment option for degenerative disc disease and discogenic pain is lumbar disc arthroplasty or total lumbar disc replacement. Unlike standard fusion procedures, the design of the disc implants allows for motion of the spine. This procedure is done using an anterior approach with a small incision made through the abdomen. The diseased disc is removed and the disc implant is inserted between the vertebral bodies. The implant helps to restore normal disc space height and spinal motion. There are many contraindications for consideration of disc arthroplasty surgery, which include but are not limited to degeneration of the facet joints, active infection, diseases that affect bone quality, multilevel degeneration, and significant spondylolisthesis (Guyer & Ohnmeiss, 2008). Although lumbar disc implants have been used in Europe since the 1980s, the first total lumbar disc replacement implant to

gain FDA approval in the United States was in October, 2004. Clinical trials continue on different designs of both the cervical and lumbar disc replacement implants. The long term effects and outcomes of these implants also continue to be explored.

Spinal Deformity

For adult spinal curvature deformities such as scoliosis and kyphosis, extensive fusion with instrumentation procedures are typically necessary in order to reduce the deformity and relieve associated symptoms. The flexibility, balance, and magnitude of the spinal curve, in addition to the patient's health, are considered when deciding what type of procedure is necessary. The surgical procedures can be very lengthy. If an anterior and posterior fusion with instrumentation is being considered, the procedures may be staged or performed on separate days, several days, weeks, or months apart. The procedures can be done on the same day if they can be completed within 8 hours. If the procedures are going to take more than 12 hours, they should be staged. Procedures lasting 8 to 12 hours could be done either way; it is the surgeon's decision based on many factors (Bridwell, 1997). The instrumentation for the surgical procedures may consist of pedicle screws, intervertebral fusion cages, rods, hooks, and wires. In some cases, the instrumentation may run from the cervical to the sacral region.

Another type of spinal deformity is fixed sagittal imbalance. The imbalance occurs when a patient is not able to stand upright without bending the knees and hips. The patient presents with a forward stooped posture, causing the patient to appear as though he/she is looking at the floor. The patient may also report back pain. Often there is a surgical history of multilevel laminectomy, distal lumbar fusion, or correction of scoliosis. The imbalance can also develop due to flat-back syndrome, pseudarthrosis, or ankylosing spondylitis. In order to correct this imbalance, there are two osteotomy procedures most commonly used in conjunction with standard decompression and fusion procedures.

The first procedure is the Smith-Petersen osteotomy. This procedure loosens the posterior column of the spine by removing portions of the spinous processes and the facet joints of two adjacent vertebrae (see Figure 3-19). This allows space for the vertebrae to be tipped back against each other, pinching the newly cut surfaces together. In the anterior column of the spine, the two vertebral bodies are then spread wider apart, which helps to adjust the spine into a more correct lordotic position. However, due to the lengthening of the anterior column, there can be a significant risk of injuring the anterior vascular and neural structures (Bridwell, Lewis, Lenke, Baldus, & Blanke, 2003).

The other procedure is a pedicle subtraction osteotomy or transpedicular wedge resection. Just as its name implies, this procedure removes a wedge of bone that includes the pedicles (see Figure 3-20). The wedge is narrow in the anterior column, gradually grows wider as it passes through the middle column, and it is widest in the posterior column. The vertebra above the osteotomy level is able to be closed down posteriorly, against the newly cut surface. Because the

Figure 3-19
Smith-Petersen Osteotomy

Bone removed from the posterior column allows the anterior column to stretch open, actually lengthening it. This helps to restore lordosis, but the anterior lengthening may cause neural and vascular structures to stretch, resulting in injury.

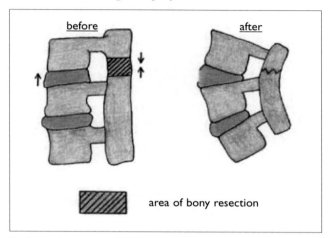

before   after

area of bony resection

Reprinted with permission from Dr. Keith Bridewell.

wedge is narrow in the anterior column, there is only a small adjustment that occurs anteriorly, thus decreasing the risk of injuring the vascular and neural structures. The posterior column is shortened, allowing the spine to adjust into a more correct lordotic position (Bridwell et al., 2003). Care is taken to ensure that the posterior neural structures are free of injury. This is a very technically challenging surgery to perform. The goals of the osteotomy procedures are to restore sagittal balance and decrease back pain. This allows the patient to stand upright with their head centered over their sacrum, without having to bend their hips and knees.

Depending on where the anterior approach is located, it may be necessary for the surgeon to deflate a lung in order to reach the spine. This will require the patient to have a chest tube after the surgery to reinflate the lung. Patients may also require intensive monitoring after these long procedures, so they may be admitted to a critical care unit postoperatively.

Lumbar Fractures

Fractures of the lumbar spine most often occur in the upper segments. Common lumbar fractures include compression fractures, burst fractures, and Chance fractures. A compression fracture is an injury caused by a flexion force, causing crushing and disruption of the anterior portion of the vertebral body (Levine, 1999). An example of a compression fracture is when someone slips on ice: the feet come out from under the body, causing the individual to land hard on the buttocks as the upper body is propelled forward. In the elderly, especially those with osteoporosis, compression fractures may also occur spontaneously or may be caused by a simple activity such as reaching forward to lift an object (Zigler & Strausser, 2002).

A compression fracture causes a loss of vertebral height. The posterior aspect of the vertebral body and posterior ligaments are usually unaffected. A compression fracture is typically a source of back pain, but is usually stable and does not cause neurologic deficits. After a course of conservative treatment including the use of a brace, analgesics, and bed rest, pain may still be intense and persistent. At this point, painful osteoporotic vertebral compression fractures may be treated with a procedure called vertebroplasty. Over the last 15 years, vertebroplasty has offered a minimally invasive treatment option to help stabilize osteoporotic vertebral compression fractures and reduce pain (Phillips et al., 2003). Vertebroplasty is performed by the percutaneous insertion of a large needle into the fractured vertebra, allowing for bone cement to be injected into the center of the vertebral body. Patients can experience pain relief soon after the procedure. Pain relief leads to increased mobility which helps to reduce the risk of morbidity associated with conventional treatments (Gross, 2002).

Although vertebroplasty helps to decrease pain, it does not restore normal vertebral body height. Kyphoplasty is a newer procedure used to treat unrelieved pain associated with osteoporotic vertebral compression fractures. By reducing the compression fracture and restoring the vertebral body closer to the original height, kyphoplasty also helps to correct spinal deformity at the fracture site (Phillips et al., 2003). Kyphoplasty is a percutaneous procedure performed by inserting a small instrument into a fractured vertebra that allows a small balloon to be inserted and inflated to create a cavity into which bone cement is injected. Although cement leakage around the neural elements does not happen often, it is the most common complication from vertebroplasty and kyphoplasty.

Figure 3-20
Pedicle Subtraction Osteotomy

The removed wedge of bone starts narrow, then gradually widens out through all three columns. In addition to the closure of the middle and posterior columns, the anterior column is able to close slightly on itself. This helps to reduce anterior lengthening, thus minimizing neural and vascular injury, while still restoring lordosis.

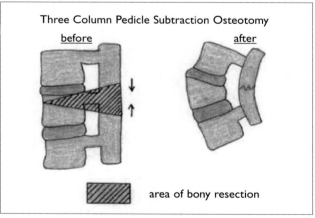

Three Column Pedicle Subtraction Osteotomy

before   after

area of bony resection

Reprinted with permission from Dr. Keith Bridewell.

Figure 3-21
Lateral View of Anterior Lumbar Corpectomy in Progress

The discs have been removed and vertebral body is being bitten away.

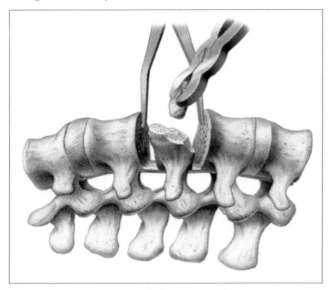

Reproduced with permission from DePuy AcroMed™.

Burst fractures are typically the result of a flexion and compression injury, such as jumping or falling off a high surface and landing on the feet. The torso is propelled forward, while the body makes an abrupt stop that compresses the spine downward. The vertebral body breaks apart with loss of height both anteriorly and posteriorly. A burst fracture is considered stable when the posterior ligaments are intact and there is no neural compression from the fracture pieces. Conservative treatment for a burst fracture is consistent with that of a compression fracture. Bracing can last as long as 3 to 6 months.

Unstable burst fractures involve the total disruption of the posterior elements of the vertebra (Goldstein, Cunningham, & McAfee, 1999). The neural structures in the spinal canal are at great risk because fragments of bone can be pushed against them with the destruction of the posterior elements. Burst fractures can be extremely unstable injuries and require internal fixation to prevent further compression of the spine (Goldstein et al., 1999). One common surgical procedure for this injury is an anterior lumbar corpectomy (see Figure 3-21). The goals of surgical intervention are anatomic reduction of the deformity, rigid fixation, and neural decompression (Levine, 1999).

A Chance fracture is considered a flexion and distraction injury. It is best exemplified by an auto accident in which the victim is wearing a lap seat belt and is hit head-on. The pelvis is secured by the safety belt, but the upper body is propelled forward, tearing the vertebra apart. Chance fractures that extend only through bone have an excellent prognosis for healing with nonsurgical treatment (Connolly

et al., 1997). Typical treatment includes bed rest and immobilization in a hyperextension cast or brace for several months. If the Chance fracture involves disruption of the ligaments and disc, it is considered unstable and should be treated surgically with a posterior fusion and instrumentation.

Tumors of the Spine

Disruption of bony, vertebral structures can also be caused by tumors and infections. Spinal tumors are frequently metastatic lesions from other primary malignancies; the occurrence of a primary tumor in the spine is extremely low. The thoracolumbar region is the most common location for skeletal metastases, accounting for about 70% of all lesions (Aboulafia & Levine, 2002). Tumors most likely to metastasize to the spine include lung, prostate, breast, renal, and gastrointestinal (Heller & Pedlow, 1997). Since metastatic spine lesions are found in the vertebral body 85% of the time, the lesions can have a profound effect on the structural integrity and stability of the spine (Heller & Pedlow, 1997). Vertebral collapse and neural impingement are always a concern. Although posterior decompression can be done to relieve neural compression, it does not provide adequate access to the vertebral body. Patients experiencing neural deficits have an anterior tumor approximately 70% of the time (Aboulafia & Levine, 2002). An anterior approach affords the most direct tumor access and allows decompression, anterior column reconstruction, and spinal stabilization in the appropriate patients (Heller & Pedlow, 1997).

Spinal Infections

Medical conditions that cause bacteremia may eventually lead to the development of vertebral osteomyelitis. Back pain is the most consistent symptom. Most patients report relentless pain at night, not associated with activity. Approximately 10% of patients with vertebral osteomyelitis present with neurological complications. Staphylococcus aureus is the most common organism, accounting for 30-55% of vertebral osteomyelitis found in adults (Jacofsky & Currier, 2002). Over the last decade, gram-negative bacteria have also become a more prevalent cause of vertebral osteomyelitis.

Nonoperative treatment may consist of intravenous antibiotics followed by oral antibiotics. Pain management strategies include analgesic medication, bed rest, and bracing. Among other factors, neural compression, substantial destruction of the vertebral body, and significant deformity are all indicators to proceed with surgical intervention. An anterior surgical approach to the spine is most common because isolated posterior infections are extremely rare (Jacofsky & Currier, 2002). This allows direct access to the infected tissue and adequate debridement, enabling stabilization of the spine with bone grafting, promoting rapid healing without collapse, and facilitating rehabilitation (Currier & Eismont, 1999). The debridement of necrotic tissue often includes a corpectomy, which may warrant a posterior instrumentation and fusion for stability. It is suggested that the surgeries be separated by 1-2 weeks to minimize contamination or seeding of the incisional area by the necrotic tissue (Levine & Heller, 1997).

Table 3-2

Nursing Diagnoses, Outcomes, and Interventions for the Lumbar Spine

Diagnoses	Outcomes	Interventions
A. Physical mobility, impaired	• Patient verbalizes understanding of activity requirements and restrictions • Patient complies with activity requirements and restrictions	• Instruct patient to walk a comfortable distance several times a day • Instruct patient to limit sitting in a chair to 20 to 30 minutes at a time • Instruct patient to avoid bending at the waist, twisting, or lifting greater than 10 pounds • Instruct patient to limit daily tasks to light duty activities
B. Neurologic status, altered postoperative	• Patient's neurologic status remains unaltered	• Assess patient's neurological status as ordered • Notify physician about deviations from the patient's norm immediately
C. Knowledge, deficient	• Patient verbalizes understanding of healing process	• Assess patient's knowledge of healing process related to lumbar spine surgery • Provide additional information as necessary
D. Coping, ineffective	• Patient verbalizes decreased anxiety related to healing process	• Provide encouragement to patient

Nursing Considerations for the Lumbar Spine

As the patient's ability to ambulate postoperatively can greatly impact recovery (see Table 3-2), it is imperative to mobilize this population of patients. Typically, walking is one of the only physical activities that spine patients can participate in to build strength and stamina after surgery. Some patients cannot tolerate sitting in a chair postoperatively because it exacerbates leg pain. For patients who can tolerate sitting, limiting it to 20 to 30 minutes at a time is usually recommended so as not to stress the back muscles and nerves for a prolonged period of time.

A potentially devastating neurological event that can occur in the lumbar spine is cauda equina syndrome. A patient is at risk when the cauda equine nerve plexus experiences pressure caused by a large lumbar disc herniation, postoperative hematoma, infection, or tumor. Symptoms include the sudden loss of bowel and bladder control, numbness and weakness in both legs, rectal pain, numbness of the perineum, and paralysis of the anal sphincter (Williams & Park, 2003). This syndrome typically warrants immediate evaluation and probable surgical intervention. Loss of bowel and bladder control may become a permanent dysfunction if the signs of the syndrome are not recognized soon enough. It is crucial to be aware of the cardinal signs of cauda equina syndrome when caring for postoperative lumbar spine patients.

Urinary retention and constipation are common postoperative concerns in most patient populations, but require a heightened awareness with postoperative lumbar spine patients. It is important to understand the patient's normal elimination patterns in order to identify a change from the baseline. The patient should be assessed for a history of urinary retention or incontinence. While medications and anesthesia contribute to urinary retention, retention can be a symptom of a more significant problem. If the patient requires catheterization, it is important to assess tactile sensation. If the patient reports decreased sensation on the inner thighs or cannot feel the catheterization, further evaluation may be necessary. If a spinal anesthetic was used during the surgery, the patient should be able to confirm when the spinal has worn off. It is important to differentiate decreased motor function and sensory perception related to anesthesia, versus pathologic alterations. Assess the patient's pre-surgical and post-surgical neurologic status to assure there are no new deficits.

Other surgical complications that may develop during the extended period of postoperative healing may include, but are not limited to, dural tear, infection of the surgical or graft site, loosening of the plate or screws, pseudarthrosis, and permanent spinal cord or nerve injury.

Generally, after lumbar spine surgery, patients are instructed to restrict bending, lifting more than 5-10 pounds, and twisting for a period of several weeks to several months. Physical therapy may be ordered by the physician to help the patient strengthen their back muscles. Returning to work will depend on the physical demands of the job and an employer's ability to accommodate activity restrictions.

General Nursing Considerations for Spine Patients

After spine surgery, patients are often anxious about persistent symptoms (see Tables 3-1 and 3-2). Although patients should be instructed about reasonable postoperative expectations of symptom relief, many assume that symptoms experienced prior to surgery will be relieved immediately after surgery. Most often, symptoms have improved but may not be completely resolved. Neuronal healing time is lengthy and may take months to be completed. Recurrent symptoms may produce considerable anxiety for some patients. Unfortunately, spine surgery often provides symptomatic relief but is not a cure and does not return the spine back to a normal state (Williams & Park, 2003). Patients require education about the healing process, the importance of maintaining activity restrictions, and following postoperative instructions.

The potential for tearing of the dural layer of the meninges during any type of spinal procedure is always present. Some procedures such as myelography or spinal anesthesia require the dura to be punctured. Most punctures will seal spontaneously. No matter how the breach of the dura occurs, cerebral spinal fluid escapes. The goal is to minimize the amount of fluid loss. Tears that occur during surgery may be repaired with fibrin glue or sutures. Persistent leaks may require placing a small amount of the patient's blood over the leak to form a blood patch. Occasionally, patients become symptomatic as a result of the loss of cerebral spinal fluid. A patient may report a severe headache when attempting to sit up in bed that is only relieved by lying down flat. Nausea and vomiting may accompany the headache. A headache of this type is referred to as a spinal headache.

The occurrence of a spinal headache should be communicated to the physician. Treatment of symptoms may include bedrest for 12 to 48 hours, administration of additional intravenous fluids, and pain and antiemetic medications. Bed rest minimizes the pressure changes experienced by the brain as a result of the loss of fluid. Increasing fluid volume will help to hydrate the body and aid in the replacement of the cerebral spinal fluid. Pain and antiemetic medications will help the patient control discomfort and nausea.

Summary

The spine is integral to every movement of the body. Degenerative processes, acute injuries, and debilitating deformities diminish the spine's strength and stability. There are many factors to consider when determining the appropriate treatment options for cervical and lumbar spine disorders. Improvements in diagnostic testing, surgical techniques, and surgical devices continue to evolve.

Orthopaedic nurses serve as a vital resource for spine patients navigating through their health care experience. Having a clear understanding of spine anatomy, common spine conditions, treatments, complications, and realistic outcomes is invaluable. This knowledge facilitates the orthopaedic nurse's ability to provide thorough patient care, identify and respond to potential patient complications, and to deliver accurate patient education. Possessing the necessary information to better understand the patient's experiences will enhance care that focuses on the patient's individual needs.

References

Aboulafia, A. J., & Levine, A. M. (2002). Musculoskeletal and metastatic tumors. In D. F. Fardon, S. R. Garfin, J. Abitbol, S. D. Boden, H. N. Herkowitz, & T. G. Mayer (Eds.), *Orthopaedic knowledge update: Spine 2* (pp. 411-430). Rosemont, IL: American Academy of Orthopaedic Surgeons.

Amundson, G., Edwards, C. C., & Garfin, S. R. (1999). Spondylolisthesis. In H. N. Herkowitz, S. R. Garfin, R. A. Balderston, F. J. Eismont, G. R. Bell, & S. W. Wiesel (Eds.), *The spine* (4th ed., Vol. 1, pp. 835-885). Philadelphia: W. B. Saunders.

Balderston, R. A. (1997). Spondylolisthesis. In S. R. Garfin, & A. R. Vaccaro (Eds.), *Orthopaedic knowledge update: Spine* (pp. 155-160). Rosemont, IL: American Academy of Orthopaedic Surgeons.

Bell, G. R., & Ross, J. S. (1997). Imaging studies of the spine. In S. R. Garfin, & A. R. Vaccaro (Eds.), *Orthopaedic knowledge update: Spine* (pp. 41-54). Rosemont, IL: American Academy of Orthopaedic Surgeons.

Bridwell, K. H. (1997). Adult idiopathic and degenerative scoliosis. In S. R. Garfin, & A. R. Vaccaro (Eds.), *Orthopaedic knowledge update: Spine* (pp. 161-172). Rosemont, IL: American Academy of Orthopaedic Surgeons.

Bridwell, K. H, Lewis, S. J., Lenke, L. G., Baldus, C., & Blanke, K. (2003). Pedicle subtraction osteotomy for the treatment of fixed sagittal imbalance. *The Journal of Bone and Joint Surgery, 85*(3), 454-463.

Charuk, G. E. (2006). Interventional Diagnostic Imagery. In J.M. Spivak, & P.J.Connolly (Eds.), *Orthopaedic knowledge update: Spine 3* (pp. 69-76). Rosemont, IL: American Academy of Orthopaedic Surgeons.

Connolly, P. J., Abitbol, J., Martin, R. J., & Yaun, H. A. (1997) Spine: Trauma. In S. R. Garfin, & A. R. Vaccaro (Eds.), *Orthopaedic knowledge update: Spine* (pp. 197-218). Rosemont, IL: American Academy of Orthopaedic Surgeons.

Currier, B. L., & Eismont, F. J. (1999). Infections of the spine. In H. N. Herkowitz, S. R. Garfin, R. A. Balderston, F. J. Eismont, G. R. Bell, & S. W. Wiesel (Eds.), *The spine* (4th ed., Vol. 2, pp. 1207-1258). Philadelphia: W. B. Saunders.

Fischgrund, J. S., & Herkowitz, H. N. (1997). Cervical degenerative disease. In S. R. Garfin, & A. R. Vaccaro (Eds.), *Orthopaedic knowledge update: Spine* (pp. 75-86). Rosemont, IL: American Academy of Orthopaedic Surgeons.

Floman, Y. (2008). Surgical management of isthmic, dysplastic, and degenerative spondylolisthesis. In C. W. Slipman, R. Derby, F. A. Simeone, & T. G. Mayer (Eds.), *Interventional spine: An algorithmic approach* (pp. 1099-1108). Philadelphia: W. B. Saunders.

Goldstein, J. A., Cunningham, B. W., & McAfee, P. C. (1999). Spine trauma in adults: Spinal instrumentation for thoracic and lumbar fractures. In H. N. Herkowitz, S. R. Garfin, R. A. Balderston, F. J. Eismont, G. R. Bell, & S. W. Wiesel (Eds.), *The spine* (4th ed., Vol. 2, pp. 1037-1070). Philadelphia: W. B. Saunders.

Gross, K. A. (2002). Vertebroplasty: A new therapeutic option. *Orthopaedic Nursing, 21*(1), 23-29.

Guyer, R. D., Delmarter, R. B., Fulp, T., & Small, S. D. (1999). Surgical management of cervical disc disease: Complications of cervical spine surgery. In H. N. Herkowitz, S. R. Garfin, R. A. Balderston, F. J. Eismont, G. R. Bell, & S. W. Wiesel (Eds.), *The spine* (4th ed., Vol. 1, pp. 540-551). Philadelphia: W. B. Saunders.

Guyer, R. D., & Ohnmeiss, D. D. (2008). Disc replacement. In C. W. Slipman, R. Derby, F. A. Simeone, & T. G. Mayer (Eds.), *Interventional spine: An algorithmic approach* (pp. 1389-1396). Philadelphia: W.B. Saunders.

Hai, Y. (2004). Classification,natural history, and clinical evaluation. In H. N. Herkowitz, J. Dvorak, G. R. Bell, M. Nordin, & D. Grob (Eds.), *The lumbar spine* (3rd ed., pp. 464-471). Philadelphia: Lippincott, Williams, & Wilkins.

Heller, J. G., & Pedlow, F. X. (1997). Tumors of the spine. In S. R. Garfin, & A. R. Vaccaro (Eds.), *Orthopaedic knowledge update: Spine* (pp. 235-256). Rosemont, IL: American Academy of Orthopaedic Surgeons.

Hickey, J.V. (1997). *The clinical practice of neurological and neurosurgical nursing* (4th ed., pp. 441-442, 457-462). Philadelphia: Lippincott-Raven.

Jacofsky, D., & Currier, B. L. (2002). Infections of the spine. In D. F. Fardon, S. R. Garfin, J. Abitbol, S. D. Boden, H. N. Herkowitz, & T. G. Mayer (Eds.), *Orthopaedic knowledge update: Spine 2* (pp. 431-442). Rosemont, IL: American Academy of Orthopaedic Surgeons.

Inamasu, J., & Guiot, B. H. (2006). Initial evaluation and management of spinal trauma . In J.M. Spivak, & P.J.Connolly (Eds.), *Orthopaedic knowledge update: Spine 3* (pp. 179-187). Rosemont, IL: American Academy of Orthopaedic Surgeons.

Jenkins, D. B. (Ed.). (2009). *Hollinshead's functional anatomy of the limbs and back* (9th ed., p. 241). St. Louis: W. B. Saunders.

Johnson, R. M., Murphy, M. J., & Southwick, W. O. (1999). Surgical approaches to the spine. In H. N. Herkowitz, S. R. Garfin, R. A. Balderston, F. J. Eismont, G. R. Bell, & S. W. Wiesel (Eds.), *The spine* (4th ed., Vol. 2, pp. 1463-1572). Philadelphia: W. B. Saunders.

Kim, D. H., & Vaccaro, A.R. (2008). Surgical treatment of cervical myelopathy. In C. W. Slipman, R. Derby, F. A. Simeone, & T. G. Mayer (Eds.), *Interventional spine: An algorithmic approach* (pp. 753-766). Philadelphia: W.B. Saunders.

Kirshblum, S., & Benevento, B. (2009). Understanding spinal cord injury and advances in recovery. In S. A. Sisto, E. Druin, & M. M. Sliwinski (Eds.), *Spinal cord injuries: Management and rehabilitation* (pp. 1-17). St. Louis: Mosby.

Levine, A. M. (1999). Spine trauma in adults: Surgical techniques for the treatment of thoracic, thoracolumbar, lumbar, and sacral trauma. In H. N. Herkowitz, S. R. Garfin, R. A. Balderston, F. J. Eismont, G. R. Bell, & S. W. Wiesel (Eds.), *The spine* (4th ed., Vol. 2, pp. 1003-1036). Philadelphia: W. B. Saunders.

Levine, M. J., & Heller, J. G. (1997). Spinal infections. In S. R. Garfin, & A. R. Vaccaro (Eds.), *Orthopaedic knowledge update: Spine* (pp. 257-272). Rosemont, IL: American Academy of Orthopaedic Surgeons.

Linville, D. A. (2003). Other disorders of the spine. In S. T. Canale (Ed.), *Campbell's operative orthopaedics* (10th ed., Vol. 2, pp. 2061-2121). Philadelphia: Mosby.

Mayer, T. G. (1999). Lumbar musculature: Anatomy and function. In H. N. Herkowitz, S. R. Garfin, R. A. Balderston, F. J.Eismont, G. R. Bell, & S. W. Wiesel (Eds.), *The spine* (4th ed., Vol. 1, pp. 75-82). Philadelphia: W. B. Saunders.

Mignucci, L. A., & Bell, G. R. (1999). Differential diagnosis of sciatica. In H. N. Herkowitz, S. R. Garfin, R. A. Balderston, F. J. Eismont, G. R. Bell, & S. W. Wiesel (Eds.), *The spine* (4th ed., Vol. 1, pp. 89-108). Philadelphia: W. B. Saunders.

Mirkovic, S., Cybulski, G., Montgomery, D. M., Wang, A., Wesolowski, D. P., & Garfin, S. R. (1999). Spinal stenosis: Clinical evaluation and differential diagnosis. In H. N. Herkowitz, S. R. Garfin, R. A. Balderston, F. J. Eismont, G. R. Bell, & S. W. Wiesel (Eds.), *The spine* (4th ed., Vol. 1, pp. 799-806). Philadelphia: W. B. Saunders.

Perry, A., Kim, C. W., & Garfin, S. R. (2008). Fusion Surgery. In C. W. Slipman, R. Derby, F. A. Simeone, & T. G. Mayer (Eds.), *Interventional spine: An algorithmic approach* (pp. 11121-1128). Philadelphia: W.B. Saunders.

Phillips, F. M., Pfiefer, B. A., Lieberman, I. H., Kerr, E. J., Choi, I., & Paziznos, A. G. (2003). Minimally invasive treatments of osteoporotic vertebral compression fractures: Vertebroplasty and kyphoplasty. In D. C. Ferlic (Ed.), *Instructional course lectures* (Vol. 52, pp. 559-567). Rosemont, IL: American Academy of Orthopaedic Surgeons.

Rao, R. D., & Bagaria, V. (2006). Pathophysiology of degenerative disk disease and related symptoms. In J.M. Spivak, & P.J.Connolly (Eds.), *Orthopaedic knowledge update: Spine 3* (pp. 35-41). Rosemont, IL: American Academy of Orthopaedic Surgeons.

Upham, K.L. (2007). Musculoskleletal assessment. In *NAON core curriculum for orthopaedic nursing* (pp. 37-70). Chicago: Pearson.

Russell, M. E., & Hanley, E. N. (1999). Surgical management of spinal stenosis: Indications, techniques, and results of decompressive laminectomy. In H. N. Herkowitz, S. R. Garfin, R. A. Balderston, F. J. Eismont, G. R. Bell, & S. W. Wiesel (Eds.), *The spine* (4th ed., Vol. 1, pp. 806F-806M). Philadelphia: W. B. Saunders.

Vocaturo, L. C. (2009). Psychological adjustment to spinal cord injury. In S. A. Sisto, E. Druin, & M. M. Sliwinski (Eds.), *Spinal cord injuries: Management and rehabilitation* (pp. 104-120). St. Louis: Mosby.

Wiesel, S. W. (1997). Spondylosis: Degenerative process of the aging spine. In S. R. Garfin, & A. R. Vaccaro (Eds.), *Orthopaedic knowledge update: Spine* (pp. 71-74). Rosemont, IL: American Academy of Orthopaedic Surgeons.

Williams, K. D., & Park, A. L. (2003). Lower back pain and disorders of intervertebral discs. In S. T. Canale (Ed.), *Campbell's operative orthopaedics* (10th ed., Vol. 2, pp. 1955-2028). Philadelphia: Mosby.

Wisneski, R. J., Garfin, S. R., Rothman, R. H., & Lutz, G. E. (1999). Lumbar disc disease. In H. N. Herkowitz, S. R. Garfin, R. A. Balderston, F. J. Eismont, G. R. Bell, & S. W. Wiesel (Eds.), *The spine* (4th ed., Vol. 1, pp. 613-680). Philadelphia: W. B. Saunders.

Yoganandan, N., Halliday, A. L., Dickman, C. A., & Benzel, E. C. (2005). Practical anatomy and fundamental biomechanics. In E. C. Benzel, (Ed.), *Spine surgery: Techniques, complications, avoidance, and management* (2nd ed., Vol. 1, pp. 109-135). Philadelphia: Elsevier.

Yu, W. D., & Williams, S. L. (2006). Spinal imaging: Radiographs, computed tomography, and magnetic resonance imaging. In J.M. Spivak, & P.J.Connolly (Eds.), *Orthopaedic knowledge update: Spine 3* (pp. 57-67). Rosemont, IL: American Academy of Orthopaedic Surgeons.

Zdeblick, T. A. (1997). Spinal instrumentation. In S. R. Garfin, & A. R. Vaccaro (Eds.), *Orthopaedic knowledge update: Spine* (pp. 55-62). Rosemont, IL: American Academy of Orthopaedic Surgeons.

Zigler, J. E., & Strausser, D. W. (2002). The aging spine. In D. F. Fardon, S. R. Garfin, J. Abitbol, S. D. Boden, H. N. Herkowitz, & T. G. Mayer (Eds.), *Orthopaedic knowledge update: Spine 2* (pp. 123-134). Rosemont, IL: American Academy of Orthopaedic Surgeons.

Chapter 4

Care of the Patient with Knee Problems

Maureen P. Cooper, MSN, RN, CS, ONC®

Objectives

- Identify the structures and function of the knee.

- Review pathophysiology and treatment options for common conditions of the knee.

- Outline nursing interventions for patients with common conditions of the knee.

Key Terms

Active range of motion (AROM): active muscle contraction, muscle stretch, and joint range of motion facilitated by an outside force, usually the physical therapist.

Anterior cruciate ligament: ligament of the knee that prevents excessive rotation of the knee.

Apprehension test: a test to evaluate patellar instability; examiner applies lateral pressure on the patella while flexing the knee; marked discomfort or apprehension by the patient indicates instability.

Articular cartilage: a layer of dense connective tissue that provides shock-absorbing properties at the ends of synovial joints.

Bursa(e): small fluid-filled sac that reduces friction between tendons, bones, and ligaments.

Condyles: rounded projection of bone, usually for articulation with another bone.

Crepitus: squeaking, creaking, or grating with joint movement.

Femur: bone that articulates with the proximal tibia of the knee joint; also known as the thigh bone.

Lateral meniscus: crescent-shaped cartilage on the outer aspect of the knee.

Medial meniscus: crescent-shaped cartilage on the inner aspect of the knee.

Nonsteroidal anti-inflammatory drugs (NSAIDs): medications commonly used for mild to moderate arthritic pain.

Osteoarthritis (OA): a non-inflammatory degenerative joint disease marked by the degeneration of articular cartilage, hypertrophy of bone at the margins, and changes in the synovial membrane accompanied with pain and stiffness.

Passive range of motion (PROM): an outside force is used to move the joint or stretch the muscle.

Patella: the knee cap; protects the knee joint and provides greater leverage for muscles of the leg.

Pes anserine Bursitis: painful inflammation of the three conjoined tendons of the hamstring muscles and/or bursae of the medial knee.

Proximal tibial osteotomy (PTO): a surgical procedure involving the removal of a wedge of bone in order to realign the knee joint.

Recurvatum deformity: hyperextension; results in the knee bending backward beyond normal extension.

Rheumatoid arthritis (RA): chronic, systemic, progressive disease characterized by inflammation of connective tissue with unexplained periods of remissions and exacerbations.

Synovial joint: a joint in which synovial fluid acts as a lubricant to reduce friction between joint surfaces and distributes stress in the joint due to impact and motion.

Tibia: bone of the lower leg that articulates with the proximal femur of the knee joint; also known as the shin bone.

Total knee arthroplasty (TKA): surgical procedure of the knee joint in which surfaces of the femur, tibia, and patella are replaced with metal alloys and polyethylene plastic.

Unicompartmental knee arthroplasty (UKA): surgical procedure of the knee joint in which the medial aspect of the proximal tibia and distal femur are replaced with metal alloys; also called a partial knee replacement.

Valgus deformity: knock-kneed; may be the result of uneven wear of the knee.

Varus deformity: bow-legged; may be inherited or the result of uneven wear of the knee.

The knee is the largest joint in the body and is comprised of various complex structures, which make it particularly susceptible to injury. The knee can be exposed to forces 3-4 times the weight of the body during normal activities, thereby exposing it to high-energy injuries.

Pain is the most common reason for seeking medical care in order to obtain symptom relief and because of its effect on activities of daily living (Collyott & Vasquez-Brooks, 2008). The knee is one of the most frequently treated body parts by orthopaedic surgeons. Approximately 19.4 million annual visits are made to physician offices due to knee problems (American Academy of Orthopaedic Surgeons (AAOS), 2007). The purpose of this chapter is to provide an overview of the knee anatomy, common knee injuries/conditions and their treatment options.

Arthritis and injury can damage the articular cartilage, resulting in acute pain and limited mobility. Although there are several types of arthritis, osteoarthritis (OA), rheumatoid arthritis (RA), (see Chapter 5, *Care of the Patient with Hip, Foot and Ankle Problems*, for further discussion of these disorders), and post-traumatic arthritis are the most common types of arthritis leading to knee joint destruction. Post-traumatic arthritis is caused by resultant damage to the cartilage and may develop years after a fracture, ligament injury, or meniscus tear.

Anatomy

The knee joint consists of three bones: the femur, the tibia, and the patella (see Figure 4-1). The distal femur includes the medial and lateral condyles, the medial and lateral epicondyles, the femoral trochlear groove, and the intercondylar notch. The femoral condyles articulate with the proximal tibia to form a hinge joint. The proximal tibia is comprised of the medial and lateral condyles, the medial and lateral plateaus, and the intercondylar eminence. The patella (knee cap) is a sesamoid bone embedded in the tendon of the quadriceps femoris muscle (Evans, 2007).

Articular cartilage covers the end of the femur, the tibia, and the underside of the patella. It functions to distribute the forces applied to the articulating surfaces, reducing stress, wear, and tear within the joint. The articular cartilage is mainly avascular and therefore has limited reparative qualities.

The knee is a synovial joint that is lubricated by both glycoprotein molecules that cover the cartilage and by fluid extracted from articular cartilage when force is applied to the joint. The suprapatellar and prepatellar bursae also help to reduce friction between adjacent tissues such as tendons and ligaments by lubricating tissues with synovial fluid, facilitating movement of the joint.

The bony anatomy of the knee itself provides minimal stability to the knee. The soft tissues that surround the knee joint including ligaments, muscles, tendons, and menisci provide stability and function. Ligaments are strong, fibrous tissues that connect bone to bone in order to provide strength and stability to the knee joint. There are four major ligaments in the knee: medial collateral ligament (MCL), lateral collateral ligament (LCL), anterior cruciate ligament (ACL), and posterior cruciate ligament (PCL) (see Figure 4-2). These ligaments resist valgus and varus stress and anterior/posterior translation of the tibia in relation to the femur. Of the four major ligaments, the ACL and MCL are the most commonly injured in sports (AAOS, 2007). The MCL extends from the medial

Figure 4-1
Picture of a Knee Joint

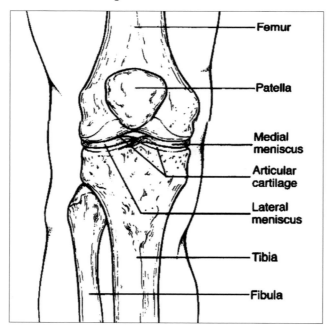

Reprinted with permission from Maher, A.B., Salmond, S.W., & Pellino, T.A. (2002). *Orthopaedic nursing* (p. 169). Philadelphia: W.B. Saunders.

Figure 4-2
Bony Anatomy and Major Ligamentous Structures of the Flexed Knee Joint (posterior view)

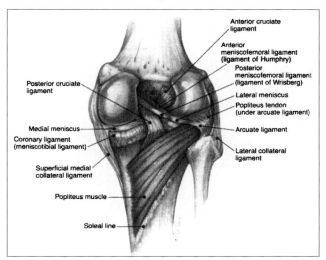

Reprinted with permission from Thibodeau, G.A., & Patton, K.T. (1996). *Anatomy and physiology* (p.292). St. Louis: Mosby.

femoral epicondyle to the proximal border of the tibia just below the medial tibial plateau to prevent excessive valgus rotation of the knee. The LCL extends from the lateral femoral epicondyle to the head of the fibula and prevents excessive varus rotation and external rotation of the knee. The ACL extends posterolaterally from the tibia and inserts on the lateral femoral condyle to prevent anterior translation and rotation of the tibia relative to the femur. The PCL extends anteromedially from the tibia posterior to the medial femoral condyle to prevent posterior subluxation of the tibia on the femur (Abate, 2008).

The menisci are two crescent-shaped cartilaginous structures attached to the proximal tibia and function to decrease stress on articular cartilage and allow the femur and tibia to turn in many directions. The medial meniscus is located on the inner aspect of the knee, and the lateral meniscus is located on the outer aspect of the knee (see Figure 4-3). The menisci transmit 50% of the total load when the knee is in extension and up to 90% of the load when in flexion. The medial meniscus is firmly attached along the entire peripheral edge of the joint capsule. The lateral meniscus is attached to the posterior capsule but there is a posterolateral region where it is not firmly attached. Consequently, the medial meniscus has less mobility and therefore makes it more vulnerable to tears when trapped between the femoral condyles and tibial plateau (McMahon & Kaplan, 2006).

The muscles and tendons are the dynamic restraints of the knee. The muscles are divided into those that extend (knee extensors) and flex (knee flexors) the knee. The extensor mechanism of the knee is comprised of the quadriceps muscle group, quadriceps tendon, patella, patellar retinaculum, patellar ligament and adjacent soft tissues. The quadriceps muscle group (also known as quadriceps femoris) is comprised of four large muscles: rectus femoris, vastus lateralis, vastus medialis, and vastus intermedius. The rectus femoris is the only muscle that crosses the hip joint at the anterior inferior

Figure 4-3
Posterior Aspect of the Knee Joint

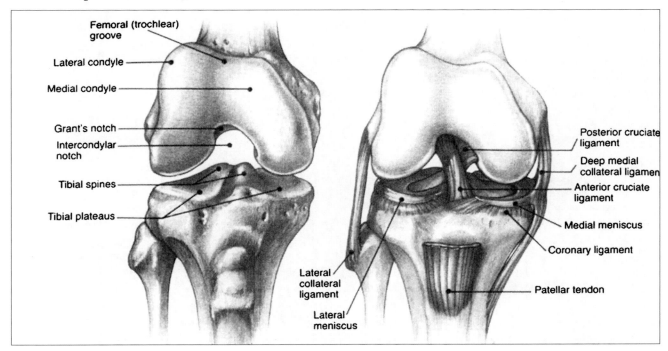

Reprinted with permission from Wiesel, S.W., & Delahey, J.N. (2002). *Essentials of orthopaedic surgery* (p. 254). Philadelphia: W.B. Saunders.

Figure 4-4
Flexor Mechanism

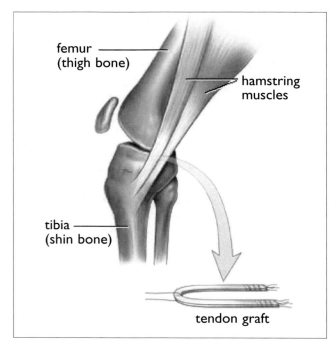

femur
(thigh bone)

hamstring
muscles

tibia
(shin bone)

tendon graft

Courtesy of ACLsolutions.com.

iliac spine. The rest of the quadriceps muscle group originates on the femoral shaft. The vastus medialis can be subdivided into the vastus medialis longus and the vastus medialis obliquus (VMO) and is located on the medial side of the femur. The vastus lateralis is located on the lateral side of the femur. The vastus intermedius is located between the vastus lateralis and the vastus medius on the front of the femur. These four muscles are attached to the patella via the quadriceps tendon. The patellar tendon extends from quadriceps femoris over the patella to the tibial tuberosity to form the medial and lateral patellar retinaculum. The primary flexors of the knee are the hamstring muscles – the semimembranosus, semitendinosus and biceps femoris, and the sartorius and gracilis (Evans, 2007). The hamstrings are proximally attached to the ischial tuberosity and distally attach to the posteromedial and posterolateral proximal tibia. The sartorius originates from the anterorsuperior iliac spine and the gracilis originates from the pubis. Both the satorius and gracilis, along with the semitendinous, insert into the proximal medial tibia in the pes anserine. The gastrocnemius and popliteus knee flexor muscles extend from the posterior femoral condyles to the calcaneus and proximal tibia (Figure 4-4).

Assessment

The initial step in assessing an individual with a musculoskeletal complaint is to obtain a comprehensive health history that includes a detailed account of the presenting problem and its effect on functional ability. Primary techniques used in musculoskeletal examination include inspection, palpation, range of motion (ROM), and special tests such as the anterior drawer test (Collyott & Vasquez-Brooks, 2008).

Inspection of the knee begins with comparing both knees for general appearance, symmetry, edema, effusion, muscle atrophy, skin changes, and knee alignment. Joint alignment should be observed during gait and with the patient in a standing position. Alignment assessment includes observations for varus (bow-legged), valgus (knock-kneed), and hyperextension (recurvatum) malalignment, instability of the joint, and alignment of the patella. The evaluation should include observation of gait in which normal gait involves ROM from 0-65 degrees of flexion with smooth, equal strides (Evans, 2007).

The knee joint can be palpated and mobilized to assess for pain, tenderness, swelling, warmth, ROM, and instability (Timby & Smith, 2007). Palpation of bony structures and soft tissues should be performed with the knee in both the flexed and the extended positions, as well as during ROM techniques. Crepitus, a grinding sensation between the patella and femoral trochlear groove, may be associated with chondromalacia patella (also referred to as patellofemoral syndrome).

Crepitus can be palpated by flexing the knee with the hand over the patella. The medial and lateral joint structures are palpated with the knee extended and flexed to assess for tenderness that may suggest meniscal injury. The patient can lie prone to assist in assessing the posterior knee structures such as the popliteal fossa, popliteal artery and vein, and the presence of swelling or decreased circulation. The patella should be gently palpated in all directions with the leg extended and should be pain free.

ROM includes active and passive techniques. Active ROM is assessed by having the patient independently flex (bend) and extend (straighten) the knee. To assess active flexion, the patient should be asked to perform a deep knee bend while standing. Active extension is evaluated with the patient sitting at the edge of the chair or table, and fully extending their legs. Active internal rotation and external rotation is performed by having the patient turn their foot inward and outward. Passive ROM is achieved using the same techniques noted above, but the examiner passively moves the joint. Normal ROM of the knee joint is 0-130 degrees flexion and 0-15 degrees extension (Upham, 2007) (see Table 4-1). Inability to fully bend or straighten the knee is referred to as locking of the knee and may be the result of a loose body, large effusions, or prior ligament injuries (Evans, 2007).

The cruciate and collateral ligaments can be assessed by placing the patient's foot between the examiner's elbow and

Table 4-1
Normal Range of Motion for Knee Joint

Flexion	0-130 degrees
Extension	0-15 degrees
Medial Rotation	20-30 degrees
Lateral Rotation	30-40 degrees

Adapted with permission from the National Association of Orthopaedic Nurses (2001), *NAON Core curriculum for orthopaedic nursing* (6th Ed., p. 44). Boston: Pearson.

hip and utilizing both hands to palpate the joint. The examiner places varus and valgus stress on the knee to determine laxity. Typically, the knee has a small amount of laxity in the MCL and LCL (McMahon & Kaplan, 2006). Menisci are examined by palpating the outer margin along the joint line at the proximal tibia.

Neurovascular and muscle strength assessment are essential to detect changes in circulation, sensation, or mobility of the joint especially in high energy injuries such as knee dislocations. Both extremities must be assessed and compared in order to accurately discern changes. See Chapter 1, *Musculoskeletal Anatomy and Neurovascular Assessment*, for discussion of neurovascular assessment.

Common Knee Conditions and Injuries

Osteochondritis Dissecans

Osteochondritis dissecans occurs when an area of bone next to the articular cartilage becomes avascular and eventually separates from the underlying bone. The exact cause is unknown but there may be a familial predisposition (Hosalkar & Wells, 2007). Although the knee is the most commonly affected joint, it may also occur in the elbow, hip or ankle (Childs, 2002). Repetitive microtrauma causes a lack of blood supply to the bone that eventually leads to avascular necrosis. It most commonly affects the medial aspect of the lateral femoral condyle; however, it can occur at any of the condylar surfaces.

Osteochondritis dissecans typically occurs during bone growth in childhood but can occur during adolescence or early adulthood. The primary complaint is usually vague non-localized knee pain (Evans, 2007). Additional findings on physical exam include crepitus of the medial knee, popping, giving way and occasional locking of the knee. Radiographs in early stages may show small defects of the medial condyle. If the condition progresses, it may lead to loosening or separation of fragments causing pain and articular defects. Initial management in children with open growth plates includes close observation with enough activity restriction to allow symptoms to abate. Typically, most children can return to sports and the conservative treatment is sufficient to resolve symptoms. Stage I and II lesions are treated with activity modification, isometric exercises and knee immobilizer (Hosalkar & Wells, 2007). However, if symptoms continue or if the defect is larger than 1 cm or located in a weight-bearing area, arthroscopy is indicated. Arthroscopic surgery may be limited to drilling the fragment for intact lesions; however, if the lesion is loose or separated, drilling of the fragment and pin fixation is required. If the fragment is detached, excision of the lesion is warranted (Davis & Abbate, 2007).

Osgood-Schlatter Disease

Osgood-Schlatter disease is pain over the tibial tubercle in a growing child. The patellar tendon inserts into the tibial tubercle which extends from the proximal tibial epiphysis. It is traction apophysitis of the knee, where a muscle group pulls on an open growth plate, causing overload and resultant inflammation of local tissues (Evans, 2007). The condition affects males more often than females and is frequently associated with activities or sports that include repetitive knee flexion, such as jumping. The ossification area (apophysis) is vulnerable to repetitive stress at the patellar tendon insertion. Most commonly after a growth spurt, it is thought that stress from quadriceps contraction extends to the patellar tendon and tibial tuberosity which can result in tendonitis and avulsion fractures of the tibial tubercle. As a result, bony overgrowth may persist and cause a bony prominence.

Symptoms of Osgood-Schlatter disease include pain associated with activities such as climbing up or down stairs, running, jumping or squatting. Local swelling and tenderness is noted over the tibial tuberosity. Pain can be reproduced during physical examination by either forced knee extension against resistance or when squatting in full knee flexion. Osgood-Schlatter is primarily a clinical diagnosis; however if imaging studies are utilized such as radiographs or MRI, they are more for differential diagnosis. The disease is usually self-limiting and the key to successful treatment includes activity restriction and activity modification until the growth plate is closed. Ice after activity and occasional use of a compression knee sleeve can be beneficial. Surgical excision is rare but may be indicated for a skeletally mature patient (Hawk & Bailie, 2007).

Pes Anserine Bursitis

Pes anserine bursitis or pes tendonitis is painful inflammation of the tendons and/or bursae of the medial knee. The pes anserine bursa is located between the tibia and the three conjoined tendons of hamstring muscles (the sartorius, gracilis and semitendinosus) along the proximal medial aspect of the tibia. These three muscles are the primary knee flexors and allow for knee flexion and protect the knee against rotational stress. Pes tendonitis is common in middle-aged, obese women and often seen in younger athletes. It can also result from overuse, trauma or degenerative changes from osteoarthritis or medial meniscus tear. However, the most common cause of pes tendonitis is hamstring tightness which places additional stress on the bursae. Pain and tenderness over the proximal medial tibia at the insertion of the pes anserine, approximately 2-5 centimeters below the anteromedial joint line of the knee is a common symptom (AAOS, 2007). Additionally, the patient may complain of painful extension/flexion of the knee such as with stair climbing. On physical examination, the pes anserine can be palpated distal to the tibial tubercle, sometimes with notable warmth, swelling and complaint of pain in the region. Examination should also include careful evaluation of the hamstrings to determine if hamstring tightness is contributing to the condition.

Treatment is directed at identifying the underlying cause but includes rest and ice to reduce acute inflammation and swelling; Non-steroidal anti-inflammatory medications (NSAIDs) can be effective for pain management. Intra-articular cortisone injections or injections directly into the pes tendon may provide pain relief. Modification of activities coupled with hamstring stretching and a quadriceps strengthening program is very beneficial. In rare cases, surgical excision of the bursa may be performed in situations of prolonged disability, as with an athlete who is disabled for 6-8 weeks (Glencross & Little, 2008).

Extensor Mechanism Injuries

Patellar dislocation

Patellar dislocations are usually the result of a direct blow to the patella or twisting of the knee and are commonly associated with sports such as soccer, hockey and gymnastics. The mechanism of injury is due to the quadriceps tendon, along with other ligament stabilizers of the patella, contracting forcefully as the knee is rotating resulting in the patella sliding, most often laterally, out of the patellofemoral groove (Dath, Chakravarthy, & Porter, 2006). Females are more susceptible to patellar dislocation, particularly young female athletes (Palmu, Kallio, Donell, Helenius, & Nietosvaara, 2008). Patella malalignment, as a result of malformation of the patellofemoral joint, is a condition in which the patella is situated abnormally higher than normal and can be a predisposing factor to patellar dislocation (Buchner, Baudendistal, Sabo, & Schmitt, 2005). The vastus medialis obliquus (VMO) muscle is a knee stabilizer; however, if weakened can lead to patellar instability and dislocation.

Patellar dislocations are associated with severe swelling and impaired mobility of the knee. On physical examination of the knee, a positive apprehension test is noted when the patella is pushed laterally or medially when the knee is flexed at 30 degrees. Tenderness upon palpation is usually noted along the medial/lateral retinaculum. Diagnostic tests may include radiographs to assess for position of the patella and any bony fracture fragments. Fractures of the patella and lateral femoral condyle can occur due to the force of the patellar dislocation. An MRI may be indicated to assess for soft tissue injuries such as meniscus or retinacular tears which can occur as a result of the dislocation. Surgical treatment (arthroscopy or open repair) is usually suggested if other structures of the knee are severely damaged or if there is osteochondral injury or gross instability. If these factors are not present, research indicates that conservative treatment is preferable when possible (Shea, Nilsson, & Belzer, 2006).

Figure 4-5
Patellar Fracture

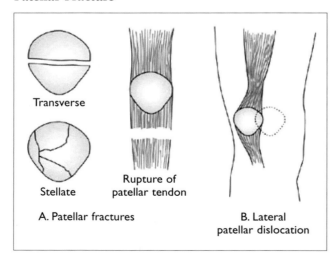

Transverse

Stellate

Rupture of patellar tendon

A. Patellar fractures

B. Lateral patellar dislocation

Reprinted with permission from LeBlond, R., DeGowin, R., & Brown, D. (2009). *DeGowin's diagnostic examination* (9th ed.). New York: McGraw-Hill.

Immediate treatment includes elevation and ice to reduce swelling, reduce dislocation if still present at the time of presentation, and pain management with NSAIDs and/or narcotic analgesics. Compression bracing for 2-4 weeks may offer comfort and stability while soft tissues are healing (Davis & Abbate, 2007).

Physical Therapy is usually offered for both conservative and surgical treatments due to high risk of patellar re-dislocations. Initial focus of rehabilitation includes isometric hamstring and quadriceps strengthening to restore normal function, progressing to full ROM, increased activities such as jogging at 6-8 weeks and possible return to sports by the 12th week.

Knee dislocations

True knee dislocation is rare but is considered a very serious injury due to potential popliteal artery disruption (Wissman, Verma, Kreeger, & Robertson, 2009). The popliteal artery is located at the proximal tibia near the interosseous membrane making it vulnerable to injury. The incidence of popliteal artery injuries is more common in posterior knee dislocation than anterior knee dislocation due to the high energy necessary to cause this type of dislocation. Pulse deficit and ischemia are noted; however, clinical findings can be misleading since the presence of distal pulses does not rule out arterial injury. There is some controversy as to whether to obtain an arteriogram since the incidence of popliteal artery injury is so high and testing may delay vascular reconstruction. There are sources who recommend arteriography if there is a confirmed knee dislocation, whereas others suggest that clinical confirmation should be sufficient to determine if arteriography or surgical intervention is warranted (Steele & Glaspy, 2004).

Patellar fractures

Patellar fractures are the most common traumatic injury of the knee extensor mechanism and are typically caused by either a direct fall or blow to the patella or ruptured quadriceps or patellar tendons. Symptoms of patellar fracture include pain, swelling and hemarthrosis. Asking the patient to extend the knee against resistance or to do a straight leg raise (lifting the foot from the exam table into the air) assesses the function of the quadriceps muscle. If unable to extend the knee or to do a straight leg raise suggests disruption to the quadriceps tendon, patella or patellar tendon (Davis & Abbate, 2007). See Figure 4-5. Radiographs are obtained to determine the type of fracture and extent of displacement.

Initial treatment of a patellar fracture includes rest, ice, compression and elevation (RICE). Non-displaced or mildly displaced patellar fractures are treated by bracing the knee in extension for 6 weeks. However, if there is displacement, an open reduction and internal fixation is recommended (Delahey & Sauer, 2007).

Quadriceps and Patellar Tendon Rupture

The quadriceps and patellar tendons are part of the extensor mechanism of the knee, which are responsible for straightening the knee and for activities such as kicking. In order for knee extension to occur, the quadriceps muscle contracts with force transmitted through the quadriceps tendon across the patella, through the patellar tendon. The quadriceps and patellar tendons are strong, thick fibrous tissues meant to transmit the pulling force of the quadriceps muscle. Quadriceps tendon ruptures occur more often over the age of 40, whereas patellar tendon ruptures occur in those younger than 40 years of age (McMahon & Kaplan, 2006). Quadriceps and patellar tendon ruptures usually result from either landing from a jump which causes excessive load, or falling onto a partially bent knee. Findings on the physical examination usually include a diagnostic triad which includes complaint of acute pain, inability to straight leg raise or extend the knee, and swelling. There may be a notable suprapatellar gap at the rupture site since most ruptures occur between 0-2 cm above the patella. Additional symptoms include instability and weakness of the knee and the inability to weight bear. Radiographs will demonstrate abnormal position of the patella and any bony avulsion. A MRI may be ordered to evaluate whether there is partial or complete rupture of the tendon, so that a course of treatment can be determined. Initial management includes ice, elevation and immobilization. Partial tears can be treated conservatively with bracing in extension for approximately 1 month followed by a quadriceps strengthening program. In severe or complete tears, surgical repair and re-attachment of the tendon to the patella is performed. The most common complications after quadriceps tendon repair are loss of knee motion and extensor weakness and atrophy (Ilan, Tejwani, Keschner, & Leibman, 2003).

Ligament sprains/strains

The four ligaments of the knee, MCL, LCL, ACL, and PCL provide stability to the knee joint. However, these ligaments are commonly injured, especially in sports. Ligament injuries usually result from hyperextension or abnormal rotation of the knee ranging from mild to severe sprains/strains of the ligament. The most common grading system for ligament injuries is: grade I –ligament is stretched, but no detectable instability; grade II- ligament is further stretched with detectable instability; and grade III – ligament is completely disrupted (McMahon & Kaplan, 2006).

Injuries to the MCL commonly occur when the foot is firmly planted, while sustaining valgus (on the lateral side of the knee) stress. MCL injury can also be associated with ACL and medial meniscus tears. Upon examination, there is complaint of medial knee pain and instability noted with valgus stress. Radiographs may be performed to identify any avulsion fractures of the femur or tibia. Initial treatment includes RICE, bracing, and pain management. For a grade I or II tear, conservative management includes refraining from sports for 6-12 weeks, depending on the type of sport or severity of injury. Arthroscopy may be indicated for grade III injuries and with other ligament or soft tissue injuries (Davis & Abbate, 2007).

LCL injuries are relatively uncommon but can occur when there is a varus stress such as a direct blow to the medial side of the knee. A pop or snap may be felt at the time of injury with lateral knee swelling and pain. Surgery for isolated LCL injuries is not usually necessary. However, if the LCL is injured as a result of significant trauma or in conjunction with other ligament injuries such as the PCL, surgical repair may be required to prevent future instability.

ACL injuries are the most common ligament injury especially in high demand sports such as soccer, football, lacrosse and basketball which require sudden turns. It typically occurs when there is sudden pivoting, causing excessive rotational forces on the ligament. Often, a pop with severe pain is felt at the time of injury with immediate swelling to the joint. Symptoms may also include the feeling of the knee giving out. Findings on the physical examination of the knee should include noting any swelling and assessing for any associated injuries such as medial or lateral meniscus tears. Lateral meniscus tears are more common with acute ACL injury, whereas medial meniscus tears are more commonly associated with chronic ACL tears. Radiographs may be ordered to assess for bony injury, however, a MRI is usually ordered to identify ACL injury. Initial treatment as with the other ligament injuries includes RICE, bracing, and physical therapy with quadriceps and hamstring strengthening. Surgery is indicated for failed conservative management, for those who plan on returning to aggressive sports, or if there are injuries to the menisci or posterolateral corner of the knee.

Surgical repair of ACL tears involves arthroscopic reconstruction of the ligament. Either autograft or allograft tissues can be utilized to reconstruct the ACL. Two of the most common autologous grafts for ACL reconstruction are the patellar and hamstrings tendons. Autograft typically involves harvesting the patellar tendon with bone block on the ends. Hamstring muscle may be inserted but there is not bone-to-bone contact. There is no rejection risk; however, there is often pain from the donor site.

Allograft is cadaver graft of patellar tendon with bone or soft tissue and can be utilized without donor site pain but there is a small risk of viral or bacterial infection. Surgical repair is achieved by placing drill holes into the attachment sites of the ligament on the tibia and femur. The graft is pulled through the drill holes into the joint to replace the ACL and secured with biodegradable or metal screws. Full recovery from ACL repair has moved from greater than a year in the 1970's to 4 to 9 months today. While there is no consensus on timing, surgical techniques and rehabilitation, studies indicate that early and progressive rehabilitation does not adversely affect outcomes (Roi et al., 2005). Postoperatively, early ROM is recommended to restore strength and motion within 2 days of surgery followed by a quadriceps strengthening program. Crutches are often used for the first 7-10 days but may be stopped when comfortable. A knee brace may be used if associated with ACL or posterolateral corner injuries (Davis & Abbate, 2007).

Meniscal Injuries

The medial and lateral meniscus are c-shaped cartilage structures that function to absorb shock during weight bearing activities. Meniscus tears most commonly occur due to traumatic injury such as when the knee is bent and then twisted. Meniscal injuries often cause the knee to lock and prevent full extension. Pain and swelling may be noted upon palpation on the medial or lateral joint line. Radiographs may be ordered to assess for arthritis or degenerative changes. An MRI is typically ordered to identify the type of tear. There are different types of tears including vertical or horizontal, longitudinal, transverse, oblique and complex (including degenerative tears). Vertical longitudinal or oblique tears tend to occur in younger patients, whereas complex and degenerative tears occur more commonly in those 50 years or older. Bucket handle tears are when a portion of the meniscus is torn from the tibia and forms a flap that resembles a bucket handle. A flap tear is when a portion of the meniscus has torn and flipped up. Linear tears are across the length of the meniscus. Degenerative tears are when edges of the menisci become jagged or frayed. Treatment depends on the type of tear, age of the patient and response to conservative management. Conservative management is typically for small or degenerative tears. The inner two thirds of the meniscus are avascular and when torn, usually will require resection. Tears in the outer areas of the meniscus, if small, may heal without surgery because there is a blood supply.

Meniscus injuries are the most common reason for arthroscopic surgery. Arthroscopic surgery aims to preserve and repair the meniscus, in lieu of menisectomy, in order to reduce the risk of developing knee arthritis and maintaining kinematics (Schoen, 2007). A partial meniscectomy has excellent results in patients with normal knee stability and without any degenerative changes. Postoperatively, exercises aimed at ROM and strengthening are initiated immediately (McMahon & Kaplan, 2006).

Chondral Defects

Articular injury is a common injury, yet repair of articular cartilage defects is one of the most challenging procedures in orthopaedic surgery (Ochi et al., 2004). Since cartilaginous tissues are avascular, arthroscopic chondroplasty has been the traditional surgery. Subchondral bone is either drilled, burred or microfractured in order to stimulate bleeding, inflammatory response, and eventual scar tissue. However, scar tissue in comparison to hyaline cartilage does not have load-bearing capabilities and eventually degrades. In the 1990s, cellular therapy approaches with autologous chondrocyte implantation emerged as a possible option for cartilage defects of the femoral condyle. The clinical application of chondrocyte implantation was first developed in Sweden and has been in use in the United States and Europe. In 1997, Carticel®, an autologous chondrocyte implantation product, was the first cellular product to be approved by the Food and Drug Administration. This product was approved for repair of symptomatic cartilage defects of the femoral condyle that were not responsive to other surgeries (Wood et al., 2006). The autologous chondrocyte implantation technique is done by harvesting autologous chondrocytes from a non load-bearing area such as the intercondylar notch or the superior aspect of the medial or lateral femoral condyles. The chondrocytes are grown and then placed back into the patient at the site of the injury. The cells are kept in place by suturing a flap of periosteum to the surrounding cartilage tissue with the

intent of proliferating the cells under the flap to create a replacement cartilage. Studies have demonstrated varying results with early encouraging results reported; however, similar results were found with placement of the periosteal flap alone. The surgery is technically challenging and further research is needed to improve cartilage repair including improvement in surgical techniques and cellular biology.

Conservative Management of Patients with Knee Problems

The initial treatment of knee pain usually includes conservative management strategies including activity modification, oral analgesics and NSAIDs, intra-articular injections, and assistive devices. There is increasing evidence that persons with osteoarthritis benefit from physical therapy, muscle strengthening, and aerobic exercise. Additional, non-pharmacological management with local heat or ice may be beneficial to decrease pain and stiffness (Roberts, 2007). Biologic products that may be beneficial in alleviating osteoarthritis (OA) symptoms in the knee are glucosamine and chondroitin. OA prevalence is expected to double in the next 20 years and along with NSAID-related gastrointestinal symptoms, the investigation of disease-modifying treatment options are growing in orthopaedics. Glucosamine (GH) and chondroitin sulfate (CS) are both naturally occurring body substances that have cartilage constituents. They have been used for arthritis treatment in Europe and Asia for more than 20 years, with increased public interest in the United States since the late 1990s. Several studies have been conducted about their effect on joint space narrowing, functionality, and pain but have been criticized due to study design. However, meta-analysis concluded that GH and CS have some efficacy in treating symptoms of OA (Vangsness, Spiker, & Erickson, 2009). Some studies have also demonstrated that those who take CS for mild to moderate OA, achieve pain relief similar to that of NSAIDs but take longer to return to work (Roberts, 2007). Glucosamine is an amino sugar synthesized by chondrocytes and is a substrate for cartilage synthesis. Chondroitin is a glycosaminoglycan which is found in the cartilage matrix and helps prevent cartilage breakdown and stimulate cartilage repair. Glucosamine is obtained from crustacean shells and chondroitin is obtained from bovine tissues. Oral glucosamine appears to be well-tolerated, with minimal adverse gastrointestinal symptoms and does not elevate blood glucose levels (Hughes & Barrows, 2009).

Topical agents such as salicylates and capsaicin are relatively effective and inexpensive options to reduce OA pain. Capsaicin is extracted from a pepper plant. Its therapeutic effect is believed to be the result of the stimulation of nociceptors that inhibit slower pain signals. Capsaicin cream has been found to be effective in diminishing knee pain when used concomitantly with arthritis medication (Roberts, 2002). Multiple applications of the topical cream are necessary to obtain therapeutic effect.

Intra-articular steroid injections have been frequently used for treatment of OA in the knee. In patients with OA that have moderate to severe knee pain and signs of joint inflammation, aspiration and intra-articular glucocorticoid injection(s) may be beneficial. However, the effects are only temporary and vary from patient to patient (Geier, Keeperman, Sproul, Roth, & Reynolds, 2002). Side effects of intra-articular injections include local reactions and infection. Intra-articular corticosteroids may provide relief for up to 6 months (Baird, 2001). Typically, intra-articular steroid injections are given 3 to 4 months apart to decrease the possibility of residual cortisone build-up which might damage the joint. If a patient requires more than four injections in one year, alternative interventions should be considered (Roberts, 2002).

Viscosupplementation with hyaluronic acid (HA) has gained popularity in recent years. Multiple studies have been conducted to evaluate the efficacy of hyaluronic acid injections. Several peer-reviewed studies have shown little difference between steroid injections, hyaluronic acid, and NSAID therapies. Others studies have shown significant improvement with HA, especially in relation to pain and function (Peters & Crofoot, 2008). Hyaluronan is a polysaccharide known as glycosaminoglycan which is an essential element of synovial fluid. Injecting hyaluronan may possibly restore properties of synovial fluid in the osteoarthritic joint and provide an anti-inflammatory function similar to NSAIDs by inhibiting release of prostaglandins (Geier et al., 2002). The most common side effect of HA therapy is injection site inflammation and pain. If there is a known allergy to eggs, HA should be administered with caution because it is manufactured from rooster comb. A series of weekly injections are administered into the affected knee joint. Patients should be instructed that pain relief following viscosupplementation might not occur until several weeks after the last injection. Pain relief may last up to 10 months but the exact mechanism of action is unknown (Namba, Skinner, & Gupta, 2006).

Exercise can help diminish symptoms of OA and may delay progression of the disease by strengthening the muscles that stabilize the joint and help reduce pain and improve functional ability. Low-impact exercises such as swimming, walking, stationary bicycling, and water aerobics are not only beneficial in reducing pain but also help to maintain flexibility and strength. Attempts to maintain function can be helped through non–weight bearing strengthening, especially of the quadriceps (Amy & Micheo, 2008). Mind-body exercises such as tai chi have been found to release muscle tension which can help with improving flexibility (Roberts, 2007).

Additional alternative treatments include meditation, biofeedback, and acupuncture. Meditation has been utilized for centuries to help reduce stress and manage pain, and is an acceptable adjunct to exercise and medication for treating arthritis pain. Biofeedback is a relaxation technique involving the use of sensory equipment to measure heart rate, blood pressure, and muscle response to help control involuntary responses to pain and muscle spasms. Acupuncture, a technique in existence for thousands of years, has gained renewed interest as a treatment of osteoarthritis. A National Institutes of Health randomized controlled study found acupuncture to be effective as adjunctive therapy for reducing pain and improving function in patients with knee osteoarthritis (Hochberg, Lixing , Bausell, Langenberg, & Berman, 2004).

Oftentimes, it is an automatic reflex to rub a painful joint. The analgesic effect of massage is related to the release of endorphins into the bloodstream (Weinrich, Haddock, & Robinson, 1999). Massage was once believed to increase blood flow, but studies do not support this premise. Nonetheless, massage is a harmless and simple technique that can be utilized to relieve tension and relax muscles.

Obesity or being overweight can increase mechanical stress on cartilage of the knee joint. While age is a primary risk factor of osteoarthritis due to wear and tear to the joint, obesity is a significant risk factor as well. Studies have shown that osteoarthritis is 4-5 times more common in those who are overweight as compared to those who are of normal weight (Eustace & Eustace, 2009). Patients should be encouraged to lose weight, which will reduce biomechanical stress on the joint and retard the progression of OA. A loss of 5 kilograms can reduce symptomatic OA in women by 50% (Wilkins & Phillips, 2008). Health care professionals often recommend a weight reduction plan that focuses on lifestyle changes rather than on diet alone.

Adjustment in activities of daily living reduces the pain of OA and maintains stamina throughout the day. Incorporating

Figure 4-6
Proximal Tibial Osteotomy

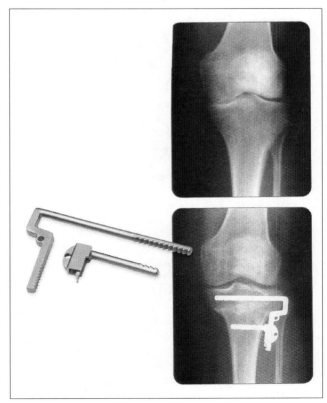

Courtesy of Stryker Howmedica Osteonics.

rest periods into daily routines may be an effective means of maintaining independence. When simple activities such as dressing, bathing, and getting in and out of cars become difficult to perform, a referral to an occupational therapist may be beneficial. Adaptive equipment such as an elevated toilet seat, shoe horn, sock aide, reacher, and dressing stick may assist with activities of daily living. Most patients can tolerate pain and weakness associated with arthritis before resorting to an assistive device for walking. However, a cane or walker should be considered to enhance functional ability and safety once a patient begins to consistently ambulate with a limp.

Surgical Management

When conservative options fail to relieve the symptoms of knee injuries, OA, RA, and post-traumatic arthritis, and there is radiographic evidence of advanced arthritis, surgical intervention may be considered. The goal of surgery for the patient with knee problems is to eliminate pain and improve function. Surgical options for osteoarthritis include proximal tibial osteotomy, unicompartmental knee arthroplasty, and total knee arthroplasty.

Proximal Tibial Osteotomy

Patients with OA often have angular deformities, the most common being varus angulation from erosion of the medial compartment of the knee. Proximal Tibial Osteotomy (PTO), used for patients with unicompartmental arthritis of the knee, involves unloading the knee joint by correcting the malalignment and redistributing stresses within the knee (See Figure 4-6). The knee should have limited deformity of less than 15 degrees in the valgus or varus planes with no instability or subluxation. The procedure is most commonly done at the proximal tibia for medial compartment disease but may also be performed at the distal femur in lateral compartment disease (Springfield, 2005). Indications for surgery include unicompartmental involvement, patients with less than 10 degrees of fixed flexion and greater than 90 degrees of active flexion. These surgeries are best suited for young, highly active patients who have good bone stock, are not overweight, and are experiencing severe pain. Contraindications include bi-compartmental or tri-compartmental disease, ACL insufficiency, or MCL incompetence (Davis & Abbate, 2007). The surgery involves removing a wedge of bone from the lateral side of the proximal tibia to provide varus angular correction to compensate for damaged tissue. The osteotomy repositions the mechanical axis of the limb away from the diseased area. The fragments are approximated, and alignment of the limb is verified. Bone cuts are often held together with staples. The tourniquet is released, and a drain may be inserted. A compression dressing is often applied, and the patient may be placed in an immobilizer. Osteotomy is typically performed under either epidural or general anesthesia and requires a short hospital stay. Reports indicate approximately 65-85% of patients have good results after 5 years (Namba, Skinner, & Gupta, 2006). This procedure is used primarily as a temporary measure to gain 5 to 10 years before total knee arthroplasty is performed (Springfield, 2005). Non-weight-bearing or partial weight-bearing status

Figure 4-7
Unicompartmental Knee Implant

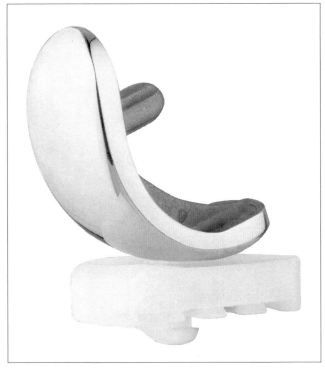

Courtesy of Stryker Howmedica Osteonics.

with crutches is instituted for 1 to 3 months, depending on the surgical technique. Resumption of full activities usually occurs at 3-6 months. It is important that physical therapy be started shortly after the procedure in order to retain joint motion (Allen, Brander, & Stuhlberg, 1998). Complications of osteotomy, while uncommon, may include peroneal nerve palsy, compartment syndrome, and delayed or non-union of bone (Roberts, 2002). Deep vein thrombosis (DVT) has also been reported; therefore, it is currently recommended that DVT prophylaxis be instituted. Infection is a possible complication, and antibiotic prophylaxis varies upon surgeon's preference. There has been a decline in the number of osteotomies with the reemergence of unicompartmental knee arthroplasty as a precursor to total knee arthroplasty (Peters & Crofoot, 2009).

Unicompartmental Knee Arthroplasty

Unicompartmental Knee Arthroplasty (UKA) can be used as an alternative to PTO or total knee arthroplasty (TKA) in patients with unicompartmental involvement. UKA can offer those with early stages of unicompartmental arthritis a resurfacing and rebalancing procedure without undergoing a total knee arthroplasty. UKA, also known as a partial knee replacement, is similar to that of a total knee arthroplasty but instead of replacing the entire knee joint as in TKA, the unicompartmental prosthesis replaces only one condyle of the joint (see Figure 4-7). UKA restores articular surfaces and provides anatomic alignment and appropriate tension to the collateral and anterior cruciate ligaments. The procedure avoids disrupting the suprapatellar pouch, reducing the need for formal postoperative physical therapy. The incision is smaller, with less removal of bone and greater preservation of the knee anatomy. Advantages of UKA are preservation of normal knee kinematics, lower perioperative morbidity, less blood loss and accelerated recovery (Borus & Thornhill, 2008). Both cruciate ligaments should be in intact and degenerative changes to the opposite compartment should be minimal. Poor flexion is not an absolute contraindication; however, poor passive extension is, particularly if the procedure cannot correct to less than 15 degrees extension. A lax MCL is a contraindication in the valgus knee with lateral compartment involvement. Varus deformity of more than 10 degrees, valgus deformity of more than 15 degrees, if not corrected by osteophyte excision, and morbid obesity are additional contraindications to the surgery (Scott, 2009). Ideal candidates for an UKA are patients older than age 60 with complete loss of the medial compartment on weight-bearing x-rays. However, younger patients undergoing UKA is increasing as a temporizing measure to TKA. One study indicated 92% survivorship of UKA after 11 year follow-up in patients under the age of 60 (Crockarell & Guyton, 2007). The UKA represents 8% of knee arthroplasty surgery (Geller, Yoon, & Macauley, 2008).

During this procedure, the patient's leg is secured in a thigh holder and a tourniquet is placed. An arthroscope is introduced to assess the articular surface of the knee joint. The surgical incision is made from the superior medial edge of the patella and extended distally. Components are cemented into the bone after irrigation and lavaged with antibiotic solution. The tourniquet is deflated, and a drain may be placed. The skin is closed with sutures and steristrips. Most patients do not require a blood transfusion after surgery. Often the patient is placed in an immobilizer before leaving the operating room. Patients who undergo UKA maintain more proprioceptive feedback from the joint and are therefore more likely to retain a normal gait pattern than those who have a TKA (Romanowski & Repicci, 2003). Nursing interventions such as pain management and hemodynamic monitoring are similar to that of the TKA.

A vast majority (95%) of unicompartmental arthritis is medial, and most patients may have this disease for more than 10 years before warranting a TKA. Only 5% of arthritis cases involve the lateral knee compartment. Lateral UKA is a different operation entirely than medial UKA because the anatomy of the lateral side is significantly different. The lateral tibia is convex rather than concave, and the alignment of the femoral component is also significantly different. Aligning the femur and tibia is more difficult to ensure full femoral contact with the lateral tibial surface. Since only 5% of the cases involve the lateral side, most surgeons do not develop expertise in performing the procedure. Although studies from the 1970s were doubtful as to the benefit of UKA, more recent studies indicate an UKA can function closer to a normal knee. Long-term outcomes studies indicate that proper patient selection and surgical technique are vital to the success of the procedure (Borus & Thornhill, 2008).

Total Knee Arthroplasty

Initial attempts to replace both femoral and tibial surfaces of the knee joint date back to the 1950s, with the initial design of hinged implants. Failure of these designs was attributed to the simplicity of the implant, which did not account for the complex nature of knee motion. Additionally, the metal-on-metal surfaces led to unacceptable high loosening rates and infection (Crockerall & Guyton, 2003). Improvements to the knee prosthesis were made in the 1970s, when Insall designed total condylar prostheses. Early criticisms of the total condylar design included the tendency to subluxate posteriorly and limited flexion of 100 degrees. During the 1980s and 1990s, increased attention was placed on reconstruction of the patellofemoral joint because this contributed to the majority of revision surgeries. Newer implant designs allow for greater patellofemoral contact (Crockerall & Guyton, 2007).

Knee prosthetics can either be unconstrained, semi-constrained, or constrained, contingent upon the amount of ligament laxity. The amount of constraint built into the artificial joint is reflective of the amount of stability the hardware provides. As such, a totally constrained joint has the femoral portion physically attached to the tibial component and requires no ligamentous or soft tissue support. The semiconstrained TKA has two separate components that glide on each other, but the physical characteristics of the tibial component prevent excessive femoral glide. The unconstrained device relies entirely on the ligaments and soft tissues to maintain the stability of the joint (Kaplan, 2008).

There are three surgical approaches for the standard TKA which include the medial parapatellar retinacular approach, the midvastus approach, and the subvastus approach. The medial parapatellar retinacular approach compromises the quadriceps tendon and can lead to more postoperative patellofemoral complications. The midvastus approach does not compromise the extensor mechanism of the knee joint. The subvastus approach also preserves the integrity of the extensor mechanism but does not expose the knee as well as the other two approaches do. TKA is most commonly performed with a midline incision that extends from the proximal patella to a few inches below it. A tourniquet is usually applied to the affected extremity to minimize blood loss and to keep the operative field clean and dry. The patient is positioned supine with the knee flexed. Bone cuts to the femur, tibia, and patella must be accurately oriented in the forward-backward, side-to-side, and rotational planes. Accurate reproducibility is achieved with the use of jigs and alignment guides to ensure proper alignment of the prosthetic components. Soft tissue is usually released to correct any valgus or varus deformities. Balancing of soft tissue is important to insure stability of the knee. The distal femur and proximal tibia are resurfaced to accommodate the femoral and tibial components. A polyethylene (plastic) button is then secured to the inner aspect of the patella after it has been resurfaced. After the prosthesis is in place, the tourniquet is released, soft tissue structures are sutured, and a suction drain may be placed. Most frequently, a staple incision is utilized for wound closure.

Figure 4-8
Total Knee Arthroplasty Implant

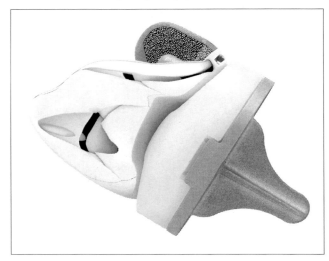

Courtesy of Stryker Howmedica Osteonics.

Despite continued research for improved implant materials, the combination of ultrahigh molecular weight polyethylene that articulates with metal alloys such as cobalt and titanium (Figure 4-8) are the prosthetic components most widely used (Harkness & Daniels, 2003). Prosthetic fixation with polymethylmethacrylate (PMMA) in total knee replacements gained widespread use in the 1970s and has continued until present. Cementless technology used in total hip replacements was extended to total knee replacements, unfortunately with lower success rates. Early failure rates related to tibial loosening, polyethylene wear, and osteolysis (resorption of bone) have been higher in cementless TKA than in cemented designs (Crockarell & Guyton, 2003).

The primary indication for a TKA is to relieve pain caused by severe arthritis (bi-compartmental or tri-compartmental) with or without associated deformity. TKA is a procedure with excellent long-term results. Several studies have reported a success rate of 93% at 10 years. Currently, there are approximately 581,000 total knee arthroplasties performed annually in the United States (AAOS, 2009). Absolute contraindications to TKA include active sepsis, absence of an extensor mechanism, and neuropathic joint. Relative contraindications include a patient's young (less than 40 years) age, and heavy demand for activity (Dutton, 2008).

Minimally Invasive Total Knee Arthroplasty

Total knee arthroplasty is a major surgery and recovery can be difficult. There is often substantial postoperative pain which must be endured during aggressive physical therapy required for optimal outcomes. In addition, reliance on assistive devices and narcotic analgesics may be required for several weeks. Consequently, there has been increased interest in less invasive total knee arthroplasty approaches. Several different procedures or techniques aimed at utilizing smaller incisions with less disruption to the extensor mechanism and joint capsule during surgery have been put

under the minimally invasive surgery (MIS) category. Proposed advantages include less postoperative pain, shorter hospitalization, earlier quadriceps control and shorter recovery time. While there is limited evidence that there is better long term function over traditional approaches, most surgeons believe that benefits are limited to the recuperative period. Of the studies conducted, few were randomized and they examined different methods or aspects of the MIS procedure, therefore limiting the ability for comparison (Leopold, 2009).

Relative contraindications to MIS include previous open knee surgery, severe osteoporosis, rheumatoid arthritis, obesity and severe joint deformity. In the traditional approach, an anterior longitudinal incision of 6-9 inches is made through the quadriceps tendon, whereas the MIS typically uses a shorter anteromedial incision along the medial border of the patella, extending distally to the tibial tubercle (see Figure 4-9). In addition, MIS avoids quadriceps dissection by opening the medial capsule and extends proximally and obliquely into either the midvastus or subvastus plane. Unlike the traditional approach in which the patella is everted, the patella is retracted laterally and not everted in MIS. Regardless of approach, attention to ligament balancing and protecting neurovascular structures is paramount (Watson & Haas, 2009).

Length of postoperative recovery can vary, but length of stay for MIS is typically one day shorter than traditional TKA. Physical therapy begins on the day of surgery with emphasis on range of motion and gait training. While recovery time may vary, a walker is usually used for 10-14 days, followed by transition to a cane. The cane is discontinued once the patient feels steady enough to walk without an assistive device. Complications of MIS are similar to those of traditional TKA and include infection, deep vein thrombosis (DVT), nerve injuries and prosthetic failure. Some studies of MIS suggest inferior alignment of the prosthetic components, impaired wound healing, and longer surgical duration. The studies fail to validate earlier recovery times for MIS verses traditional TKA. Since MIS is a relatively new approach, long term

Figure 4-9
MIS Incision

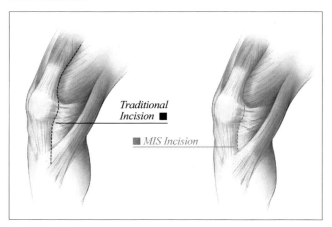

Traditional Incision ■

■ *MIS Incision*

Courtesy of Zimmer.

Table 4-2
Common Nursing Diagnoses, Outcomes, and Interventions for Patients with Problems of the Knee

Diagnoses	Outcomes	Interventions
Pain, acute	Patient is comfortable	– Assess pain level – Encourage use of pain medication – Elevate and ice extremity
Physical mobility, impaired	Knee motion is restored and weight bearing is maintained	– Promote range of motion – Encourage exercise program – Instruct on use of continuous passive motion machine (CPM) – Discuss potential problems of over exercising
Knowledge, deficit	Patient has knowledge of diagnosis, surgical procedure, postoperative expectations and complications	– Provide patient teaching on diagnosis and surgical procedure – Assess and explain expectations related to pain, function and rehabilitation. – Assess and reinforce understanding of potential complications such as infection, bleeding, and deep vein thrombosis – Patient and family education for rehabilitation
Infection, risk for	Patient will remain free of infection	– Observe for signs and symptoms of infection such as redness, swelling, drainage, odor, temperature and increased pain. – Vigilant universal precautions – Administer prophylactic antibiotics – Monitor laboratory results (CBC) – Remove invasive lines/ urinary catheters as soon as possible following surgery – Instruct patient on importance of long-term prophylaxis for dental procedures and invasive procedures (TKA)
Tissue perfusion, altered	Tissue perfusion will remain intact	– Assess for signs of deep vein thrombosis, and neurovascular compromise – Promote early mobilization – Teach patient signs of decreased tissue perfusion to report to physician – Teach mechanical and pharmacological prevention of deep vein thrombosis
Fluid volume, deficit	Patient will not exhibit signs and symptoms of hemorrhage or dehydration	– Monitor hemodynamic status – Measure and record accurate intake and output – Monitor vital signs – Assess skin turgor – Observe for mental status changes

Adapted with permission from National Association of Orthopaedic Nurses (2007), *NAON Core curriculum for orthopaedic nursing* (6th ed., pp. 560-561). Boston: Pearson.

outcomes and formal guidelines have yet to be established (Leopold, 2009).

Preoperative Evaluation Prior to Total Knee Arthroplasty

Preoperative education is vital for a successful outcome to any surgery. Risks and benefits of surgery must be reviewed with the patient to allow an informed decision regarding the procedure. Many hospitals offer interdisciplinary preoperative programs for patients and caregivers, enabling the patients and families to become more active participants in the recovery process, recognize potential postoperative complications, and recover more quickly (NAON, 2009).

A comprehensive preoperative medical evaluation is essential to prevent potential complications that may threaten the patient's outcome. A complete history including medical and surgical history, allergies, medications, family and social history must be conducted preoperatively. Comorbidities must be considered, especially with the increased number of elderly patients undergoing surgical procedures. Patients with multiple medical risk factors have been shown to require

longer hospitalization. Smokers, in particular, tend to have longer operative times and increased hospital charges after undergoing joint arthroplasty. Patients must have adequate cardiopulmonary reserve to withstand anesthesia and blood loss; consequently, consultants should further evaluate patients with a history of coronary artery disease, pulmonary disease, and peripheral vascular disease. Routine chest x-rays are not cost-effective but should be considered in patients with cardiopulmonary disease (Crockarell & Guyton, 2007). Lab work-up includes complete blood cell count, electrolytes, and urinalysis. Routine coagulation studies are not usually performed except in patients with a history of bleeding or coagulopathy. Patients should be instructed as to when to stop anticoagulants and NSAIDs prior to surgery. Most surgeons recommend discontinuing these medications 1-2 weeks preoperatively. Pain medications with acetaminophen (Tylenol®) may be used to replace NSAIDs for pain management.

Patients may donate 1-2 units of their own blood preoperatively for possible reinfusion after a TKA. This practice is not as common with unicompartmental or PTO surgery. Patients must have a hemoglobin level of 11 grams to be eligible to donate their own blood. The only true contraindication to autologous blood donation is bacteremia; however, if a patient has a history of seizures, severe respiratory disease or cardiac comorbidities in which decreasing the oxygen carrying capacity may be deleterious, autologous blood donation may also be contraindicated (Barnett & Strickland, 2007). See Chapter 8, *Complications Associated with Orthopaedic Conditions and Surgeries*, for further discussion of blood management strategies.

The preoperative anesthetic evaluation is an integral component in the planning phase of TKA. As the population ages, patients with concurrent medical conditions such as coronary artery disease, hypertension, chronic obstructive pulmonary disease, diabetes, and cerebral vascular disease are increasingly prevalent. The most common anesthesia options for TKA are spinal or general anesthesia. The decision as to which anesthesia method is used should be based on the patient's medical history, length of surgery, and patient preference. Although the ultimate decision lies with the anesthesiologist, input from the orthopaedic surgeon, internist, and sub-specialists involved in the patient's care should be considered. There is ongoing debate as to benefits of spinal versus general anesthesia. Cardiovascular outcomes related to both types of anesthesia have not proven to be significantly different. Controversy exists as to whether there is any effect on DVT between general and spinal anesthesia. Possible benefits of spinal anesthesia are vasodilation in the lower extremity thereby increasing blood flow with less viscosity, therefore lowering risk for DVT. Another benefit is that the epidural catheter can be left in place for 48-72 hours for pain management. Although use of spinal analgesia may require less narcotics, routine respiratory assessments are a critical aspect of epidural monitoring (Crockarell & Guyton, 2007).

Nursing Interventions for the Patient with Knee Surgery

Nursing interventions in the postoperative period for the patient having knee surgery should include pain management, proper positioning/mobilization, postoperative exercises, gait training, neurovascular assessment, deep vein thrombosis prophylaxis, hemodynamic monitoring, and incision care (NAON, 2009). See Table 4-2. See Chapter 7, *Pain Management*, for a discussion of pain management strategies and Chapter 8, *Complications Associated with Orthopaedic Conditions and Surgeries*, for an overview of postoperative complications.

Hemodynamic monitoring includes assessing the patient for any potential signs of fluid loss related to hypovolemia or blood loss. Clinical manifestations of hypovolemic shock vary with the severity of fluid loss and patient's ability to compensate. Hemodynamic monitoring includes assessment of the blood pressure, heart rate, respiratory depth and rate. Nursing assessment parameters include monitoring skin color and temperature, urine output, capillary refill, peripheral pulses, mucous membranes, and presence of pallor, cyanosis, and pain. Profound blood loss is associated with severe hypotension, tachycardia, tachypnea, decreased urine output, and delayed capillary refill (Smith-Blair, 2003). Laboratory test monitoring includes hemoglobin and hematocrit, prothrombin time, and electrolytes. TKA patients will often have a urinary catheter in place for 24 to 48 hours. The patient should be assessed

for possible signs of fluid overload or congestive heart failure including shortness of breath, crackles, increased blood pressure, and decreased oxygen saturations.

Patients undergoing orthopaedic surgery are at higher risk of deep vein thrombosis (DVT) or venous thromboembolism (VTE). Without anticoagulation, there is a 45-70% incidence of DVT after hip and knee surgery (Morris & Levin, 2007). Prevention of potentially fatal complications resulting from VTE and pulmonary embolism is essential. Routine thromboprophylaxis including the use of low molecular weight heparin, fondaparinux (Arixtra®), or adjusted dose vitamin K antagonists are recommended for elective total knee arthroplasty. Use of mechanical devices such as intermittent pneumatic compression devices are recommended for those at high risk of bleeding or as an adjunct to anticoagulation therapy; however, proper use and optimal compliance are essential for this modality to be effective (Geerts et al., 2008)

Aside from life-threatening complications, the most devastating postoperative complication for the patient with TKA is infection. The incidence of superficial or deep wound infection associated with TKA is between 1-5% (Albuhairan, Hind, & Hutchinson, 2008). The incidence is higher in patients with diabetes, hemophilia, obesity or those who had prior open knee surgery (Peters & Crofoot, 2009). Infection control begins in the operating room, with strict adherence to aseptic technique and minimized flow-through traffic. The use of laminar flow systems in the operating room, body exhaust suits for the surgical team, and prophylactic antibiotics has greatly reduced the postoperative incidence of infections in total joint arthroplasty. Gram–positive bacteria, Staphylococcus aureus and Staphylococcus epidermidis, are the most common organisms in prosthetic-related infections. These organisms are normally present in skin flora and can adhere to implants and polymers (Albuhairan et al., 2008). Consequently, a first-generation cephalosporin such as cefazolin is usually recommended for antibiotic prophylaxis. In patients with a significant penicillin allergy, vancomycin can be used (Crockarell & Guyton, 2007). Most surgeons recommend routine single-does prophylactic antibiotics preoperatively 30 minutes before skin incision (Morris & Levin, 2007). Other factors such as obesity, oral steroid use, urinary tract infection, and concurrent infections at other sites have been associated with increased incidence of postoperative infections. The optimal duration of antibiotic prophylaxis after TKA has been debated, and there is no evidence to support the administration of antibiotics beyond 48 hours. Harkness & Daniels (2003) report that 2-3 doses of postoperative antibiotic appears to be efficacious.

The most common neurologic injury after TKA is peroneal nerve palsy, which is often associated with correction of severe valgus and flexion deformities and in patients with rheumatoid arthritis (Crockarell & Guyton, 2007). Injury may also result from direct compression of the peroneal nerve, which runs along the lateral aspect of the fibular head, resulting in foot drop. The nurse must verify that the nerve is intact by assessing the sensation on top of the foot, and having the patient dorsiflex their ankle and extend their great toe. If the patient is able to perform these maneuvers, the peroneal nerve is intact. Because outcomes following peroneal nerve palsy in TKA are variable, early recognition is essential. The surgical dressing and devices such as immobilizers or continuous passive motion machines must be assessed to assure proper placement and avoid compression of the peroneal nerve.

The patient may be out of bed on the surgery day, depending on the surgeon's preference. While in bed, the patient's leg should be positioned in a neutral position. The affected leg may be elevated with pillows positioned under the lower leg to promote knee extension and prevent flexion contractures.

Postoperative physical therapy and rehabilitation greatly affects the outcome of TKA and usually begins on the first postoperative day. The therapist will dangle the patient at the bedside and assist the patient to the chair with a walker. The patient should be instructed on exercises such as ankle pumps, heel slides, and isometric muscle contractions. The surgeon may order a continuous passive motion machine (CPM), a device that passively bends and straightens the knee while the patient lies in bed (see Figure 4-10). The machine is programmed with degrees of flexion, extension, and speed as ordered by the physician. Practices vary as to the duration of use of the CPM. Orthopaedic surgeons differ in their opinions as to the efficacy of CPMs. Several studies indicate benefit in achieving early flexion, but CPMs have not been proven to be effective in long-term knee ROM or functional scores (Crockarell & Guyton, 2007). In addition to ROM exercises, the postoperative rehabilitation includes lower extremity muscle strengthening, concentrating on the quadriceps, gait training, with weight bearing as allowed by the particular knee reconstruction, and instruction in performing basic activities of daily living.

On the first postoperative day, most patients begin to walk in their room and tolerate sitting in a chair for 1 to 2 hours. The surgeon and surgical technique determine weight bearing status. Frequently, TKAs are secured with polymethylmethacrylate (PMMA), thus allowing full weight bearing. Cementless TKAs may be partial weight bearing for 4-6 weeks to allow for bony in-growth. Physical therapy is typically offered twice daily during hospitalization. Upon discharge, a physical therapist may come into the patient's home 2-3 times per week to provide therapy until the patient is able to visit an outpatient site. The patient is encouraged to use a walker or crutches for the first 3-6 weeks post-surgery and then transition to a cane to allow soft tissue healing. Weight bearing and patient safety are factors considered when selecting appropriate assistive devices. Occupational therapy may be ordered during the hospitalization to assist patients with energy conservation and activities of daily living such as dressing, showering, and getting in and out of the car.

Surgical dressings are commonly changed within 24 hours after the surgery. Surgical drains are typically discontinued at the same time but may remain in place up to 48 hours. Patients may shower 2-3 days after surgery, depending on surgeon preference. Patients must be educated regarding signs and symptoms of infection such as erythema, drainage, and elevated temperature, and the importance of keeping

Figure 4-10
Continuous Passive Motion Machine

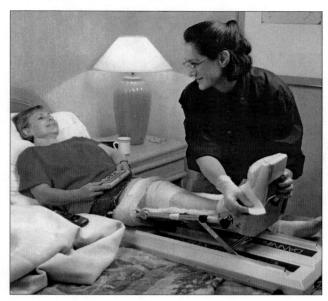

Courtesy of Orthologic.

the wound clean and dry. Typically, patients are discharged from the hospital in 2-4 days and go home or to a rehabilitation center. Staples are usually removed 10-14 days after surgery.

The recovery of the patient undergoing TKA is a multidisciplinary effort; thus, most hospitals have implemented standard protocols or clinical pathways outlining expected outcomes and length of stay. The clinical pathways may be utilized as a care map or encompass the documentation of the involved disciplines such as nursing, occupational therapy, physical therapy, and discharge planning (see Figure 4-11). In addition, the type of surgical approach will usually dictate the progression and duration of rehabilitation.

Upon discharge, it is important to educate the TKA patient regarding the need to use prophylactic antibiotics prior to certain surgical procedures. Patients should also be judicious in preventing bacterial infections including urinary tract infections or pneumonia that may result in bacteremia and possible infection of the total joint.

The need for routine prophylactic antibiotics for TKA patients undergoing dental procedures has been debated. Hematogenous infection of total joint arthroplasty patients after dental procedures has been difficult to establish. The American Academy of Orthopaedic Surgeons (AAOS) and the American Dental Association (ADA) published the first advisory statement on antibiotic prophylaxis for dental patients with prosthetic joints in 1997, and an updated advisory statement in 2003. The recommendations state that antibiotic prophylaxis is not indicated for patients with pins, screws, or plates. Antibiotic prophylaxis is not routinely indicated for most patients with TKA unless they are within two years of surgery and are undergoing high risk dental procedures. High risk procedures include dental extractions, dental implants, root canals beyond

Figure 4-11
Clinical Pathway from WBH on Total Knee Arthroplasty

CLINICAL PATHWAY

☐ TOTAL KNEE ARTHROPLASTY ☐ TOTAL KNEE REVISION ☐ UNICOMPARTMENTAL KNEE

A pathway does not represent the Standard of Care. Clinical judgment may supersede these guidelines.

PATIENT PROBLEMS	OR DAY OUTCOMES	POD #1 OUTCOMES	POD #2 OUTCOMES
Pain R/T disease process and/or surgical procedure.	Pain controlled AEB verbal and / or non-verbal indicators.	Same.	Decreased pain AEB change to PO analgesics.
Potential altered **tissue perfusion**: systemic & peripheral R/T surgical procedure.	NV status WNL AEB stable VS, good leg mobility, positive pulses and capillary refill and no numbness or tingling.	Same.	Same.
Impaired **skin integrity** R/T surgical incision.	Dressing intact & drain patent, if present.	Dressing changed.	Incision (CDI) clean dry & intact.
Altered **mobility** R/T discomfort from surgical procedure.	Pt tolerates tilt / turn Q 2° with assist.	Using proper body mechanics. Pt demonstrates ability to transfer to chair with assist, weight bear & ambulate as ordered.	Able to transfer to chair and ambulate short distances with walker and assistance.
Potential altered **elimination** R/T surgical procedure & immobility.	Urinary output adequate > 30 ml/hr.	Same.	Pt passing flatus. Pt voiding without difficulty.
Knowledge deficit R/T hospital procedures and post-op recovery.	Pt verbalizes/demonstrates understanding of post-op routine.	Pt verbalizes / demonstrates correct teaching from all disciplines.	Pt/SO verbalizes understanding of discharge instructions and Continuing Care Plan.

	OR DAY	DAY #1	Day of Discharge - DAY #2
CONSULTS	-Medical (if applicable) -Care Management -PT/OT	-Medical consult done (if applicable) -Care management consult initiated -PT/OT consult done	
TREATMENTS/ TESTS	-Post-op vitals per unit guideline -Foley to DD -Incentive spirometry 10x/hr WA -Thigh high anti-embolism stockings and/or SEQ sleeves -I & O x24hr -Empty and record hemovac -Ice to site for 30 minutes TID and PRN -Assess and document NV status of operative extremity Q 1-2hr x8, then Q 4 x24hr -Decubitus Precautions -Fall Precautions -Bleeding Precautions	-CBC with platelets in am, call if HGB < 9.0 -PT/INR in am -Basic Metabolic Panel in AM -Dressing changed/drain removed per physician -Thigh high anti-embolism stockings and/or SEQ sleeves bilaterally -X-ray of operative knee -Assess and document NV Q 4 x24hrs, then Q 8 x72hr -Ice to site for 30 minutes TID and PRN -Portable chest x-ray if ECF placement known -D/C foley at 6am per physician order -I & O (24 hours) -Empty and record hemovac -Vital signs per unit guidelines -Incentive spirometer 10 x hr while awake -Decubitus precautions -Fall precautions -Bleeding precautions	-CBC with platelets in am, call if HGB < 9.0 -PT/INR in am -Change dressing PRN -Thigh high anti-embolism stockings and/or SEQ sleeves bilaterally -Assess and document NV Q 8hr -Ice to site for 30 minutes TID and PRN -Portable chest x-ray if ECF placement known -I & O (24 hours) -Empty and record hemovac -Vital signs per unit guidelines -Incentive spirometer 10 x hr while awake -Decubitus precautions -Fall precautions -Bleeding precautions
MEDICATIONS	-IV antibiotics x24hrs -Analgesics: IV/PCA/Epidural/Stryker pump -Anticoagulation Therapy -Assess for nausea Q 2-4hrs WA	-Analgesics: IV/PCA/Epidural/Stryker pump -Anticoagulation Therapy -Assess for nausea Q 2-4hrs -Bowel Protocol	-IV to IV lock -Analgesics: IV/PO/Stryker pump -Anticoagulation Therapy -Assess for nausea Q 2-4hrs -Bowel Protocol
DIET	-Full liquid advance as tolerated (disease specific per physician order)	-Regular (disease specific per physician order)	-Regular (disease specific per physician order)
ACTIVITIES	-Overhead Trapeze -Elevate ankle higher than the knee, no pillow under knee -Turn to side Q 2hrs with assist -Weight bearing status per physician order -Dangle at bedside -Up in chair per physician order	-WB status per physician order -Bed Bath with assist -Activity initiated by RN or PT -Transfer to chair BID/Ambulate with walker PRN -PT/OT evaluation in am/PT session in PM -Assist with turning Q 2°	-WB status per physician order -Shower with assist -Pt may wear own clothes -Continue PT/OT -Transfers to chair using walker and ambulates with/without assistance 2 x/day -Daily progressive ambulation -Assist with turning Q 2°
TEACHING	-Discuss/Review Guide Through Your Hospital Stay	-Discuss Patient Daily Guidelines -Discuss and distribute Patient's Guide to Warfarin (Coumadin)	-Discharge Instructions -Review Patient Daily Guidelines -Review Patient's Guide to Warfarin (Coumadin)

3551 050709 OSB

Reprinted with permission from William Beaumont Hospital, Royal Oak, Michigan.

the apex, and prophylactic cleaning of teeth, or implants where bleeding is anticipated. After two years, only high risk patients undergoing high risk procedures should be considered for prophylaxis. High risk patients include those with previous prosthetic joint infections, hemophilia, HIV infection, Type 1 diabetes, malignancy, drug or radiation-induced immunosuppression and inflammatory arthropathies such as rheumatoid arthritis or systemic lupus erythematosus (ADA, AAOS, 2003). Recommendations for actual antibiotic regimens used for prophylaxis remain unchanged. No current guidelines exist for patients undergoing endoscopic procedures (Harkness & Daniels, 2003).

Manipulation under anesthesia

Despite improved surgical techniques and rehabilitation protocols which have contributed to improved knee function and ROM, there are a small number of patients who experience functional problems after a TKA including persistent pain, instability, and limited ROM (Seyler et al., 2007). In order to perform activities of daily living such as climbing stairs or rising from a chair, at least 90 degrees of knee flexion is required. If a patient has not been able to achieve approximately 90 degrees of flexion 8 weeks after TKA, a manipulation under anesthesia (MUA) may be performed . The procedure involves taking the patient to the operating room, and under anesthesia, manipulating the knee until there is lysis of adhesions. Typically, physical therapy is initiated within a few hours of the MUA.

Studies indicate varying criteria for MUA ranging from as early as two months following TKA to as late as 44 weeks (Keating et al., 2007). ROM criteria vary in studies, ranging from 75-90 degrees; however, all studies indicate 90 degrees or less as indication for MUA. In the literature, outcomes associated with manipulation under anesthesia after TKA vary. Some patients had a mean increase in flexion of 35 degrees after five years, with no difference in flexion between patients who were treated less than or greater than 12 weeks post-TKA. Other studies suggest initial increase of ROM following MUA, but after one year, no difference in ROM between those who underwent MUA versus those who did not (Seyler et al., 2007).

Summary

The knee is a complex joint that is commonly affected by arthritis or injury. Osteoarthritis, rheumatoid, and post-traumatic arthritis are the most common conditions affecting the knee joint. There are several non-surgical and surgical options for patients with knee arthritis. Once conservative treatment has failed, surgical intervention is usually recommended. Surgical options include proximal tibial osteotomy, unicompartmental knee arthroplasty, and standard total knee arthroplasty with or without the minimally invasive approach. The type of corrective surgery depends on multiple factors including age and severity of the arthritis. Advances in orthopaedic surgery afford patients improved quality of life and decreased pain. Advances in sports medicine have allowed athletes with knee injuries to restore function with a quick return to sports. A multidisciplinary approach to patients undergoing knee surgery optimizes patient outcomes. The orthopaedic nurse has an integral role in the care of the patient with knee problems through clinical assessment, patient teaching, and promotion of mobility and independence.

References

Abate, J. (2008). Dislocations and soft tissue injuries of the knee. In B.D. Browner, J.B. Jupiter, A.M. Levine, P.G. Trafton, & C. Krettek (Eds.), *Skeletal trauma* (pp. 2175-2189). Philadelphia: Elsevier.

Albuhairan, B., Hind, D., & Hutchinson, A. (2008). Antibiotic prophylaxis for wound infections in total joint arthroplasty: A systematic review. *The Journal of Bone and Joint Surgery, 90-B*(7), 915-919.

Allen, R. J., Brander, V.A., & Stuhlberg, S.D. (1998). *Arthritis of the hip & knee: The active person's guide to taking charge* (p. 71). Atlanta: Peachtree.

American Academy of Orthopaedic Surgeons (2007). *The Knee*. Retrieved May 28, 2009, from http://orthoinfo.aaos.org/topic.cfm?topic=A00325

American Academy of Orthopaedic Surgeons (2007). *Goosefoot (Pes Anserine Bursitis of the Knee)*. Retrieved May 30, 2009, from http://orthoinfo.aaos.org/topic.cfm?topic=A00335

American Academy of Orthopaedic Surgeons (2009). *Total Knee Replacement*. Retrieved February 20, 2010 from http://orthoinfo.aaos.org/topic.cfm?topic=A00389

American Dental Association and American Academy of Orthopaedic Surgeons (2003). Antibiotic prophylaxis for dental patients with total joint replacements. *The Journal of the American Dental Association, 134*(7), 895-899.

Amy, E., & Micheo, W. (2008). The knee and lower leg. In W.R. Frontera, J.K. Silver, & T.D. Rizzo (Eds.), *Essentials of physical medicine and rehabilitation* (pp. 345-352). Philadelphia: W.B. Saunders.

Baird, C.L. (2001). First-line treatment for osteoarthritis: Part 1: Pathophysiology, assessment, and pharmacologic interventions. *Orthopaedic Nursing, 20*(5), 17-27.

Barnett, S., & Strickland, L. (2007). Perioperative patient care. In *NAON core curriculum for orthopaedic nursing* (6th ed., pp.101-125). Boston: Pearson.

Borus T., & Thornhill T. (2008). Unicompartmental knee arthroplasty. *Journal of the American Academy of Orthopaedic Surgery, 16*(1): 9-18.

Buchner, M., Baudendistel, B., Sabo, D., & Schmitt, H. (2005). Acute traumatic patellar dislocation: Long-term results comparing conservative and surgical treatment. *Clinical Journal of Sports Medicine, 15*(2): 62-66.

Childs, S. G. (2002). Athletic performance and injury. In A.B. Maher, S.W. Salmond, & T. A. Pellino (Eds.), *Orthopaedic nursing* (pp. 674-701). Philadelphia: W.B. Saunders.

Collyott, C.L., & Vasquez-Brooks, M. (2008). Evaluation and management of joint pain. *Orthopaedic Nursing, 27*(4), 246-250.

Crockarell, J.R., & Guyton, J.L. (2003). Athroplasty of the knee and ankle. In S.T. Canale, K. Daugherty, & L. Jones (Eds.), *Campbell's operative orthopaedics* (pp.245-298). St. Louis: Mosby.

Crockarell, J.R., & Guyton, J.L. (2007). Arthroplasty of the knee. In S.T. Canale, K. Daugherty, & L. Jones (Eds.), *Campbell's operative orthopaedics* (pp. 241-299). St. Louis: Mosby.

Dath, R., Chakravarthy, J., & Porter K.M. (2006). Patella dislocations. *Trauma, 8*(1), 5-11.

Davis, J.P., & Abbate, N. (2007). The knee. In *NAON Core curriculum for orthopaedic nursing* (6th ed., pp. 556-554). Boston: Pearson.

Delahey, J. N., & Sauer, S. T. (2007). Skeletal trauma. In S.W. Wiesel, & J.N. Delahey (Eds.), *Essentials of orthopaedic surgery* (pp. 40-83). Philadelphia: W.B. Saunders.

Dutton, M. (2008). *Orthopedic examination, evaluation and intervention* (pp. 1691-1728). New York: McGraw Hill.

Eustace, C., & Eustace, R. (2009). *Obesity linked to osteoarthritis and joint replacement complications.* Retrieved from http://osteoarthritis.about.com/od/osteoarthritis101/a/obesity.htm

Evans, B.G. (2007). The knee. In S.W. Wiesel, & J.N. Delahey (Eds.), *Essentials of orthopaedic surgery* (pp. 454-471). Philadelphia: W.B. Saunders.

Geerts, W.H., Pineo, J.F., Heit, J.A, Bergqvist, D., Lassen, M.R., Colwell, C.W.,... Ray, J.G. (2008). *Prevention of venous thromboembolism: The seventh AACP conference on antithrombotic and thrombolytic therapy, 133*(6), 675-705.

Geier, K.A., Keeperman, J.B., Sproul, R.C., Roth, K., & Reynolds, H.M. (2002). Viscosupplementation: A new treatment option for osteoarthritis. *Orthopaedic Nursing, 21*(5), 25-34.

Geller J.A., Yoon R.S., & Macauley, W. (2008). Unicompartmental knee arthroplasty: A controversial history and a rationale for contemporary resurgence. *Journal of Knee Surgery, 21*(1), 7-14.

Glencross, P.M., & Little, J.P. (2008) *Pes anserinus bursitis.* Retrieved February 20, 2010 from http://emedicine.medscape.com/article/308694-overview

Harkness, J.W., & Daniels, A.U. (2003). Introduction and overview. In S.T. Canale, K. Daugherty, & L. Jones (Eds.), *Campbell's operative orthopaedics* (pp. 223-242). St. Louis: Mosby.

Hawk, D., & Bailie, S. (2007). Pediatric/congenital disorders. In *NAON Core curriculum for orthopaedic nursing* (6th ed., pp. 261-322). Boston: Pearson.

Hochberg, M., Lixing, L., Bausell , B., Langenberg, P., & Berman, B. (2004). Traditional Chinese acupuncture is effective as adjunctive therapy in patients with osteoarthritis of the knee. *Arthritis Rheumatology 2004, 50*(9), S644.

Hosalkar, H.S., & Wells, L. (2007). The knee. In R.M. Kliegman (Ed.), *Nelson textbook of pediatrics* (pp. 2796-2800). St. Louis: W.B. Saunders.

Hughes, E.F, & Barrows, K. (2009). Complimentary & alternative medicine. In J. McPhee, & M.A. Papadakis (Eds.). *Current medical diagnosis & treatment* (pp. 1502-1515). New York: McGraw Hill.

Ilan, D.I., Tejwani, N., Keschner, M., & Leibman, M. (2003). Quadricep tendon rupture. *Journal of the American Academy of Orthopaedic Surgeons, 11*(3), 192-200.

Kaplan, R.J. (2008). Total knee replacement. In W.R. Frontera, J.K. Silver, & T.D. Rizzo (Eds.), *Essentials of physical medicine and rehabilitation* (pp. 395-405). Philadelphia: W.B. Saunders.

Keating, E.M., Ritter, M.A., Harty, L.D., Haas, G., Meding, J.B., Faris, P.M., & Berend, M.E. (2007). Manipulation after total knee arthroplasty. *Journal of Bone and Joint Surgery, 89-A*(2), 282-286.

Leopold, S.S. (2009). Minimally invasive total knee arthroplasty for osteoarthritis. *New England Journal of Medicine, 360*(17), 1749-1758.

McMahon, P.J., & Kaplan, L.D. (2006). Sports medicine. In H.B Skinner (Ed.), *Current diagnosis and treatment in orthopedics* (pp. 163-186). New York: McGraw Hill.

Morris, N.S., & Levin, B. (2007). Complications. In *NAON Core curriculum for orthopaedic nursing* (6th ed., pp. 177-206). Boston: Pearson.

Namba, R.S., Skinner, H.B., & Gupta, R. (2006). Adult reconstructive surgery. In H.B. Skinner (Ed.), *Current diagnosis and treatment in orthopedics* (pp. 395-396, 396-401). New York: McGraw-Hill.

National Association of Orthopaedic Nurses (2009). In J. Foecke (Ed.), *NAON Patient education series total knee replacement* (pp. 1-29). Chicago: National Association of Orthopaedic Nurses.

Ochi, M., Adachi, N., Nobuto, H., Yanada, S., Ho, S., & Agung, M. (2004). Articular cartilage repair using tissue engineering technique - Novel approach with minimally invasive procedure. *International Journal of Artificial Organs, 28*(1), 28-32.

Palmu, S., Kallio, P.E., Donell, S.T., Helenius, I., & Nietosvaara, Y. (2008). Acute patellar dislocation in children and adolescents: A randomized clinical trial. *Journal of Bone and Joint Surgery, 90*(3), 463-470.

Peters, C.L., & Crofoot, C.D. (2008). Knee reconstruction and replacement. In J.S. Fischgrund (Ed.), *Orthopaedic knowledge update* (pp.457-471). Rosemount, IL: American Academy of Orthopaedic Surgeons.

Roberts, D. (2002). Degenerative disorders. In A.B. Maher, S.W. Salmond, & T. A. Pellino (Eds.), *Orthopaedic nursing* (pp. 468-514). Philadelphia: W.B. Saunders.

Roberts, D. (2007). Arthritis and connective tissue disorders. In *NAON Core curriculum for orthopaedic nursing* (6th ed., pp. 329-368). Boston: Pearson.

Roi, G.S., Creta D., Nanni G., Marcacci, M., Zaffagnini, S., & Snyder-Mackler, L. (2005). Return to official Italian first division soccer games within 90 days after anterior cruciate ligament reconstruction: A case report. *Journal of Orthopaedic Sports Physical Therapy, 35*(2), 52-61.

Romanowski, M.R., & Repicci, J.A. (2003). Technical aspects of medial versus lateral minimally invasive unicondylar arthroplasty. *Orthopedics, 26*(3), 289-293.

Schoen,D. C. (2007). Meniscal knee pathologies. *Orthopaedic Nursing, 26*(6), 388-391.

Scott, R.D. (2009). Unicompartmental total knee arthroplasty with conventional instrumentation. In P.A. Lotke, & J.H Lonner (Eds.), *Knee arthroplasty* (pp. 311-326). Philadelphia: Lippincott, Williams, & Wilkins.

Seyler, T.M., Marker, D.R., Bhave, A., Plater, J.F., Marulanda, G.A., Bonutti, P.M., & Mont, M.A. (2007). Functional problems and arthrofibrosis following total knee arthroplasty. *Journal of Bone and Joint Surgery, 89*(Suppl 3), 59-69.

Shea, K.G., Nilsson, K., & Belzer, J. (2006). Patellar dislocation in skeletally immature athletes. *Operative Techniques in Sports Medicine. 14*(3), 188-196.

Smith-Blair, N. (2003). Shock. In W.J. Phipps, F.D. Monahan, J.K. Sands, J.F Marek, & M. Neighbors (Eds.), *Medical-surgical nursing: Health and illness perspectives* (pp. 283-301). St. Louis: Mosby.

Springfield, D., (2005). Joint replacement surgery. In F.C. Brunicardi (Ed.), *Schwartz's principles of surgery* (pp. 1702-1706). New York: McGraw Hill.

Steele, M.T., & Glaspy, J.N. (2004). Knee Injuries. In J.E. Tintinallis (Ed.), *Emergency medicine: A comprehensive study guide* (pp. 1726 -1734). New York: McGraw Hill.

Timby, B.K., & Smith, N.E. (2007). *Introductory medical-surgical nursing* (pp. 1181-1183). Philadelphia: Lippincott, Williams, & Wilkins.

Upham, K. (2007). Musculoskeletal assessment. In *NAON Core curriculum for orthopaedic nursing* (6th ed., p. 44). Boston: Pearson.

Vangsness, C.T., Spiker, W.S., & Erickson, J. (2009). A review of evidence-based medicine for glucosamine and chondroitin sulfate use in knee osteoarthritis. *The Journal of Arthroscopic and Related Surgery, 25*(1), 86-94.

Watson, D., & Haas, S (2009). Minimally invasive total knee arthroplasty. In P.A. Lotke, & J.H. Lonner (Eds.), *Knee arthroplasty* (pp. 35-53). Philadelphia: Lippincott, Williams, & Wilkins.

Weinrich, S.P., Haddock, S., & Robinson, K. (1999). Therapeutic massage in older persons: Research issues. *British Journal of Nursing, 8*(3), 159-164.

Wilkins, A.N., & Phillips, E.M. (2008). *Osteoarthritis of the knee.* In W.R. Frontera, J.K. Silver & T.D. Rizzo (Eds.), *Essentials of physical medicine and rehabilitation* (pp. 345-352). Philadelphia: W.B. Saunders.

Wissman, R.D., Verma, S., Kreeger, M., & Robertson, M. (2009). Extensor mechanism injuries in tibiofemoral dislocations. *Journal of Computer Assisted Tomography, 33*(1), 145-149.

Wood, J.J., Malek, M.A., Frassica, F.J., Polder, J.A., Mohan, A.K., Bloom, E.T., ...Cote, T. R. (2006). Autologous cultured chondrocytes: Adverse events reported to the United States food and drug administration. *Journal of Bone and Joint Surgery, 88*, 503-507.

Chapter 5

Care of the Patient with Hip, Foot and Ankle Problems

Dottie Roberts, MSN, MACI, RN, CMSRN, OCNS-C®

Objectives

- Identify the structures and function of the hip, ankle, and foot.

- Review pathophysiology and treatment options for common conditions of the hip, ankle, and foot.

- Outline nursing interventions for patients with common conditions of the hip, ankle, and foot.

Key Terms

Articular gelling: stiffness after periods of rest or inactivity.

Autoimmunity: an immune response by a susceptible individual to his or her own tissue.

Avascular necrosis (AVN): a condition that results from circulatory compromise to bone, most commonly the femoral head.

Bone mineral density (BMD): bone mass.

Crepitus or crepitation: squeaking, creaking, or grating with joint movement.

Dysplasia: unstable hip, and/or radiographic abnormalities of the femoral head and acetabulum.

Extracapsular: occurring outside the joint capsule.

Fragility fractures: occur in individuals with osteoporosis as a result of low-trauma events.

Hallux valgus: structural deformity of the foot involving deviation of the great toe toward the smaller toes.

Hemiarthroplasty: replacement of the femoral head while retaining the natural acetabulum/acetabular cartilage.

Idiopathic osteoarthritis: occurs in a patient with no prior history of joint injury or disease.

Intracapsular: occurring inside the joint capsule.

Labrum: ring of fibrocartilage around the rim of the acetabulum.

Osteotomy: removal of a wedge of bone located near a damaged joint.

Osteophytes: loose particles of cartilage in the joint capsule.

Plantar fasciitis: painful inflammatory condition caused by excessive wear of the plantar fascia that supports the arches of the foot.

Posttraumatic osteoarthritis: occurs as a result of repetitive, high-intensity exercise or previous trauma.

Secondary osteoarthritis: occurs as a result of an identifiable cause.

Site specificity: a characteristic of osteoarthritis, in that only certain joints show high incidence of the disease.

Syndesmosis: an articulation in which adjacent bones are bound together by a ligament (i.e., tibia and fibula).

Total hip arthroplasty (THA): resection of the femoral head and neck, and preparation of the acetabulum to accept prosthetic replacement components.

Anatomy of the Hip

The hip is a diarthrodial (freely movable) ball-and-socket joint. It consists of the femur (thigh bone) and the acetabulum (socket) of the pelvis, into which the head of the femur fits (see Figure 5-1). The femur, the largest and heaviest bone in the body, is comprised of cancellous bone at its epiphyses (wide ends) and cortical bone at the diaphysis (shaft). Articular cartilage covers the surfaces of both epiphyses. The femur also is characterized by specific bony contours (see Figure 5-2) that serve as landmarks for the health care provider's description of a hip disorder. For example, a patient's fall may result in a fracture of the femoral neck.

The hip is surrounded closely and supported by an inelastic fibrous capsule. The iliofemoral, pubofemoral, and ischiofemoral ligaments of the joint capsule stabilize and limit the movement of the hip (Wasielewski, 2006). Within the capsule, the synovial membrane secretes synovial fluid to lubricate and nourish the joint. Blood vessels pass through the capsule to supply the femoral head and neck, as well as laterally to the greater trochanter. Adjacent muscles allow the hip to move in all three planes: flexion-extension, abduction-adduction, and internal-external rotation (see Table 5-1 for primary muscles and their range of motion).

Osteoarthritis

Osteoarthritis (OA), one of the most common disorders of the hip, is a slowly progressive, noninflammatory disorder marked by deterioration of articular cartilage in synovial joints. Research has proven that it is not a wear-and-tear condition occurring as a normal consequence of aging. In fact, joint changes that result from arthritis can be differentiated readily from the age-related changes in the articular cartilage of an asymptomatic older adult (Arthritis Foundation, 1999; Roberts, 2007).

Figure 5-1
The Hip Joint

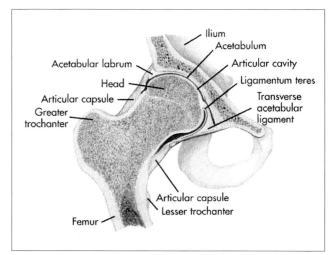

Reprinted with permission from Thibodeau, G.A., & Patton, K.T. (1996). *Anatomy and physiology* (p. 292). St. Louis: Mosby.

Figure 5-2
Femoral Markings

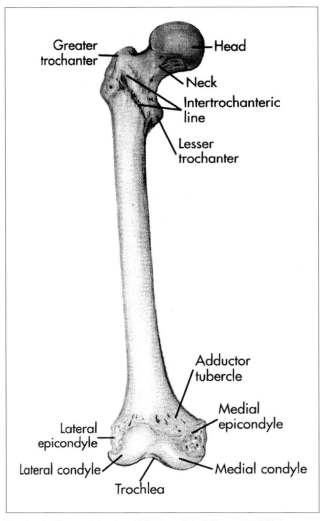

Reprinted with permission from Thibodeau, G.A., & Patton, K.T. (1996). *Anatomy and physiology* (p. 271). St. Louis: Mosby.

Etiology

Idiopathic osteoarthritis occurs in individuals with no history of joint injury or disease, or of systemic illness that may have contributed to the development of arthritis (i.e., Lyme disease, gout). In contrast, secondary osteoarthritis has an identifiable cause. Any condition or event that directly damages the articular cartilage, exposes joint surfaces to excessive or abnormal forces, or creates joint instability can cause arthritic changes. Possible causes of secondary OA are identified in Table 5-2. In particular, a greater incidence of OA has been associated with repetitive, high-intensity exercise (posttraumatic osteoarthritis). Participation in competitive sports, such as running, soccer, and football, exposes the joints of the lower extremities to increased impact and torsional stress. Even if an athlete does not have a history of specific joint injury, OA can develop from the combined effects of undetected microtraumas (Roberts, 2007).

Table 5-1
Primary Muscles of the Hip

Function and Range of Motion	Muscles
Flexion 120°	Rectus femoris
	Sartorius
	Iliopsoas
Extension 30°	Gluteus maximus
	Hamstrings
	Adductor magnus (extension assistance)
Adduction 20-30°	Adductor longus
	Adductor magnus
	Adductor brevis
	Gracilis
	Pectineus
Abduction 45-50°	Gluteus maximus
	Gluteus medius
	Gluteus minimus
	Piriformis
	Obturator externus
External rotation 45°	Gluteus maximus
	Gluteus medius
	Piriformis
	Obturator internus
	Obturator externus
	Quadratus femoris
	Gemellus superior
	Gemellus inferior
	Sartorius
Internal rotation 35°	Gluteus medius
	Gluteus minimus
	Tensor fascia lata

Adapted from ExRx, (2009). *Hip articulations*. Retrieved June 26, 2009, from http://emedicine.medscape.com/article/1232559-overview and Wasielewski, R.C. (2006). The hip. In J.J. Callahan, A.G. Rosenburg, & H.E. Rubash (Eds.), *The adult hip: Volume I* (2nd ed., pp. 51-67). Philadelphia: Lippincott, Williams, & Wilkins.

Although researchers have been unable to identify a single cause for OA, they have determined that a number of risk factors can contribute to the development and progression of the disease. Sex hormones and other hormonal factors may play a part in the onset of OA. The increased incidence of the disease in postmenopausal women, for example, is believed to be due to estrogen loss. One modifiable risk factor for development of OA is excessive weight, long recognized as a contributor to the disease. Level of activity is also a modifiable risk factor: moderate exercise has been shown to decrease both the likelihood of developing osteoarthritis and the progression of joint symptoms.

Incidence

OA is the most common articular disease, affecting approximately 33 million adults in the United States (Arthritis Foundation, 2009). It is also the leading cause of disability in older adults. OA demonstrates site specificity: only certain synovial joints show high prevalence of the disease. These include the weight-bearing joints (hips, knees); the cervical and lumbar spine; and the small joints of the hands (DIP, PIP, MCP) and feet (MTP). The hip joint is more often affected in men and the hands in women, especially after menopause (Roberts, 2007).

Clinical Manifestations

Joint pain is often the primary patient complaint and the usual reason for seeking health care. Patients often describe their joint pain as deep and aching, differentiating it from the pain of inflammatory arthritic conditions. Pain typically is localized, increasing with use but relieved by rest in the early stages of OA. As the disease progresses, night pain or pain at rest is common. The occurrence of pain may not be related to joint changes seen on x-rays; in fact, the patient may have notable radiographic joint changes and minimal pain, or severe pain with minimal joint changes apparent on x-ray.

The patient often describes joint stiffness with initial activity in the morning, generally lasting less than 30 minutes. Stiffness after periods of rest or inactivity (articular gelling) also is common, though it generally resolves within several minutes after resumption of joint movement. In addition, the patient with a stiff joint may describe a squeaking, creaking, or grating with movement (crepitus or crepitation) that could indicate fixed or loose cartilage particles (osteophytes) in the joint capsule, or uneven joint surfaces due to cartilage deterioration. Limitations in range of motion and joint locking with movement can result in part from the presence of these osteophytes. Resulting gait changes can contribute greatly to the patient's overall disability and loss of function.

Diagnosis

Diagnosis of OA almost always can be made on the basis of history and physical examination. The affected joint may be tender to palpation, range of motion may be reduced, and leg length discrepancy may be noted in advanced hip OA because of loss of joint space. Large effusions are uncommon, but some swelling may result from a local synovitis (Roberts,

Table 5-2
Causes of Secondary Osteoarthritis

Traumatic injury (i.e., sprains, strains, dislocations, fractures)

Mechanical stress from long-term participation in repetitive physical activities (recreational or occupational)

Inflammation in joint capsule with release of destructive enzymes

Joint instability from damage to supporting structures

Neurologic disorders that cause abnormal movement, weight-bearing (i.e., diabetic neuropathy)

Congenital/acquired skeletal deformities (i.e., Legg-Calvé-Perthes disease)

Hematologic/endocrine disorders (i.e., hemophilia, hyperparathyroidism)

Use of selected medications with enzymatic effects (i.e., colchicines, indomethacin, steroids)

Adapted from Roberts, D. (2007). Arthritis and connective tissue disorders. In National Association of Orthopaedic Nurses, *NAON Core curriculum for orthopaedic nursing* (6th ed., pp. 327-372). Boston: Pearson.

Table 5-3

Treatment Goals – Arthritis

- Manage joint pain and inflammation
- Maintain or improve joint function
- Stop or slow cartilage damage
- Limit disability by correcting or preventing joint deformity
- Optimize role function and independence in self-care
- Improve patient's sense of well-being
- Avoid adverse drug events

Adapted from National Institute of Arthritis and Musculoskeletal and Skin Diseases (NIAMS), (2004). Handout on health: *Rheumatoid arthritis*. Retrieved June 26, 2009, from http://www.niams.nih.gov/health_info/Rheumatic_Disease/rheumatoid_arthritis_hohipdf and Roberts, D. (2007). Arthritis and connective tissue disorders. In National Association of Orthopaedic Nurses, *NAON Core curriculum for orthopaedic nursing* (6th ed., pp. 327-372). Boston: Pearson.

Table 5-4

Patient Education – Osteoarthritis & Rheumatoid Arthritis

- Disease development and progression
- Pain management strategies (i.e., thermal applications)
- Medication use and side effects
- Exercise
- Nutritional counseling for weight management (OA)
- Energy conservation and fatigue (RA)
- Body mechanics and joint protection strategies (i.e., brace, splint)
- Stress management and coping strategies
- Complementary and alternative treatment options

Roberts, D. (2007). Arthritis and connective tissue disorders. In National Association of Orthopaedic Nurses, *NAON Core curriculum for orthopaedic nursing* (6th ed., pp. 327-372). Boston: Pearson.

2007). Routine laboratory tests help in screening for associated disorders and in identifying baseline values before initiating therapy (i.e., complete blood count for the patient taking a nonsteroidal anti-inflammatory drug [NSAIDs]). Rheumatoid factor (RF) and erythrocyte sedimentation rate (ESR) often are ordered, but positive values neither exclude nor confirm a diagnosis of OA. Synovial fluid analysis will allow the health care provider to distinguish OA reliably from inflammatory arthritis.

Radiographic studies of affected joints may help confirm a diagnosis of OA, but findings do not always correlate with the severity of the patient's symptoms. Plain x-ray films show decreased joint space as the disease progresses, reflecting the loss of articular cartilage or the progression of bone remodeling. Later radiographic changes include the formation of subchondral cysts and an altered shape of the bone ends.

Conservative Management of OA

An interdisciplinary team of health care providers collaborates with the patient to manage symptoms and progression of OA.

Primary treatment goals for all forms of arthritis are identified in Table 5-3. Most patients have some success with conservative treatment that includes physical therapy, heat and cold applications, self-care modifications, and pharmacologic interventions (i.e., viscosupplementation, intra-articular steroid injection). Patient education is the basis of effective OA management. Important topics for discussions between the patient and nurse are identified in Table 5-4.

According to the American College of Rheumatology (ACR) (2000), pharmacologic treatment should serve as an adjunct to nonpharmacologic approaches for OA management. Pain management is the first consideration, and ACR guidelines recommend treatment based on the severity of the patient's symptoms. Acetaminophen (Tylenol®) is the initial drug of choice, with dosages of up to 1000mg 4 times daily. Adverse effects from this medication generally are mild, with a very low incidence of renal and hepatic effects occurring primarily in patients who consume large amounts of alcohol. Topical capsaicin or methyl salicylate cream may be used by patients who do not respond to acetaminophen or do not wish to take systemic therapy. Nonacetylated salicylates (aspirin) or NSAIDs also are alternatives to acetaminophen. NSAID therapy typically starts with low-dose, over-the-counter products such as ibuprofen (Motrin®) or naproxen (Aleve®). If the patient is at risk for gastrointestinal side effects with the use of nonselective NSAIDs, supplemental treatment with a protective agent (i.e., misoprostol [Cytotec®]) or a proton pump inhibitor (i.e., omeprazole [Prilosec®]) may be indicated. As an alternative, the cyclooxygenase-2 (COX-2) inhibitor celecoxib (Celebrex®) may be prescribed to minimize gastrointestinal effects. In addition, diclofenac (Voltaren®) gel is available for topical treatment of arthritis, particularly in the hands and the knees (Novartis Consumer Health, Inc., 2009). Patients with moderate-to-severe pain who have contraindications to celecoxib or NSAIDs may be treated with tramadol (Ultram®) 50-100 mg in evenly divided doses 4 times daily.

Rheumatoid Arthritis

Rheumatoid arthritis (RA) is a chronic, systemic autoimmune disorder characterized by symmetrical, erosive inflammation of synovial joint tissue. The course of the disease often is marked by unexplained periods of remission and exacerbation. The most common outcomes are varying degrees of joint destruction, deformity, and disability (Roberts, 2007).

Etiology

No single cause for RA exists, but theories suggest that the disease is generated by the immune response of a susceptible individual to an antigen. Because complex genetic factors are involved in the development of RA, the antigen is probably not the same in all patients. Autoimmunity has been accepted as the cause of RA because of its association with rheumatoid factor (RF), the antibody against gamma globulin. No agent has been cultured from synovial tissue, synovial fluid, or blood with enough reproducibility to suggest an infectious cause. No risk factors have been identified for the development of RA.

Incidence

RA affects approximately 1.3 million adults and 294,000 children (Helmick et al., 2008); this is lower than previous estimates due to a change in classification of the disease. RA can occur at any time of life, but incidence tends to increase with age and peaks between the fourth and sixth decades. About 2-3 times as many women as men develop RA (Roberts, 2007). The bilateral symmetrical involvement of the small joints of the hands and feet (MCP, PIP, MTP) is characteristic of RA. Shoulders, elbows, and spine also may be affected. Elbows can become flexed and contracted in early disease, and shoulder arthritis is seen particularly with late RA. Spinal involvement generally is limited to the cervical area. In the lower extremities, RA most commonly affects the knees and feet but can develop in hip joints.

Clinical Manifestations

Joint pain and swelling are common in RA, especially in the hands and wrists. Joints are typically warm, red, and tender. The morning stiffness of RA lasts longer than that of OA, at least 1 hour and up to all day (Roberts, 2007). Characteristic deformities also develop in the small joints as the synovial damage progresses (i.e., swan-neck deformity, boutonniere deformity, claw toes). Deformities can affect the patient's independence in mobility and self-care. Involvement of the foot and ankle causes greater dysfunction and pain than upper extremity RA. The patient often complains of fatigue that begins several hours after rising. Systemic involvement also is possible in RA, particularly in the patient who is diagnosed with aggressive, early onset of the disease.

Diagnosis

As with OA, diagnosis of RA is based primarily on history and physical examination. Laboratory results are generally used to confirm diagnosis and monitor disease progression. Positive RF is seen in approximately 85% of patients, with higher occurrence found in active disease (Roberts, 2007). Elevated ESR and C-reactive protein (CRP) indicate active inflammation. Radiographic studies generally are not needed to make a diagnosis and may in fact be inconclusive in early disease. Serial films are useful, however, in monitoring disease progression and determining a prognosis if joint erosions are present.

Conservative Management of RA

General treatment goals for RA are identified in Table 5-3. Drug therapy remains the most important element in an interdisciplinary approach to RA management. Along with appropriate nonmedical therapies (i.e., physical therapy, occupational therapy) and anti-inflammatory pharmacologic interventions, the American College of Rheumatology (ACR) recommends the use of nonbiologic and biologic disease-modifying anti-rheumatic drugs (DMARDs) as a focus of RA treatment (Saag et al., 2008). Consistent use of disease-modifying anti-rheumatic drugs (DMARDs) has been shown to slow the erosive course of RA. The choice of drug depends on the disease activity. Methotrexate or leflunomide (Arava®) is recommended for all disease durations and all degrees of disease activity; other nonbiologic medications

may be prescribed based on the patient's disease activity and prognosis. Recommendations regarding use of biologic agents (also known as biological response modifiers, or BRMs) are divided by length of disease (less than or greater than 6 months). In early RA, for example, the ACR limits its recommendation for the use of biologics to patients who have not received nonbiologic DMARDs and have high disease activity. Etanercept (Enbrel®), infliximab (Remicade®), and adalumimab (Humira®) are among the recommended BRMs. Abatacept (Orencia®) or rituximab (Rituxan®) also may be indicated based on patient history. While useful for analgesic and anti-inflammatory effects, NSAIDs do not affect disease progression. Corticosteroids, which may be useful for brief periods of disease exacerbation, should not be a mainstay of RA treatment.

Patient education is critical to the success of all aspects of disease management. Important topics for discussions between the patient and nurse are identified in Table 5-4.

Developmental Dysplasia of the Hip (DDH)

A range of conditions may exist in which the femoral head abnormally relates to the acetabulum. Radiographic abnormalities that demonstrate inadequate formation of the acetabulum include dislocatable hip, subluxable hip, and dysplastic hip (shallow acetabulum with poor-fitting femoral head). Developmental dysplasia of the hip (DDH) now is preferred to "congenital dislocated hip" (CDH) as the nomenclature for this condition because hip dysplasia may be diagnosed at birth or during early development (Hawk & Bailie, 2007). Ligamentous laxity plays an important role in the occurrence of DDH. The Pavlik harness is considered the treatment of choice for infants younger than 6 months. Long-term morbidity associated with the condition is unclear, but case studies have shown incidents of leg length discrepancy, gait abnormalities, chronic pain, and osteoarthritis. Delayed complications include avascular necrosis of the femoral head in up to 12% of affected children, with the rate slightly increased if treatment is delayed (Bluth, Benson, Rawls, & Siegel, 2007). Females are more likely than males to have DDH. Rates of spontaneous resolution are high but, if abnormalities persist, surgical intervention often is necessary (Gelfer & Kennedy, 2008).

Femoacetabular Impingement (FAI)

Hip pain can result from abnormal contact between the proximal femur and the acetabulum during extremes of hip motion. This contact is caused by a structural abnormality at the femoral head-neck junction (cam type) or the acetabulum (pincer type). FAI, which usually presents in active young adults, can go undetected for years. Failure to identify the condition and restore the joint's biomechanics may lead to early onset of hip OA and possible need for early joint arthroplasty. Carefully reviewed radiographs can reveal the joint abnormality and, combined with clinical presentation, lead to timely diagnosis. Surgical treatment (i.e., femoral head-neck osteoplasty) may be indicated (Wisniewski & Grogg, 2006).

Figure 5-3
Total Hip Prosthesis

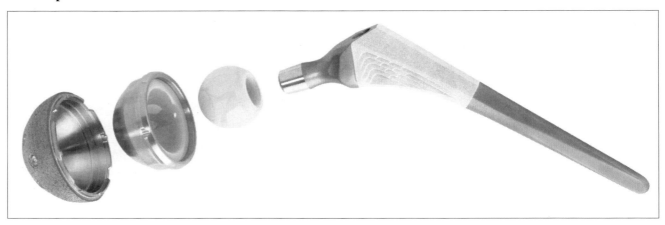

Courtesy of Stryker Howmedica Osteonics.

Labral Tears

A labral tear involves the ring of cartilage (labrum) on the rim of the acetabulum. The labrum, which helps maintain stability of the hip joint, can be damaged as a result of FAI, capsular laxity, dysplasia, or trauma. Affected patients often complain of mechanical symptoms (i.e., painful clicking) and reduced range of motion. However, complaints also may be more subtle, with symptoms of dull pain that increases with activity and fails to respond to rest. Because diagnosis is based largely on clinical presentation, misdiagnosis may occur; for example, the classic symptom of hip clicking may be attributed incorrectly to a snapping iliotibial band or a hypermobile psoas tendon. MRI and conventional radiographs are useful for definitive diagnosis. Nonoperative management, including pharmacology and physical therapy, is the cornerstone of care for labral tears. Hip arthroscopy generally is reserved for patients who do not improve with nonoperative treatment or who have clearly identifiable pathology (Ranawat & Sekiya, 2004).

Iliotibial Band Inflammation/Trochanteric Bursitis

The iliotibial (IT) band is a tendinous extension of the fascia covering the gluteus maximus and tensor fasciae muscles proximally. It descends from these muscles on the outside of the thigh to attach to the lateral condyle of the tibia; some fibers also go to the lateral aspect of the patella. The IT band, which functions primarily as a stabilizer during running, can become irritated from overuse. Under the IT band and adjacent to the trochanter on the femur are the trochanteric bursae, fluid-filled sacks that serve as a gliding surface to reduce friction between tissues. The bursae also can become inflamed and painful as a result of overuse, hip injury (i.e., fall), spine disease, leg length discrepancy, or arthritis. Trochanteric bursitis is more common in female runners than their male counterparts because they have a broader-based pelvis that makes them more susceptible to friction over the trochanter. Diagnosis is completed by

physical examination and the patient's history, with radiological studies to rule out other causes of hip and thigh pain. Initial treatment includes interventions such as activity modification, use of a walking aid, and NSAIDs. Corticosteroid injection also may be helpful in relieving symptoms. Once the condition is resolved, adequate warm up and stretching of the IT band before exercise can help prevent recurrence of bursitis (American Academy of Orthopaedic Surgeons [AAOS], 2007a).

Surgical Interventions for Hip Disorders

If conservative interventions fail to manage pain and maintain the patient's quality of life, surgical treatment may be needed. With early hip arthritis, proximal femoral osteotomy (PFO) may be indicated as an alternative to immediate total hip arthroplasty (THA) in younger patients. The candidate for femoral osteotomy has joint congruency despite the presence of arthritis, and hip motion is essentially normal. Osteotomy involves removal of a wedge of bone, usually near the lesser trochanter of the femur, to redistribute mechanical stress over less worn areas of the femoral head. The patient will have limited weight bearing for approximately 3 months after the procedure to allow complete healing (Theis & Kahn, 2007).

Hip resurfacing is an emerging procedure, most often performed in younger patients. It involves acetabular replacement similar to THA, but the femur is covered ("resurfaced") with a hemispherical component. This component spares the bone of the femoral head and neck. It is fixed to the femur with cement around the femoral head, and it has a short stem that passes into the femoral neck. Long-term success of this procedure has not been determined (AAOS, 2007b). Limited or inconsistent data support some suggested advantages of hip resurfacing, including bone conservation; improved function due to retention of the femoral head and neck, and more precise biomechanical restoration; decreased morbidity at the time of revision arthroplasty; and reduced prevalence of venousthromboembolic events due to lack of femoral instrumentation (Shimmin, Beaule, & Campbell, 2008).

Although procedures such as PFO and resurfacing may be indicated for select patients, THA remains the most common surgical procedure for hip arthritis or dysplasia. The procedure is performed by resecting the femoral head and neck, and then preparing the acetabulum (socket) to accept the prosthesis (see Figure 5-3). Total joint prostheses are now made of metallic alloys, ultra-high molecular weight polyethylene (UHMWP), and ceramics (Banchet, Fridrici, Abry, & Kapsa, 2007). In the most common type of implant, a metal femoral component articulates with a polyethylene acetabular element. Alternately, a ceramic femoral head on a titanium stem articulates with a ceramic acetabular component, or metal surfaces can be used for both components (Theis & Kahn, 2007). The use of polymethylmethacrylate (PMMA) bone cement during THA allows immediate fixation of the femoral and acetabular components. Cemented components are often used for the older patient or for the patient who has compromised bone strength because of osteoporosis or other disorders; however, component loosening occurs at about 1%-5% per year, primarily due to failure of the PMMA bone cement (Maloney, Kang, & Hartford, 2006). This failure can occur even more quickly in an overweight patient or an active patient who puts a great deal of demand on the joint.

For the younger patient or the patient who remains very active no matter what the age, noncemented components are usually indicated. These components have a porous surface that allows bony in-growth into the implant itself and may offer better long-term outcomes; however, the polyethylene under the surface of the porous coating is subject to frictional wear that may also result in prosthetic loosening. A combination of cemented and noncemented components (hybrid) also has been used in younger patients, taking advantage of the historically positive use of cemented stems and cementless sockets (AAOS, 2007b). The acetabular component is placed without cement, and the femoral component is inserted with cement. With the first cementless components implanted in the early 1980s, long-term data on their performance are lacking. The longest published average follow up is 15 years; additional experience is needed to verify the value of cementless and hybrid technology (Peters & Miller, 2006; Shen et al., 2009).

Operative Procedure

The surgeon may choose to use an anterolateral, direct lateral, transtrochanteric, or posterolateral approach when performing THA. The anterolateral and posterolateral approaches are the most common. When the surgeon uses an anterolateral approach, the patient may either be in the lateral position or may lie supine on the operating table. The operative hip then is externally rotated and extended with the knee flexed. When the posterolateral approach is used, the patient is in the full lateral position with the operative hip up and flexed, adducted, and internally rotated. The nurse must know the surgical approach in order to minimize the patient's risk for postoperative hip dislocation. By helping the patient follow appropriate activity precautions based on surgical approach, the nurse will avoid replicating the movements used by the surgeon to dislocate the femoral head before replacement.

The hip is typically exposed through an incision of approximately 10 to 12 inches in length. A minimally invasive procedure allows the surgeon to perform the replacement through one or two smaller incisions. The single incision for the minimally invasive THA will be approximately 3-6 inches in length. The two-incision surgery requires a 2-3 inch incision over the groin for placement of the acetabular component, and a 1-2 inch incision over the buttock for placement of the femoral stem; radiologic guidance may be needed to perform the two-incision procedure, which will take longer than traditional arthroplasty. The implants are the same as for traditional THA but special instruments are required to prepare the acetabulum and femur, and place the components correctly. Candidates for minimally invasive surgery generally are younger, thinner, and healthier compared to patients who undergo traditional arthroplasty (AAOS, 2007c). Because the concern during surgery is adequate visualization of the femur and acetabulum, the minimally invasive technique is not appropriate for complex procedures in which a wider exposure is necessary (i.e., revision arthroplasty, developmental dysplasia of the hip).

After dislocation of the hip, the femur is cut at the neck to expose the acetabulum. The surface of the acetabulum is then smoothed and prepared to receive the artificial component. Trial prostheses are placed and their fit evaluated before the surgeon chooses appropriately sized components. If a noncemented (press-fit) prosthesis will be used, the surgeon will press the cup firmly into place and evaluate its apposition to the bone. If a cemented prosthesis will be placed, the surgeon drills anchor holes into the iliac subchondral bone, cleans the area with a pressure-pulsed lavage, and cements the cup into place.

The intramedullary canal of the femur then is reamed to create a tunnel, and a trial prosthesis is placed to allow the surgeon to evaluate motion, stability, and length. The femoral stem of the noncemented prosthesis will be pressed into the reamed intramedullary canal. Before placement of a cemented femoral component, the femur will be cleansed and the canal plugged to keep the cement from traveling too far distally. The surgeon will fill the canal with cement, insert the femoral stem, and then place the femoral head. After the hip is reduced (femoral head replaced in acetabulum), the surgeon will perform a final evaluation. A closed wound drainage system may be placed before wound closure.

The procedure for a revision hip arthroplasty may differ slightly, depending on the surgeon's need to replace the acetabular or femoral component, or both components. Indications for revision THA include femoral shaft fracture, repeated dislocation, hardware failure, and loosening. Because of improved techniques for cement insertion and the increased use of noncemented components, loosening now occurs less often following THA. With revision arthroplasty, surgical time may be considerably longer and blood loss greater than with the primary surgery.

Postoperative Nursing Considerations

The patient's lower extremity neurovascular condition must be assessed regularly following hip procedures. The nurse should follow institution protocols or physician orders for frequency of assessment, and immediately report any deficits. See Chapter 1, *Musculoskeletal Anatomy and Neurovascular Assessment*, for a thorough discussion of parameters for evaluation.

Pain management is a major concern following THA (see Chapter 7, *Pain Management*). The nurse should assess the patient consistently using a pain-intensity scale and reassess at regular intervals to determine the efficacy of any analgesic. The patient's report of pain should never be discounted. Complaints of new or suddenly increased pain, or pain away from the surgical site should be carefully evaluated because they may suggest complications such as deep vein thrombosis (DVT), pulmonary embolus (PE), compartment syndrome, or wound infection (see Chapter 8, *Complications Associated with Orthopaedic Conditions and Surgeries*).

Early mobilization is a key to avoiding complications following hip procedures. Leg exercises (i.e., ankle pumps, quadriceps

Table 5-5
Osteoporosis Risk Factors

Gender (↑ risk for females)

Advanced age

Family history of osteoporosis

Personal history of fractures after age 50

History of fracture in first-degree relative

Current low bone mass

Thin with small frame

Caucasian or Asian ethnicity (although significant risk exists in people of all ethnic backgrounds)

Amenorrhea (abnormal absence of menses) or estrogen deficiency as a result of menopause (abnormal absence of menses)

Low testosterone (men)

Lifestyle Choices

Low lifetime calcium intake

Vitamin D deficiency

Nutritional disorders (i.e., anorexia nervosa)

Inactivity/lack of weight-bearing exercise

Smoking

Excessive alcohol use

Other Influences

Medications (i.e., corticosteroids, anticonvulsants)

Hyperthyroidism

Hyperparathyroidism

Multiple myeloma

Transplantation

Chronic disease

Adapted from National Osteoporosis Foundation (NOF) (2004). *Know your risk.* Retrieved June 26, 2009, from http://www.nof.org/awareness2/2004/nof_final_risk-assess.pdf

and gluteal sets) may have been introduced preoperatively and should be continued as soon as the patient is awake following surgery. Sometimes patients are able to sit at the bedside on the afternoon of surgery. Additional physical therapy often begins on the first postoperative day. The patient receives instruction in the use of a mobility aid, such as a walker or crutches, and should be encouraged to increasing independence with the assistive device. When transferring or ambulating the patient, the nurse always should be aware of the patient's weight bearing status. Although patients with noncemented components have been restricted from weight bearing in the past, early research on small numbers of patients indicates no adverse effects of immediate weight bearing with noncemented prosthetics (Bodén & Adolphson, 2004; Ström, Nilsson, Milbrink, Mallmin, & Larsson, 2007). The nurse and other health care providers must coach the patient to be consistent in following any weight bearing restrictions. The nurse also must follow appropriate precautions in order to minimize the patient's risk for hip dislocation postoperatively (i.e., use of an abductor pillow or dressing aids). See Chapter 9, *Body Mechanics, Mobility Techniques, and Post-Surgical Precautions*, for a discussion of assistive devices, transfers, and total hip precautions.

The patient's hemodynamic condition is monitored throughout the postoperative period. Hemoglobin and hematocrit are assessed regularly to determine the amount of perioperative blood loss and the need for transfusion. If blood replacement is needed, the patient most often receives autologous blood that was either obtained through preoperative self-donation or postoperative collection from the wound (i.e., Autovac® or other reinfusion device). (See Chapter 8, *Complications Associated with Orthopaedic Conditions and Surgeries*, for discussion of management of perioperative blood loss).

Additional postoperative care for the patient following hip procedures is similar to that of any surgical patient. The nurse closely monitors urinary output and vital signs to ensure the patient's return to baseline function. Respiratory status is assessed frequently, and the patient is encouraged to cough and deep breathe to decrease the risk for atelectasis or pneumonia.

Postoperative Discharge Needs

Planning for discharge begins even before the patient is admitted to the hospital. Many surgeons or hospitals offer total joint education programs to help the patient prepare for surgery and subsequent hospital discharge. The patient's support system and home environment are assessed, including the need for the patient to climb stairs. If the patient lives alone, has a spouse in poor health, or has not gained sufficient independence in mobility and self-care, he or she may benefit from inpatient rehabilitation, subacute care, or extended care after discharge from the acute care setting. If the patient is discharged to home, physical therapy may be continued there or in an outpatient setting. Home nursing may be ordered for the patient who is unable to self-administer an injectable anticoagulant (i.e., enoxaparin [Lovenox®]) or who needs blood work to monitor the efficacy of the oral anticoagulant warfarin (Coumadin®). Home nursing also may be needed for wound assessment and care.

The discharged patient should be instructed to avoid driving until cleared by the physician. Sexual activity can be resumed as soon as the patient is comfortable, usually 4-6 weeks after surgery, with a reminder to continue to observe appropriate dislocation precautions. The patient who has had THA should be instructed to inform the health care provider before dental procedures with a high risk of bleeding or bacteremia (i.e., cleaning, extractions, root canal, periodontal work); prophylactic antibiotics may be needed to decrease the risk of hematogenous joint infection. The at-risk population includes patients who are immunocompromised or immunosuppressed, such as those with RA, systemic lupus erythematosus (SLE), insulin-dependent diabetes mellitus, or hemophilia. Patients with a previous prosthetic infection and those who are undernourished or malnourished should also be considered at risk for joint infection with invasive procedures (AAOS, 2009).

Many physicians and health care institutions follow the long-term outcomes of their THA patients through the use of functional assessment tools (i.e., the SF-12 or SF-36) at their initial postoperative office visits, and at additional specified intervals. Information is obtained about range of motion, ability to return to previous activities, degree of pain, and work performance. A successful hip arthroplasty results in decreased pain and improvement in the patient's functional ability.

Osteoporosis

Osteoporosis, the most common metabolic bone disease, is marked by a reduction in bone mass (or bone mineral density [BMD]) and strength that occurs when bone resorption exceeds bone formation. On x-ray, bone tissue shows microarchitectural deterioration that makes it more susceptible to fracture (World Health Organization [WHO], 2003). The patient with osteoporosis is prone especially to fragility fractures from low-trauma events such as sneezing or bending to pick up a newspaper, activities that would not cause injury to healthy bone.

Etiology

The precise etiology of osteoporosis remains unknown; however, a number of contributing factors have been shown to increase the risk of developing the disease (see Table 5-5). Both men and women reach peak bone mass by about 30 years of age (National Osteoporosis Foundation [NOF], 2008c). Estrogens play an important role in preserving bone mass in women, but bone loss occurs as hormone levels decline (usually around age 50) (WHO, 2003). Rapid bone loss also can occur following surgical menopause, which results from removal of the ovaries. Men have larger, stronger skeletons than women, but they also can experience a marked decrease in BMD as they age. Because men do not experience the rapid bone loss associated with a woman's perimenopausal decline of estrogen production, their bone loss starts later in life and progresses more slowly. It often is due to undiagnosed low levels of testosterone.

Osteoporosis can also result from other medical conditions such as thyrotoxicosis, hyperparathyroidism, anorexia nervosa, and Cushing's syndrome. In addition, individuals who undergo bariatric surgery (gastroplasty) for weight reduction are at risk for developing osteoporosis because of calcium malabsorption in the altered gastrointestinal tract. Excessive alcohol intake also contributes to osteoporosis, affecting BMD in two ways: by interfering with incorporation of calcium into the bone at the cellular level, and by altering intestinal absorption of calcium. Smokers often experience menopause at an earlier age than nonsmokers and may have lower levels of estrogen, increasing their risk for osteoporosis. Finally, long-term use of medications such as thyroid hormone, anticonvulsants, a calcium-wasting diuretic such as furosemide (Lasix®), and corticosteroids can decrease BMD and increase the patient's risk for osteoporosis (Geier, 2007).

Incidence

An estimated 44 million people, or 55% of men and women age 50 or older, have osteoporosis or low bone density (NOF, 2008b). As many as 70% of women over age 80 have osteoporosis (WHO, 2003). Age is an especially important factor in the relationship between BMD and fracture risk. An addition of 13 years in age leads to an increase in hip fracture risk that is equal to a decrease of 1 standard deviation in BMD.

Clinical Manifestations

Fractures of the hip, vertebrae, and distal radius represent the most common clinical presentation of osteoporosis (WHO, 2003). The high incidence of these fractures in women is related in part to the fact that they live almost one-third of their lives after menopause. An estimated $6 billion is spent annually in the United States on direct medical treatment of patients with osteoporotic fractures (Agency for Healthcare Research & Quality [AHRQ], n.d.).

Hip fracture, the most serious consequence of osteoporosis, often occurs in the patient whose unstable gait leads to a fall. Among older women, total mortality after hip fracture is 48.1% compared with 25.1% after diagnosis of breast cancer (Bulsta & Cauley as cited in Barclay, 2007).

Approximately 33% of patients age 60 and over who sustain a hip fracture will die within 1 year following their injuries (Roche, Wenn, Sahota, & Moran, 2005). Fractures of the wrist may occur with a fall, most often on an outstretched arm, but they may not be linked readily to osteoporosis. These injuries limit a person's ability to perform self-care. Osteoporotic bone loss also can affect the mandible, leading to poorly fitting dentures or loss of teeth, and causing changes in the appearance of the face.

In addition to the impact of osteoporosis on the skeleton, the affected patient often experiences psychological distress (Australian Institute of Health and Welfare, 2008). The patient often describes decreasing involvement with family and friends and acknowledges that the ability to participate in valued social activities has been influenced by painful osteoporotic conditions.

Diagnosis

In many cases, the diagnosis of osteoporosis is made after a fracture has occurred. The patient with a vertebral

Table 5-6
Medications for Prevention and Treatment of Osteoporosis

MEDICATION	AVAILABLE FORMS	ACTION	ADMINISTRATION GUIDELINES
Bisphosphonates alendronate (Fosamax®) ibandronate (Boniva®) risedronate (Actonel®) zoledronic acid (Reclast®)	**Tablets** alendronate: 5-10 mg daily or 35-70 mg weekly (also available in oral solution taken weekly) ibandronate: 150 mg once monthly risedronate: 5 mg daily, 35 mg weekly, 75 mg twice monthly (on 2 consecutive days), or 150 mg monthly ibandronate also available as 3mg IV dose given every 3 months zoledonic acid 5 mg IV annually	Inhibit osteoclast-mediated bone resorption.	Because bisphosphonates are poorly absorbed from the GI tract, oral forms must be taken with 6-8 oz plain water 30 minutes before first food, drink, medication of day; pt must remain upright 30 minutes after morning dose. *Warning:* concomitant use of bisphosphonates and estrogen not recommended because of uncertain interaction potential.
Selective estrogen receptor modulator (SERM) raloxifene (Evista™)	**Tablets** 60 mg daily	Exerts estrogen-like protective effects by binding to estrogen receptors in bone.	*Warning:* raloxifene has not been evaluated in combination with any form of estrogen that comes in a pill, patch, or injection, and should not be taken with any of these forms of estrogen. It should not be given to women at risk for stroke, including those with previous stroke, transient ischemic attack, atrial fibrillation, or uncontrolled hypertension.
Parathyroid hormone (PTH) teriparatide (Forteo®)	Self-administered as daily injection from pre-loaded pen	Anabolic that rebuilds bone and significantly increases bone mineral density, especially in the spine.	Drug is taken for a maximum of 2 years; most experts recommend then placing patient on an antiresorptive medication.
Calcitonin (Fortical®, Miacalcin®)	Injectable (subcutaneous or intramuscular): dosage varies Nasal spray: 200 IU daily in alternating nostrils	Blocks effects of parathyroid hormone on bone resorption. Possible analgesic effect on pain of osteoporotic fractures.	Approved for women at least 5 years beyond menopause. Drug should be administered with adequate calcium and vitamin D. Teach injection technique if parenteral form prescribed. Refrigerate nasal spray if in use for more than 14 days. Rhinitis possible with nasal spray. May need to discontinue drug for 6-12 months before resuming therapy because some people develop resistance to salmon-calcitonin.

Adapted from National Osteoporosis Foundation (NOF) (2008a). *Medications to prevent and treat osteoporosis.* Retrieved June 28, 2009, from http://www.nof.org/patientinfo/medications.htm

compression fracture, for example, may complain of a sudden onset of severe back pain that increases with movement and is relieved by rest. Vertebral fractures may also be discovered accidentally, either on routine x-rays or from radiologic evaluation of suspected pneumonia. The standard x-ray examination does not, however, reveal changes of osteoporosis until approximately 30% of bone mass has been lost (Geier, 2007).

Dual energy x-ray absorptiometry (DEXA) is the "gold standard" for diagnosis of osteoporosis. The spine and the hip are the sites most commonly measured. Results are reported as a T-score, the difference between the patient's BMD and that of a normal young adult of the same gender, expressed as standard deviations above or below the normal result. A patient with a T-score of -2.0, for example, has a BMD that is two standard deviations below the normal value.

BMD measurement can also be done at sites such as the heel or finger. Quantitative ultrasound (QUS) devices and peripheral DEXAs are smaller and less expensive; however, their use in screening before an actual measurement has been done by DEXA is not cost-effective (WHO, 2006). Diagnostic studies also may include analysis of serum and urinary markers of

bone remodeling. Serum calcium and phosphorus typically are normal in the presence of osteoporosis, but urinary calcium may be elevated. Osteocalcin, which is synthesized by the osteoblasts and is therefore a biochemical marker of bone formation, is increased during rapid bone turnover. Urinary alkaline phosphatase is one biochemical marker of bone resorption. The level of such markers offers some information about changes in bone remodeling within a relatively short time after they occur, and before changes in BMD can be detected. Unfortunately, marker levels do not indicate bone mass and cannot predict fracture risk.

Conservative Management of Osteoporosis

Estrogen has been commonly prescribed in postmenopausal women for the prevention or treatment of osteoporosis; however, findings of the Women's Health Initiative Hormone Program led to the recommendation that hormone replacement therapy should not be routinely prescribed for postmenopausal women (National Institutes of Health, 2005). Instead, women are encouraged to talk to their health care providers about their personal risks and benefits from any therapy. Benefits should be weighed against any risk of heart disease, stroke,

Table 5-7
Risk Factors for Falls and Hip Fracture

Intrinsic Factors
History of falls
Increasing age
Female gender
Ethnicity (Caucasian)
Weakness/impaired mobility and gait
Sedentary behavior with associated muscle disuse/atrophy
Fear of falling
Medication Use
Diuretics, laxatives
Benzodiazepines
Psychotropics
Class Ia anti-arrhythmics
Sedatives/hypnotics
Excessive alcohol
**Concommitant use of 4 or more medications, regardless of type, increases fall risk.
Pathologic Conditions
Circulatory disease
Chronic obstructive pulmonary disease
Depression
Arthritis
Diabetes
Nutritional deficiencies
Impaired cognition
Visual impairments
Foot disorders (i.e., bunions, calluses)
Extrinsic Factors
Loose/poorly fitting clothing or footwear
Living alone
Inappropriate walking aids or assistive devices
Environmental hazards
Loose carpeting or rugs
Slippery floors, tubs
Inadequate lighting
Irregular walking surface (i.e., streets or sidewalks)

Adapted from World Health Organization (WHO) (2004). *What are the main risk factors for falls amongst older people and what are the most effective interventions to prevent these falls? Health Evidence Network Report.* Retrieved June 28, 2009, from http://www.euro.who.int/document/e82552.pdf

and breast cancer. Health care providers should identify other options for osteoporosis prevention and treatment when appropriate (see Table 5-6). Although not a treatment for osteoporosis, calcium is necessary to promote bone health. Recommended intake of calcium is 1000 mg daily for adults ages 19-50, and 1200 mg daily for those age 51 and older. Vitamin D supplementation (400-1000 IU) may be needed to maximize calcium absorption in the person who does not get adequate exposure to sunlight (NOF, 2008d).

The patient with decreased BMD may be reluctant to use allopathic or mainstream therapies prescribed by health care providers, avoiding estrogen replacement in particular because of its link to cancer and its potentially unpleasant effects. An alternative, soy isoflavones, are nonsteroidal molecules with a chemical structure similar to the selective estrogen receptor modulator (SERM) raloxifene (Evista®). However, the efficacy of soy isoflavones has not been demonstrated in randomized clinical trials. These products seem to have a favorable effect on BMD in menopausal women, but the effects on bone fracture and the safety of long-term supplementation have not been determined (Atmaca, Kleerekoper, Bayratkar, & Kucuk, 2008).

Conventional exercise, particularly weight bearing exercise such as walking, is known to have a positive effect on bone mass. However, the patient with osteoporosis may wish to avoid the physical stress of conventional exercise because of perceived risk to fragile bones. As an alternative, he or she may prefer to practice tai chi. This ancient form of Chinese exercise can enhance flexibility, improve balance, and reduce the risk of falls in older adults. The meditative aspects of tai chi also may be beneficial to patients with a chronic disease such as osteoporosis.

Surgical Interventions for Osteoporosis
Painful vertebral compression fractures are initially treated conservatively with rest, analgesics, and occasional bracing. Surgical treatment options include vertebroplasty and kyphoplasty (see Chapter 3, *Care of the Patient with Spine Problems*). Surgical interventions for hip fractures are identified after the following discussion of trauma.

Trauma
An estimated 350,000 hospital admissions and 60,000 nursing home admissions occur each year as a result of hip fractures (AAOS, 2008). Most hip fractures are due to falls, which occur as a result of combined intrinsic and extrinsic risk factors (see Table 5-7).

Figure 5-4
Common Types of Hip Fractures

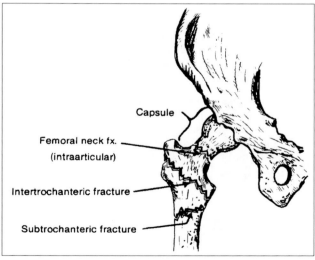

Capsule
Femoral neck fx.
(intraarticular)
Intertrochanteric fracture
Subtrochanteric fracture

Reprinted with permission from *An Introduction to Orthopaedic Nursing* (2004). In C. Mosher (Ed.), (3rd ed., p. 149). Chicago, IL: National Association of Orthopaedic Nurses.

Hip fractures involve the proximal portion of the femur. They are described as either intracapsular or extracapsular, depending on whether they are located within or outside the joint capsule. Figure 5-4 depicts the general types of hip fractures. Various combinations of these fractures can occur. Further classification is based on the extent of displacement of the fracture fragments. Femoral neck fractures are more common in older women or frail elders. They generally are associated with osteoporosis or other conditions affecting bone strength (i.e., osteomalacia, diabetes, alcoholism), and often involve minimal trauma. Extracapsular fractures, more often seen in males or vigorous elders, are typically associated with a greater traumatic force. Clinical manifestations include rotation (external or internal, depending on fracture location), shortening of the affected extremity, pain, and an inability to walk or to move the injured leg when lying supine (Theis & Kahn, 2007).

The older adult with a hip fracture typically enters the health care system through the emergency department, where goals of care include pain management and anxiety reduction, immobilization of the affected leg, and assessment of other conditions that may impact the patient's perioperative course (i.e., pre-existing chronic health problems). X-rays will be taken to confirm the diagnosis. The nurse should coordinate radiologic studies with the technologist to minimize the patient's movement and discomfort. Neurovascular assessment is a priority, and the affected extremity is compared to the unaffected leg to determine the patient's baseline condition. The nurse also must determine the extent of any soft tissue bruising or skin breakdown, and ensure that pressure is minimized over bony prominences. Before surgery, the affected extremity should be maintained in a position of comfort or in light traction (5 pounds of Buck's traction) to decrease associated muscle spasms at the hip.

The nurse should obtain a complete patient history, including the circumstances of injury. How did the fall occur? Did the patient experience a long "lie time" before emergency personnel transported him or her to the hospital? What was the patient's pre-injury mental and functional status? What is the meaning of the event to the patient and family or caregiver? Is this the first fall for the patient, or has injury occurred previously from a fall? How successful was rehabilitation after a previous fracture?

A nondisplaced or stable fracture may be treated conservatively with bed rest followed by bed-to-chair transfers. For a majority of older adults, a hip fracture should be considered a surgically urgent condition. Patients who are medically stable should proceed to surgery as soon as practically possible. If a patient's medical condition is unstable, surgery may be delayed until the patient is at his or her best possible health; available evidence suggests that waiting up to 72 hours to allow stabilization of existing medical conditions does not affect health or functional outcomes adversely (Whinney, 2005). If possible, the patient should receive preoperative teaching regarding pulmonary hygiene measures (i.e., coughing and deep breathing, use of incentive spirometer) as well as ankle-pumping exercises to

decrease clot risk. However, the patient who is anxious, in pain, and possibly confused following injury may not be able to comprehend such instructions.

Surgical Interventions for Hip Fracture

Impacted and nondisplaced femoral neck fractures generally are repaired by open reduction and internal fixation (ORIF) with nail, pin, or compression screw. Displaced fractures are repaired either by ORIF or hemiarthroplasty (replacement of the femoral head while retaining the natural acetabulum/acetabular cartilage). Total hip arthroplasty may be appropriate for the patient with marked hip arthritis before the fracture. Intertrochanteric fractures are all treated with ORIF. See Chapter 1, *Musculoskeletal Anatomy and Neurovascular Assessment*, for examples of fracture fixation.

Postoperative Nursing Considerations

Postoperative nursing care following fracture repair is similar to that provided to the patient who has undergone THA. Neurovascular assessment, pain management, hemodynamic monitoring, and anticoagulation remain nursing priorities. Early mobilization is also critical. Weight bearing has been restricted historically following ORIF of a hip fracture, though many experts now order early weight bearing according to the patient's tolerance of pain (Cassel, Leipzig, Cohen, Larson, & Meier, 2003).

Potential complications following fracture repair include those typical after THA. The patient who had a hemiarthroplasty may need to follow precautions to avoid prosthesis dislocation (see Chapter 9, *Body Mechanics, Mobility Techniques, and Post-Surgical Precautions*); precautions are not required for the patient who underwent ORIF for fracture repair. In addition, postoperative delirium (acute confusional state) is nearly universal in patients with pre-existing cognitive impairment, but also occurs in patients who have no prior history of confusion. Its presence is associated with increased hospital mortality, length of stay, and post-hospital institutionalization. See Chapter 8, *Complications Associated with Orthopaedic Conditions and Surgeries*, for a discussion of delirium.

The patient with a hip fracture is also at risk for nonunion or malunion and avascular necrosis (AVN). Nonunion, the failure of fracture fragments to unite, is relatively rare. If the femoral head fragment of an intracapsular fracture is a shell containing the fragile cancellous bone of osteoporosis, however, it will provide poor anchorage for a fixation device. This condition increases the probability of nonunion or malunion (poor or incomplete healing). Treatment by bone grafting across the fracture site may be indicated.

Disruption of the blood supply to the femoral head also can occur at the time of injury, increasing the risk for AVN. AVN results in bone death with the resultant ischemia causing microfractures and bone collapse. Early diagnosis and treatment of AVN are essential in preventing irreversible damage. X-rays may show evidence of collapse of the femoral head. Treatment of AVN varies contingent upon the patient's age, stage of disease, and cause. Conservative management, such as protected weight bearing and

Figure 5-5
Lateral View of the Ankle Joint of the Right Foot

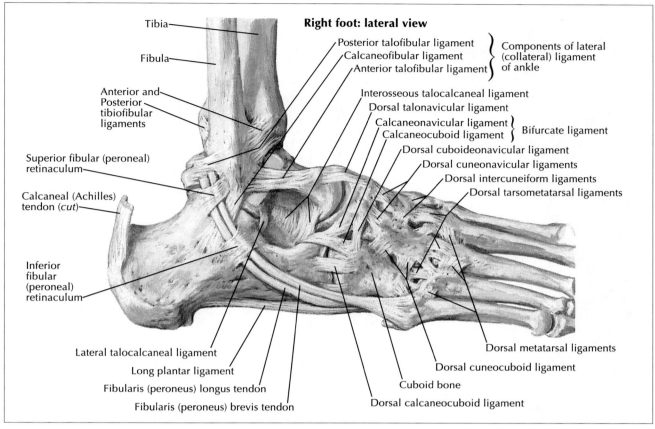

Right foot: lateral view

Tibia

Fibula

Anterior and Posterior tibiofibular ligaments

Superior fibular (peroneal) retinaculum

Calcaneal (Achilles) tendon (*cut*)

Inferior fibular (peroneal) retinaculum

Posterior talofibular ligament
Calcaneofibular ligament
Anterior talofibular ligament
} Components of lateral (collateral) ligament of ankle

Interosseous talocalcaneal ligament
Dorsal talonavicular ligament
Calcaneonavicular ligament }
Calcaneocuboid ligament } Bifurcate ligament
Dorsal cuboideonavicular ligament
Dorsal cuneonavicular ligaments
Dorsal intercuneiform ligaments
Dorsal tarsometatarsal ligaments

Dorsal metatarsal ligaments
Dorsal cuneocuboid ligament
Cuboid bone
Dorsal calcaneocuboid ligament

Lateral talocalcaneal ligament
Long plantar ligament
Fibularis (peroneus) longus tendon
Fibularis (peroneus) brevis tendon

analgesics, often is utilized. Total hip arthroplasty is the most reliable method for treatment of AVN in order to restore function and decrease pain.

Postoperative Discharge Needs

Assessment in the emergency department actually begins the discharge planning process for the patient with a hip fracture. As with the patient who has undergone THA, the support system and home environment must be evaluated. The older adult with a hip fracture may benefit from inpatient rehabilitation, subacute care, or extended care. For the patient who is discharged to home, physical therapy may be continued there or in an outpatient setting.

Anatomy of the Foot and Ankle

The ankle joint contains three articulating structures: the tibiotalar, the fibulotalar, and the tibiofibular joints (Figure 5-5). Movement is minimal at the tibiofibular joint, with only 1-2 mm of spread during dorsiflexion. The tibiotalar and fibulotalar joints together comprise the hinged talocrural joint, which only allows flexion and extension. Forces across the ankle exceed twice a person's body weight when he or she is standing, and more than five times the body weight when ambulating (Burton & Tierney, 2007).

The hindfoot contains the subtalar joint, an articulation of the talus and calcaneus. This gliding joint allows the foot and ankle to invert and evert. The midfoot is comprised of five bones: navicular, cuboid, and three cuneiform bones (lateral, middle, medial). The forefoot contains five metatarsals, five proximal phalanges, four middle phalanges, and five distal phalanges. Flexor, extensor, and peroneal tendons facilitate movement; all have synovial sheaths. The retinacula are thick, fibrous bands that hold the tendons in position. The arches of the foot allow its varied function during weight bearing.

Ankle Sprain

An ankle sprain is a stretched or torn ligament, often due to overuse or trauma. The lateral ankle is affected more commonly, with 85% of all ankle sprains due to inversion forces. Torn ligament fibers initiate an inflammatory response that causes swelling and pain. Bleeding and bruising may occur as well, and joint stability may be compromised depending on the extent of the injury. In early treatment, the concern is managing pain and decreasing inflammation. This is done through prescription of anti-inflammatory medications as well as use of RICE intervention. Compression is accomplished through supportive bandaging or bracing.

Figure 5-6
Displaced Trimalleolar Ankle Fracture, Posterior Malleolus Fracture and Medial Malleolus Fracture

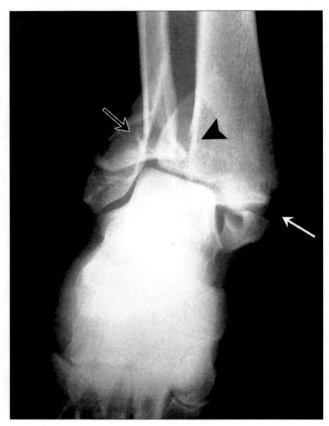

Reprinted with permission from Grantham, S.A. (1990). *Trimalleolar ankle fractures and open ankle fractures.* Instructional Course Lecture, *39,* 105-111.

Assistive ambulatory devices may be indicated if weight bearing is restricted, but early range of motion is important. During the next phase of treatment, cryotherapy continues and range of motion is increased, often through muscle strengthening exercises. In particular, the ankle stabilizer muscles are targeted through calf raises and inversion/eversion exercises. Proprioceptive training also is initiated. During the third phase of treatment, a specific exercise program is designed to return the individual to his or her former activity level; this phase of rehabilitation is critical for the athlete. In order to return to athletic activity, the affected person must be able to walk, run forward and backward, perform figure eights or zigzags, and negotiate a one-foot hop without pain. No swelling can remain in the affected extremity. Immobilization of the ankle through bracing or casting is discouraged, and surgery is only warranted for the severely unstable ankle (Burton & Tierney, 2007).

Fractures of the Lower Leg, Foot, and Ankle

Lower leg fractures involve injuries to the tibia and fibula, which articulate at the tibia-fibular syndesmosis. The tibia is the only weight bearing bone, and the most common site of long bone fractures. Fractures of the tibia often are accompanied by fibular fracture because the traumatic force is transmitted across the intraosseous membrane to the fibula. In addition, because the skin over the anterior and medial tibia is very thin, fractures to this area often are open. Mechanisms of injury for tibial/fibular fractures either can be low-energy (i.e., ground-level falls, athletic injuries) or high-energy (i.e., motor vehicle/pedestrian injuries, gunshot wounds). In addition, twisting injuries can result in tibial/fibular fractures. Stress fractures also can occur due to repetitive stresses from participation in athletics, and often are related to a change in training routine. Fractures of the tibia can involve the tibial plateau, tibial tubercle, tibial eminence (insertion site of anterior cruciate ligament), proximal tibia, tibial shaft, and tibial plafond (end of shin bone, just above the ankle). Radiographs are indicated, though computed tomography (CT) may be used in patients who are unable to get diagnostically sufficient plain films of the knee. CT also can help in evaluation of tibial plateau and plafond fracture. Plain films usually reveal stress fractures after 2-8 weeks of symptoms; they often are not sensitive during early stages of symptoms. However, bone scan and MRI are more sensitive than radiographs in diagnosing stress fractures.

Nondisplaced fractures are immobilized and the patient typically remains non-weight bearing, at least until swelling resolves; a walking cast or crutches may be indicated at that time. Intra-articular fractures generally require open reduction and internal fixation, though external fixation also may be used. In addition, patients who experience open fractures may require immunization or booster with tetanus immune globulin (Norvell & Steele, 2008).

Ankle fractures refer to injuries of the distal tibia and fibula, talus, or calcaneus. The primary motion of the true ankle, which is composed of the tibia, fibula, and talus, is dorsiflexion and plantar flexion. Inversion and eversion occur at the subtalar joint. Excessive inversion stress is the most common cause of ankle injury, due in part to the fact that the medial malleolus is shorter than the lateral malleolus and also to the stronger support offered the medial ankle by the deltoid ligament (compared to the thinner lateral ligaments) (see Figure 5-6). Evaluation of a suspected ankle fracture should include the mechanism of injury (i.e., inversion, plantar flexion) and associated vascular or ligamentous injury. Posterior malleolar fractures often are associated with other fractures and ligamentous disruption, while transverse malleolar fractures generally represent an avulsion injury only. A pilon fracture occurs at the distal tibial metaphysis and is combined with disruption of the talar dome; pilon fractures account for up to 10% of all tibial fractures. The Pott fracture, a bimalleolar injury, is considered unstable. Both the pilon and Pott fracture require urgent orthopaedic attention for possible ORIF. Unrecognized or undertreated open injuries are at high risk of infection, including local infection as well as osteomyelitis and sepsis (Iskyan & Aronson, 2008).

The calcaneus is the most frequently fractured tarsal bone. It functions as a lever arm for the gastrocsoleus complex, providing support for a person's body weight and maintaining the lateral column of the foot. Thus, any unresolved injury to

Figure 5-7
Lateral View of the Hindfoot

Lateral view of the hindfoot with fractures of both talus and calcaneus.

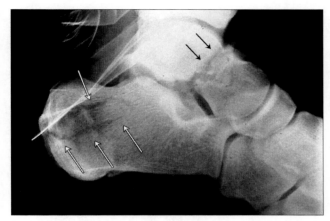

Reprinted with permission from Levine, A.M. (1996). *Orthopaedic knowledge update: Trauma* (pp. 191-209). Rosemont, IL: American Academy of Orthopaedic Surgeons.

this area will affect a person's gait. Calcaneal fractures often result from a fall from a height, a twisting injury, or pathology such as osteoporosis. Because there is no obvious deformity, however, they may remain undiagnosed clinically. While the patient's history is helpful, radiographic examination is essential for accurate diagnosis. Management of intra-articular calcaneal fractures and any associated soft tissue injury remains somewhat controversial. Displaced intra-articular fractures typically are treated through ORIF with a lateral plate. Extra-articular fractures often are managed conservatively with RICE intervention (rest, ice, compression, and elevation); vigorous exercises are prescribed after swelling resolves in order to help the patient regain subtalar and ankle movement (Khan, Rahim, Irion, & MacDonald, 2008) (see Figure 5-7).

Fractures of the foot are common, with metatarsals among the bones most frequently injured. They often result from dropping heavy objects on the foot or from the stress of repetitive trauma. Acute fractures, which are recognized easily, may be transverse, oblique, or comminuted. However, stress fractures may be more difficult to recognize, especially in early stages when a periosteal reaction may be the only evidence. A Jones fracture, caused by inversion of the foot, is a transverse fracture at the base of the fifth metatarsal; this type of injury is prone to nonunion. A Lisfranc fracture-dislocation occurs at the tarsometatarsal joints, often as result of falling from a height, falling downstairs, or stepping off a curb. Stress fractures of the foot (also called marcher's fractures) can occur from abnormal stress on normal bone; other predisposing factors include injury to adjacent bones, neuropathic disease, and RA. Although casting and weight-bearing restrictions are successful in many cases, surgery may be needed to repair more serious metatarsal injuries. Early diagnosis and treatment are critical to prevent complications, including nonunion or malunion, arthritis, and chronic pain disorders (Rajiah & Karthikeyan, 2008).

Ankle Arthroplasty

As with similar surgeries on other joints, total ankle arthroplasty may be considered if arthritis pain and mobility limitations affect a patient's quality of life. However, some clinicians and insurers still consider the procedure investigational. First-generation total ankle arthroplasty designs had unacceptably high complication and failure rates compared with ankle fusion (arthrodesis). Surgical techniques have improved and second-generation prosthetics seem better designed. However, Spirt, Assel, and Hansen (2004) identified a high rate of reoperation with the newer prosthetics and noted the functional outcome of the procedure could not be determined. For ankle arthroplasty, a tibial component replaces the socket-like portion of the ankle, and a talar component replaces the top of the talus. The tibial component is made of two parts: a flat metal piece attached directly to the tibia and a plastic cup that fits on the metal piece, forming a socket. The talar component is made of metal and fits into the socket of the tibial component. Cement is used to attach the metal components after the patient's bones have been shaped to accommodate them, and screws are commonly used to stabilize the joint. In addition, bone is grafted between the tibia and fibula to create fusion between these bones.

Because younger, active patients tend to place too much demand on current ankle prosthetics, patients under age 50 still are offered ankle fusion surgery. Ankle fusion also is suggested for patients over age 50 who remain active and place relatively high demand on the joint. Patients who are overweight or obese are not considered good candidates for ankle arthroplasty because excess weight increases the burden on the implanted joint. Other patients who should avoid ankle replacement include patients with ankle infections, peripheral vascular disease, and severely abnormal alignment or stability of the ankle.

Patients undergoing ankle arthroplasty generally spend 1 night in the hospital after surgery. A mobility aid (walker or crutches) is used and toe-touch weight bearing is observed for several weeks to decrease pressure on the operative ankle. Complete rehabilitation from ankle arthroplasty takes approximately 4-9 months.

Achilles Tendon Rupture

The Achilles tendon extends from the distal aspect of the tibia (origin) to the calcaneus (insertion). Injury to this tendon becomes more likely with a person's increased participation in recreational and competitive sports. Achilles tendon rupture is an overuse syndrome that most often occurs in persons ages 35-45. Injuries occur most often because of rapid loading of the tendon, generally from push-off with the foot in plantar flexion as the knee is flexed simultaneously; rupture can also result from sudden, unexpected dorsiflexion of the foot accompanied by powerful calf muscle contraction. Direct impact accounts for less than 10% of Achilles injuries. Repetitive stresses cause microtraumas and, if regenerative processes cannot keep pace with the injuries, tendon rupture results. Patients with Achilles tendon rupture often describe feeling as if they had

Figure 5-8
Bunion Deformity

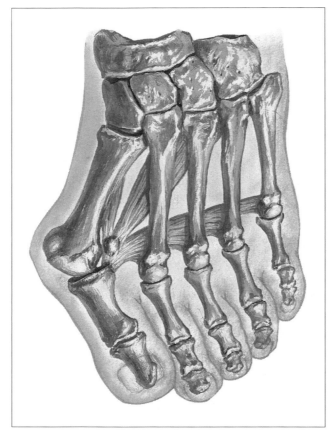

been struck in the calf. Pain is intense, generally accompanied by a crack or popping sound. Physical examination reveals a palpable gap in the tendon which may not be readily visible due to hematoma. Strength of plantar flexion typically is decreased or lost completely, and the foot often is externally rotated as well. Most ruptures can be diagnosed clinically, but ultrasound (US) or MRI may facilitate diagnosis and determine treatment selection. Nonoperative immobilization with a cast is no longer justified because of risk of muscle atrophy, loss of proprioception, and joint stiffness that result from cast treatment. If MRI or US reveals a persisting gap of the tendon ends, surgery is necessary (Thermann & Becher, 2009). While operative treatment may provide stronger repair and faster rehabilitation, however, it carries risks of operative morbidity. Alternately, nonoperative treatment may include use of an equinus ankle cast, rehabilitation in a boot with a heel lift, and full weight bearing as soon as tolerated (Weber, Niemann, Lanz, & Müller, 2003).

Plantar Fasciitis

The plantar fascia extends from the calcaneus to the metatarsal heads, serving as a support to the longitudinal arch of the foot. Irritation and microtears near the calcaneal insertion typically start the inflammation process, which involves the plantar fascia and periosteum. Plantar fasciitis can be precipitated by trauma or overuse; risk factors include a sudden increase in activity, poor shoe support, training errors (i.e., inadequate stretching), rigid pes planus (flatfoot) or pes cavus (high arch), and sudden weight gain. Plantar fasciitis is a common cause of plantar heel pain, which can be especially severe when the person walks barefoot or when taking the first step of the morning. The pain, which may extend into the Achilles tendon, can be replicated with passive dorsiflexion of the toes or the foot. Local tenderness also is common. Diagnosis generally is done based on clinical presentation, through x-rays may be done for an ambiguous presentation. While approximately 60% of films show a bone spur at the insertion site, that is an associated finding and not the underlying cause of pain. Immobilization, NSAIDs, stretching exercises, and use of orthotics or heel cups may be indicated. Surgery is a last resort if conservative therapy fails (Burton & Tierney, 2007).

Hallux Valgus

The bunion deformity, or hallux valgus, is caused by a lateral deviation of the great toe on the first metatarsal head (MTP joint) (See Figure 5-8). The bunion is the callus, thickened bursa and excess bone that results from the lateral deviation of the proximal phalanx in the great toe and the medial prominence of the MTP head. Its development often is linked to wearing narrow-toed, high-heeled shoes. Other foot pathologies that contribute to hallux valgus include severe flatfoot deformity, chronic Achilles tendon tightness, spasticity, RA, and family history of the condition. Pain and gait changes can result from hallux valgus, making the change to a wider shoe necessary to allow adequate space for the forefoot (Burton & Tierney, 2007). Orthotics and steroid injections of the MTP joint also may be considered. If severe, progressive hallux valgus affects the function of the remaining toes, surgical alignment of the great toe may be needed to correct the deformity and improve the mechanics of the foot. Choice of procedure (i.e., osteotomy, fusion of MTP joint) is based on the degree of deformity and the surgeon's preference. The goal is pain reduction and restoration of the foot's normal anatomy.

Table 5-8
Nursing Diagnoses for the Patient with Lower Extremity Problems

Pain: acute or chronic
Impaired physical mobility
Self-care deficit (bathing/hygiene, dressing/grooming)
Impaired skin integrity
Disturbed body image
Altered sexuality pattern
Ineffective role performance
Ineffective individual/family coping

Hammer/Claw/Mallet Toe Deformities

Hammer toe deformity is the most commonly occurring deformity of the lesser toes. It is primarily a flexion deformity of the PIP joint of the toe, with hyperextension of the MTP and DIP joints. Incidence of the condition is unknown, but it is correlated strongly with the presence of a length disparity among the toes. Ill-fitting shoes can compound the problem. The patient with symptomatic hammer toe typically complains of pain over the dorsal surface of the PIP joint as well as over the plantar head of the MTP joint. Assessment should be done with the patient standing to determine the functional significance of the deformity. Nonoperative treatment includes taping (for flexible deformity) and the use of footwear with a toe box of adequate depth (for fixed deformity). Surgical correction is indicated if the pain is disabling or does not improve with conservative treatment. The patient undergoing correction of hallux valgus also should have correction of an asymptomatic hammer toe to minimize the likelihood of recurrence (Watson, 2009).

The term "claw toe" probably reflects the digit's similarity in appearance to the claw of an animal or talon of a bird. This deformity is characterized by dorsiflexion of the proximal phalanx on the lesser MTP joint and the concurrent flexion of the PIP and DIP joints; this involvement of both the MTP and DIP joint differentiates the condition from hammer toe, which cannot have MTP hyperextension co-existing with DIP plantar flexion. Claw toe is seen most frequently in people in the seventh and eighth decades of life, with women affected 4-5 times more often than men. There is no specific underlying disease responsible for the deformity. Conservative treatment includes avoiding high-heeled, narrow-toed shoes, which produce impingement as they crowd the toes against each other. Metatarsal pads can be used for additional comfort in shoes with a wide toe box. Because such treatments do not reverse the claw toe position, surgery may be needed (De Orio, 2008).

A mallet toe is a fixed or flexible deformity of the DIP joint of the lesser toes. Pain, either from callus or pressure on the nail, may be the patient's presenting symptom when the DIP joint develops abnormal flexion. Inappropriate shoe wear, trauma, neuromuscular disorders, and pes cavus can contribute to development of this deformity. Painful deformity is the justification for surgery, though cosmesis also may be raised as a rationale for operative treatment. Nonoperative treatment focuses on relieving the pressure under the tip of the toe, usually with footwear with an extra-depth toe box. Soft orthotics or toe protectors also can be useful (Brown & Cullen, 2009).

Summary

Lower extremity disorders occur in all ages. Caring for affected patients requires a combined understanding of age-specific needs and the principles of orthopaedic nursing. See table 5-8 for common nursing diagnoses for patients with lower extremity problems. An interdisciplinary plan of care developed by the patient or family, the physician, the nurse, rehabilitation therapists, and others will ensure an optimal level of function for the patient.

References

Agency for Healthcare Research and Quality (n.d.). FY 2004: *Research on health costs, quality and outcomes.* Retrieved June 26, 2009, from http://www.ahrq.gov/about/cj2004/hcqo04a.htm

American Academy of Orthopaedic Surgeons (AAOS). (2007a). *Hip bursitis.* Retrieved June 26, 2009, from http://orthoinfo.aaos.org/topic.cfm?topic=a00409

American Academy of Orthopaedic Surgeons (AAOS). (2007b). *Hip implants.* Retrieved June 26, 2009, from http://orthoinfo.aaos.org/topic.cfm?topic=A00355

American Academy of Orthopaedic Surgeons (AAOS). (2007c). *Minimally invasive total hip replacement.* Retrieved June 26, 2009, from http://orthoinfo.aaos.org/topic.cfm?topic=A00404

American Academy of Orthopaedic Surgeons (AAOS). (2008). *Hip fractures in seniors: A call for health system reform.* Retrieved June 28, 2009, from http://www.aaos.org/about/papers/position/1144.asp

American Academy of Orthopaedic Surgeons (AAOS) (2009). *Dental work after a joint replacement.* Retrieved June 26, 2009, from http://orthoinfo.aaos.org/topic.cfm?topic=A00226

American College of Rheumatology (ACR) Subcommittee on Osteoarthritis Guidelines (2000). Recommendations for the medical management of osteoarthritis of the hip and knee: 2000 update. *Arthritis & Rheumatism, 43*(9), 1905-1915.

Arthritis Foundation. (1999). *National arthritis action plan: A public health strategy.* Atlanta: Author.

Arthritis Foundation. (2009). *What is osteoarthritis?* Retrieved June 26, 2009, from http://www.arthritistoday.org/conditions/osteoarthritis/all-about-oa/what-is-oa.php

Atmaca, A., Kleerekoper, M. Bayratkar, M., & Kucuk, O. (2008). *Soy isoflavones in the management of postmenopausal osteoporosis.* Retrieved June 28, 2009, from http://www.medscape.com/viewarticle/580688

Australian Institute of Health and Welfare. (2008). A picture of osteoporosis Australia. *Arthritis Series No. 6,* Cat. No. PHE 99. Canberra, Australia: Author.

Banchet, V., Fridrici, V., Abry, J.C., & Kapsa, P. (2007). Wear and friction characterization of materials for hip prosthesis. *Wear, 263*(7-12), 1066-1071.

Barclay, L. (2007). *Mortality greater for hip fracture than breast cancer in elderly women.* Retrieved June 28, 2009, from http://www.medscape.com/viewarticle/556768

Bluth, E.I., Benson, C.B., Ralls, P.W., & Siegel, M.J. (2007). *Ultrasound: A practical approach to clinical problems* (2nd ed.). New York: Thieme Medical Publishers, Inc.

Bodén, H., & Adolphson, P. (2004). No adverse effects of early weight bearing after uncemented total hip arthroplasty: A randomized study of 20 patients. *Acta Orthopaedica Scandinavica, 75*(1), 21-29.

Brown, C., & Cullen, N. (2009). *Mallet toe.* Retrieved June 30, 2009, from http://emedicine.medscape.com/article/1236338-overview

Burton, N., & Tierney, C.D. (2007). Foot and ankle. In National Association of Orthopaedic Nurses, *NAON Core curriculum for orthopaedic nursing* (6th ed., pp. 575-601). Boston: Pearson.

Cassel, C. K., Leipzig, R. M., Cohen, H. J., Larson, E. B., & Meier, D. E. (2003). *Geriatric medicine: An evidence-based approach* (4th ed.). New York: Springer-Verlag.

DeOrio, J.K. (2008). *Claw toe.* Retrieved June 30, 2009, from http://emedicine.medscape.com/article/1232559-overview

ExRx. (2009). *Hip articulations.* Retrieved June 26, 2009, from http://www.exrx.net/Articulations/Hip.html#anchor850108

Geier, K.A. (2007). Metabolic bone conditions. In National Association of Orthopaedic Nurses, *NAON Core curriculum for orthopaedic nursing* (6th ed., pp. 373-394). Boston: Pearson.

Gelfer, P., & Kennedy, K.A. (2008). Developmental dysplasia of the hip. *Journal of Pediatric Health Care, 22*, 318-322.

Hawk, D., & Bailie, S. (2007). Pediatric/congenital disorders. In National Association of Orthopaedic Nurses, *NAON Core curriculum for orthopaedic nursing* (6th ed., pp. 259-326). Boston: Pearson.

Helmick, C.G., Felson, D.T., Lawrence, R.C., Gabriel, S., Hirsch, R., Kwoh, C.K., ...Stone, J.H., for the National Arthritis Data Workgroup. (2008). Estimates of the prevalence of arthritis and other rheumatic conditions in the United States: Part I. *Arthritis & Rheumatism, 58*(1), 15-25.

Iskyan, K., & Aronson, A.A. (2008). *Fracture, ankle.* Retrieved June 3, 2009, from http://emedicine.medscape.com/article/824224-overview

Khan, A.N., Rahim, R., Irion, K.L., & MacDonald, S. (2008). *Calcaneus fractures.* Retrieved June 30, 2009, from http://emedicine.medscape.com/article/388031-overview

Maloney, W.J., Kang, M.N., & Hartford, J.M. (2006). The cemented femoral component. In J.J. Callahan, A.G. Rosenberg, & H.E. Rubash (Eds.), *The adult hip: Volume 1* (2nd ed., pp. 917-945). Philadelphia: Lippincott, Williams, & Wilkins.

National Institute of Arthritis and Musculoskeletal and Skin Diseases (NIAMS) (2004). Handout on health: *Rheumatoid arthritis.* Retrieved June 26, 2009, from http://www.niams.nih.gov/Health_Info/Rheumatic_Disease/rheumatoid_ arthritis_hoh.pdf

National Institutes of Health (2005). *Facts about menopausal hormone therapy.* Retrieved June 28, 2009, from http://www.nhlbi.nih.gov/health/women/pht_facts.pdf

National Osteoporosis Foundation (NOF) (2004). *Know your risk.* Retrieved June 26, 2009, from http://www.nof.org/awareness2/2004/nof_final_risk-assess.pdf

National Osteoporosis Foundation (NOF) (2008a). *Medications to prevent and treat osteoporosis.* Retrieved June 28, 2009, from http://www.nof.org/patientinfo/medications.htm

National Osteoporosis Foundation (NOF) (2008b). *Osteoporosis: Fast facts.* Retrieved June 26, 2009, from http://www.nof.org/osteoporosis/diseasefacts.htm

National Osteoporosis Foundation (NOF) (2008c). *Osteoporosis: Men.* Retrieved June 26, 2009, from http://www.nof.org/men/index.htm

National Osteoporosis Foundation (NOF) (2008d). *Prevention: Calcium.* Retrieved June 28, 2009, from http://www.nof.org/prevention/calcium2.htm

Norvell, J.G., & Steele, M. (2008). *Fracture, tibia and fibula.* Retrieved June 30, 2009, from http://emedicine.medscape.com/article/826304-overview

Novartis Consumer Health, Inc. (2009). *About Voltaren® gel.* Retrieved July 12, 2009, from http://www.voltarengel.com/consumer/VoltarenGelIndication.jsp

Peters, C.L., & Miller, M.D. (2006). The cementless acetabular component. In J.J. Callahan, A.G. Rosenberg, & H.E. Rubash (Eds.), *The adult hip: Volume 1* (2nd ed., pp. 946-967). Philadelphia: Lippincott, Williams, & Wilkins.

Ranawat, A.S., & Sekiya, J.K. (2004). *Hip labral tears.* Retrieved June 26, 2009, from http://www.aana.org/labralhiptears.Aspx

Rajiah, P., & Karthikeyan, S. (2008). *Metatarsal fractures.* Retrieved June 30, 2009, from http://emedicine.medscape.com/article/399372-overview

Roberts, D. (2007). Arthritis and connective tissue disorders. In National Association of Orthopaedic Nurses, *NAON Core curriculum for orthopaedic nursing* (6th ed., pp. 327-372). Boston: Pearson.

Roche, J.J.W., Wenn, R.T., Sahota, O., & Moran, C.G. (2005). Effect of comorbidities and postoperative complications on mortality after hip fracture in elderly people: Prospective observational cohort study. *British Medical Journal*, doi:10.1136/bmj.38643.663843.55 (published 18 November 2005).

Saag, K.G., Teng, G.G., Patkar, N.M., Anuntiyo, J., Finney, C., Curtis, J.R., ...& Furst, D.E. (2008). American College of Rheumatology 2008 recommendations for the use of nonbiologic and biologic disease-modifying antirheumatic drugs in rheumatoid arthritis. *Arthritis & Rheumatism, 59*(6), 762-784.

Shen, B., Yang, J., Wang, L., Zhou, Z., Kang, P., & Pei, F. (2009). Midterm results of hybrid total hip arthroplasty for treatment of osteoarthritis secondary to dysplasia of the hip: Chinese experience. *The Journal of Arthroplasty.* Advance online publication. doi:10.1016/j.arth.2009.07.002

Shimmin, A., Beaule, P., & Campbell, P. (2008). Metal-on-metal hip resurfacing arthroplasty. *Journal of Bone and Joint Surgery – American, 90*, 637-654.

Spirt, A.A., Assal, M., & Hansen, S.T. (2004). Complications and failure after total ankle arthroplasty. *The Journal of Bone and Joint Surgery, 86*, 1172-1178.

Ström, H., Nilsson, O., Milbrink, J., Mallmin, H., & Larsson, S. (2007). Early migration pattern of the uncemented CLS stem in total hip arthroplasties. *Clinical Orthopaedics and Related Research, 454*, 127-132.

Theis, L.M., & Kahn, B. (2007). The hip, femur, and pelvis. In National Association of Orthopaedic Nurses, *NAON Core curriculum for orthopaedic nursing* (6th ed., pp. 533-554). Boston: Pearson.

Thermann, H., & Becher, C. (2009). Nonoperative management of acute ruptures. In J.A. Nunley (Ed.), *The Achilles tendon: Treatment and rehabilitation* (pp. 41-53). New York: Springer.

Wasielewski, R.C. (2006). The hip. In J.J. Callahan, A.G. Rosenberg, & H.E. Rubash (Eds.), *The adult hip: Volume 1*(2nd ed., pp. 51-67). Philadelphia: Lippincott, Williams, & Wilkins.

Watson, A. (2009). *Hammertoe deformity.* Retrieved June 30, 2009, from http://emedicine.medscape.com/article/1235341-overview

Weber, M., Niemann, M., Lanz, R., & Müller, T. (2003). Nonoperative treatment of the acute rupture of the Achilles tendon. *American Journal of Sports Medicine, 31*, 685-691.

Whinney, C.M. (2005). *Do hip fractures need to be repaired within 24 hours of injury?* Retrieved June 28, 2009, from https://www.clevelandclinicmeded.com/medicalpubs/ccjm/march05/whinney.htm

Wisniewski, S.J., & Grogg, B. (2006). Femoroacetabular impingement: An overlooked cause of hip pain. *American Journal of Physical Medicine & Rehabilitation, 85*, 546-549.

World Health Organization (WHO) (2003). *Prevention and management of osteoporosis: WHO Technical Report Series 912.* Geneva, Switzerland: Author.

World Health Organization (WHO) (2004). *What are the main risk factors for falls amongst older people and what are the most effective interventions to prevent these falls? Health Evidence Network Report.* Retrieved June 28, 2009, from http://www.euro.who.int/document/e82552.pdf

World Health Organization (WHO) (2006). *What evidence is there for the prevention and screening of osteoporosis? Health Evidence Network Report.* Retrieved June 28, 2009, from http://www.euro.who.int/Document/HEN/HENReport_Osteoporosis.pdf

Chapter 6

Care of the Patient with Traumatic Orthopaedic Injuries

Cathy A. Murray, MSN, RN, OCNS-C®
Mary Catherine Rawls, BSN, RN-BC, MS, ONC®

Objectives

- Identify common mechanisms of trauma which result in musculoskeletal injuries.

- Describe assessment strategies for the patient with traumatic injuries.

- Describe treatment options and nursing interventions associated with traumatic injuries.

- Describe nursing assessment and care of patients in traction, casts, and external fixators.

Key Terms

Blast Injury: any injury to the body that is the result of an explosive that is detonated.

Comminuted Fracture: fracture in which the bone breaks into more than two pieces.

Compound Fracture: fracture in which penetration of the skin has occurred and there is communication with outside air (also referred to as open fracture).

Compression: squeezing together of structures.

Crush Injury: forceful compression of any extremity or part of the body that causes fracture, damage to muscle tissue, hemorrhage and/or neurologic compromise.

Elasticity: the quality of returning to original size and shape after compression or stretching.

External fixation: an immobilization method that uses percutaneous transfixing pins or wires attached to a rigid frame to stabilize a fracture.

Osteogenesis Imperfecta: an inherited connective tissue disorder characterized by defective bone matrix and calcification.

Paget's Disease: a disturbance of osteoblast and osteoclast activity resulting in the formation of disorganized bone which easily fractures.

Pathological Fracture: a break occurring at the site of pre-existing bone disease or a result of malignancy.

Penetrating Injury: injury to the body as a result of a foreign object, such as a bullet or debris, being forced through the dermis and into underlying tissues, structures, or organs.

Percutaneous: surgical procedure performed through the skin without a surgical incision.

Reduction: the restoration or correction of fracture fragments to normal anatomic relationships; the relocation of bones after dislocation of a joint.

Residual Limb: the part of the extremity that remains after surgical or traumatic amputation.

Shearing: twisting and tearing of tissues when structures slip relative to one another.

Simple Fracture: a closed fracture.

Skeletal Traction: application of a pulling force directly to the bone using pins, wires or screws.

Tensile Strength: amount of stretch tension a tissue can bear until it gives.

Traction: application of a pulling force to a part of the body.

Trauma is the result of injury to the human body through numerous mechanisms. The body can be harmed through violent assaults; extrinsic exposure such as thermal, chemical, electrical, or radiation; or lack of life sustaining elements such as oxygen or heat. The impact of trauma is physical, psychological and economic. Trauma can result in an alteration to a previous lifestyle or health state, with a degree of physical, mental, or socioeconomic disability. Musculoskeletal trauma ranges from strains and sprains to multiple fractures and soft tissue injuries. Causes of trauma are numerous and include motor vehicle accidents, falls, sports injuries, bullet and stabbing injuries, burns, blasts, water accidents, and severe temperature variations. The risk of traumatic injury to the musculoskeletal system can vary with age, gender, race, income, and environment (Weigelt, Brasel, & Klein, 2009).

Risk Factors

Trauma is listed as the fifth most common cause of death in the United States by the Center for Disease Control and Prevention (CDC, 2006). It is the leading cause of death for 15-24 year olds due to their participation in high-risk activities. Males suffer more injuries and death than females, although women are more likely to be victims of fatal domestic violence. For the elderly, death and injury rates from falls are high, often compounded by medical co-morbidities. The elderly may suffer greater physical injury from lesser traumatic events than younger adults. The potential and severity of musculoskeletal injury is increased by alcohol and drug use (CDC, 2006).

Unintentional injury rates are higher in low income areas and more fatal to Native Americans than other races, while African Americans have the highest homicide rate, and Caucasians and Native Americans the highest suicide rates. Asian Americans have the lowest rate of death from unintentional injuries, homicides and suicide. In times of economic depression, the numbers of suicides and homicides increase while motor vehicle crashes decrease; and in higher income areas, death rates from trauma are lower (CDC, 2006).

In rural settings, the mortality rates from farming accidents, such as machinery injuries, and motor vehicle accidents may be higher than in urban areas. This is related to the time it takes to be transported to the nearest trauma center.

Table 6-1
Open Fractures

Severity	Description
Grade I	Wound < 1 cm; minimal contamination
Grade II	Wound > 1 cm; moderate contamination
Grade III	Wound > 6-8 cm; extensive damage to soft tissue, nerve, and tendon; high degree of contamination

Adapted from Black, J.M. (1997). Nursing care of clients with musculoskeletal trauma or overuse. In J.M. Black, & E. Matassarin-Jacobs (Eds.), *Medical-surgical nursing: Clinical management for continuity of care* (5th ed., pp. 2129-2170). Philadelphia: W.B. Saunders.

Intentional injuries, such as homicides, are higher in urban settings while unintentional injuries such as falls can occur in either environment (CDC, 2006).

Trauma Evaluation

The American College of Surgeons has developed a process for a systematic evaluation in the Advanced Trauma Life Support and Advanced Trauma Care for Nurses guidelines. These guidelines outline a process for the primary survey that includes the ABCDEs of assessment in trauma patients:

Airway – assess airway for ineffective airway clearance and airway obstruction

Breathing – assess ineffective breathing patterns and impaired gas exchange

Circulation – assess decreased cardiac output, impaired tissue perfusion and decreased fluid levels

Disability – assess level of consciousness and neurologic status

Exposure – assess all body surfaces for injury and protect from hypothermia (Bongiovanni, Bradley, & Kelley, 2005)

The secondary survey is a head-to-toe examination of the entire patient to identify additional and potential injuries (Weigelt et al., 2009). The tertiary survey typically occurs within 24 hours of admission, after initial resuscitation and treatment, and is a comprehensive, formal review of the lab data, radiographs, primary and secondary surveys, mechanism of injury, co-morbidities and medical record to date. The purpose is to identify any missed injuries or delayed diagnoses (Petersen, 2003).

In emergency situations, the basic principles of trauma care must be observed. If there is an indication of cervical spine trauma, the neck must be stabilized until injury is ruled out by radiographic examination. In individuals who are unconscious, the inability to communicate makes the need for a more detailed assessment critical. Nursing assessment of other injuries, fractures, soft tissue damage, and neurovascular function is essential. Stabilizing fractures with splints and minimizing the risk of infection by covering open wounds will reduce discomfort and facilitate the patient's long-term recovery (see Table 6-1 for classification of open fractures).

Mechanisms of Injury

Awareness of the mechanism of injury helps the trauma team identify the patterns of injury the patient is likely to have suffered. Injuries can be blunt or penetrating. The type of injury, speed with which it occurred, and location in the body help predict the extent and severity of the injury to the patient (Weigelt et al., 2009).

Blunt Trauma

Blunt trauma is caused by a combination of forces: compression, deceleration, acceleration, shearing, or crushing. Blunt trauma results in multiple, life-threatening injuries with diagnoses that are complex and less obvious than injuries from penetrating trauma. The age of the patient must be considered as children experience different patterns of injury than adults because of their size (Weigelt et al., 2009).

Compression is the most common type of blunt trauma. Injury depends upon the length of time of the compression, the force of compression, and the areas/tissues compressed. Compressive resistance is the ability of tissue or a structure to resist squeezing forces or inward pressure. Skeletal injury often results from compression forces.

Shearing is another example of blunt trauma and involves the twisting and tearing of tissue which occurs when structures slip relative to one another. Tensile strength is the amount of stretch tension a tissue can bear until it gives. Elasticity is the property of tissue to return to its original shape and size after being stretched. Tissues have limits to the amount of tension or energy they can absorb; the energy is dissipated through the tissues to protect underlying organs and structures. When that energy limit is exceeded, tissue damage occurs (Weigelt et al., 2009).

Another example of blunt trauma is a motor vehicle crash (MVC) which involves three separate impacts: 1) the vehicle strikes an object; 2) the occupant collides with the inside of the vehicle; and 3) the occupant's internal organs collide with the rigid structures of the body. Restrained drivers decelerate with the vehicle rather than meeting the obstacle of the windshield or road and consequently suffer fewer injuries and less mortality than unrestrained drivers. Other important considerations include the speed at which the vehicle was traveling, and the direction of the impact: frontal, T-boned, rear-ended, or rollover. Whether the driver/passenger had to be extricated from the car may be a predictor of the degree of injury (Weigelt et al., 2009).

If the patient was involved in a motorcycle/bicycle accident, it is important to note whether they were riding or driving the bike, if they were helmeted, if thrown from the bike or crushed during impact, and whether loss of consciousness was experienced. For pedestrian accidents, it is important to be aware of whether the patient was hit from the side, head-on, thrown, or run over (Weigelt et al., 2009).

Falls are another form of blunt trauma often resulting in skeletal injuries or fractures. Height, position upon impact, and cause of the fall determine the impact of the trauma (Weigelt et al., 2009).

Penetrating Trauma

Penetrating trauma occurs through the introduction of a foreign object into the body. The severity of the wound is defined by the amount of tissue damage. The velocity of the object plays a major role in the extent of the injury. Bullet injuries are an example of penetrating trauma. A low-velocity bullet causes less damage than a high-velocity bullet because less energy dissipates into the tissues (Weigelt et al., 2009).

Traumatic Orthopaedic Injuries

Strains and Sprains

A strain is the excessive stretching or tearing of a tendon or muscle which may occur as a result of a fall, heavy lifting, exercise, or inappropriate use of body mechanics. Strains are classified according to their severity: a mild (first degree) strain is defined as an inflamed muscle with little bleeding; a moderate (second degree) strain involves partial tearing of the tendon or muscle; and a (third-degree) severe strain is consistent with a ruptured muscle; or separation of the tendon from muscle, muscle from muscle, or tendon from bone. Therapeutic interventions for strains include the intermittent applications of cold or heat, and rest. Pharmacologic intervention may include anti-inflammatory medications and muscle relaxants. Surgical repair of the muscle or tendon may be required in third-degree strains (Murray, 2009).

Sprains involve excessive stretching or tearing of a ligament that may occur from a fall or twisting motion during a sporting activity. Like strains, they are classified by either degrees or severity. A mild (first-degree) sprain involves torn ligament fibers without joint impairment. Second-degree or moderate sprains involve additional ligament fibers with maintenance of joint stability. In a third-degree or severe sprain, the ligament injury results in joint instability. Treatment includes rest, the application of ice for 24-48 hours, compression, and elevation. Second- and third-degree sprains require immobilization with compression bandages, immobilizers, braces, splints, or casts for up to 6 weeks, or until healing occurs. For some third-degree sprains, surgery may be necessary to restore joint stability (Murray, 2009).

Dislocations

Dislocations are joint injuries in which bone ends are forced from their normal position as a result of trauma (falls, sports injuries, motor vehicle crashes). These injuries can occur in the shoulders, hips, knees, elbows, ankles, fingers, thumbs, and toes. Immediate consequences of a joint dislocation are severe and sudden pain with joint deformity, which constitute an orthopaedic emergency. Surrounding nerves may be involved resulting in a loss of feeling or inability to move. Joint immobilization and the application of ice may temporarily reduce pain, swelling, and the extravasation of fluid into the joint space. Physical examination, X-rays and MRI can assist in confirming the dislocation and reveal additional injuries such as fractures, soft tissue and joint damage. Interrupted blood supply to the joint may lead to osteonecrosis while cartilage damage may result in joint arthritis. Treatment is based on the extent of the injury and can range from gently maneuvering the bones back into position (a reduction) with or without anesthesia; joint immobilization for several weeks with a sling, splint or traction; or surgical intervention. Healing is gradual and may require several months for a return to function. Once dislocated, the joint is more susceptible to future dislocations. Focused strength and stability exercises may decrease the possibility of reoccurrences (AAOS, 2007; Mayo Clinic, 2008).

Stress Fractures

Stress fractures are a type of overuse or repetitive use injury commonly seen in people of all ages who participate in sports such as running, tennis, track and field, gymnastics, and basketball. Repetitive impact on hard playing surfaces or use of improper footwear or equipment are contributing

Table 6-2
Methods of Fracture Classification

Fracture Pattern/Appearance	
Burst	Results in multiple pieces of bone; often occurs at ends of bones or in vertebrae
Comminuted	More than one fracture line, more than two bone fragments; fragments may be splintered or crushed
Complete	Break across the entire section of bone, dividing it into distinct fragments; frequently displaced
Displaced	Fragments out of normal position at fracture site
Incomplete	Fracture occurs through only one cortex of the bone; usually nondisplaced
Linear	Fracture line is intact; fracture results from minor to moderate forced applied directly to the bone
Longitudinal	Fracture line extends in the direction of the bone's longitudinal axis
Nondisplaced	Fragments aligned at the fracture site
Oblique	Fracture line occurs at approximately a 45 degree angle across the longitudinal axis of the bone
Spiral	Fracture line results from twisting force; forms a spiral encircling the bone
Stellate	Fracture lines radiate from one central point
Transverse	Fracture line occurs at a 90 degree angle to the longitudinal axis of the bone
General Description	
Avulsion	Bone fragments are torn away from the body of the bone at the site of attachment of a ligament or tendon
Compression	Bone buckles and eventually cracks as the result of unusual loading force applied to its longitudinal axis
Greenstick	Incomplete fracture in which one side of the cortex is broken and the other side flexed but intact; usually occurs in children, whose bones are still soft and pliable
Impacted	Telescoped fracture, with one fragment driven into the other
Pathologic	Fracture occurring from minimal trauma after bone has been weakened by underlying disorder, such as osteoporosis or tumor
Stress (fatigue)	Fracture results from repeated stress on a bone, as with metatarsal injuries from endurance activities
Anatomic Location	
Articular	Fracture involves a joint surface
Extracapsular	Fracture occurs outside the joint capsule
Intracapsular	Fracture occurs within the joint capsule
Supracondylar	Fracture occurs above the condyle of the Humerus after a fall on extended or flexed elbow
Transcondylar	Fracture occurs at or close to the condyle of the Humerus and partially within the joint capsule
Eponym	
Colles'	Fracture within the last inch of the distal radius; distal fragment is displaced in a position of dorsal and medial deviation
Pott's	Fracture of the distal fibula, seriously disrupting the tibiofibular articulation; a piece of the medial malleolus may be chipped off due to rupture of the internal lateral ligament

Adapted from Black, J.M. (1997). Nursing care of clients with musculoskeletal trauma or overuse. In J.M. Black, & E. Matassarin-Jacobs (Eds.), *Medical-surgical nursing: Clinical management for continuity of care* (5th ed., pp. 2129-2170). Philadelphia: W.B. Saunders and Maher, A.B. (1996). Trauma. In S.W. Salmond, N.E. Mooney, & L.A. Verdisco (Eds.), *Core curriculum for orthopaedic nursing* (3rd ed., pp. 415-450). Pitman, NJ: National Association of Orthopaedic Nurses.

factors to stress fractures. As muscles become too fatigued to absorb additional shock from an increased amount or intensity of activity, the stress load is transferred to the bone resulting in a small crack termed a stress fracture. Over half of stress fractures occur in the weight-bearing bones of the lower leg and foot. Female athletes may experience this condition more frequently than males, especially if there are also issues with osteopenia. Pain with activity that subsides with rest is a common symptom of a stress fracture. Diagnosis is made through an evaluation of a patient's risk factors, X-rays, or a CT or MRI. Treatment includes resting

from the activity responsible for the fracture for 6-8 weeks to allow for healing. Braces or shoe inserts may also be used. Early resumption of causative activities may result in re-injury and lead to chronic problems. Prevention of stress fractures can be achieved by gradually increasing activity when participating in a new sport, cross-training to accomplish fitness goals, maintaining a healthy diet, and using proper equipment. If pain or swelling occur related to specific activities, cessation of the activity with several days of rest is recommended (American Academy of Orthopaedic Surgeons (AAOS, 2007).

Fractures

Fractures most often occur as a result of excessive external force applied to the body. The amount of force needed to fracture a bone can vary considerably. A careful history will determine if the fracture resulted from a direct blow, a fall from a height, a motor vehicle accident, or from twisting, crushing, penetrating or compression forces (Weigelt et al., 2009).

A fracture is a partial or complete structural break in bone continuity. One way to classify fractures is to differentiate between simple (closed) or compound (open) fractures. Table 6-2 describes a variety of fracture classification systems. The most common system describes the appearance of bone ends at the fracture line (e.g. spiral) and notes the anatomical locations of the damage (e.g. metaphyseal). Eponyms can be used to define both the appearance and location of breaks (e.g. Colles' fracture- distal radius).

When bone is weakened or diseased, pathological fractures can occur. These types of fractures are the result of minimal force that would not typically injure healthy bone. Conditions such as Paget's disease or osteoporosis alter biologic factors, resulting in changes in bone structure and strength that can increase the risk for fracture. Osteogenesis Imperfecta (OI), an inherited condition of the connective tissue in which bones fracture easily, is characterized by defective bone matrix that does not provide a satisfactory framework for normal calcification (Taber, 2005). Bone fractures can be the precursor to a diagnosis of cancer or bone cysts. Adverse response of bone to medical treatments such as steroid or radiation therapies can weaken bone sufficiently to cause fractures.

Other conditions that significantly alter bone strength from loss of calcification are disuse and malnutrition. Wolff's Law states that bone modeling and remodeling occur as a response to forces acting upon it (Nelson & Blauvelt, 2007). When osteoblasts are stimulated by increased physical load and supported by an adequate intake of vitamin D, they lay down new bone in a way that perfects its ability to withstand stress or load and thereby maintain adequate bone density. Bone growth occurs where stress forces are applied. When these forces are reduced or absent, bone is resorbed. Lack of activity (prolonged bed rest, extended care, comatose patients, or wheelchair users), restricted weight bearing (casted patients), or time spent in non-gravitational forces (space travel) will lead to osteoporosis and increased risk of fracture. Individuals of all ages should be instructed about regular weight bearing exercise, healthy eating, adequate intake of calcium and vitamin D, and injury prevention to maintain healthy bones.

Malnutrition from lack of dietary intake, improper breakdown or absorption of nutrients, and/or poor distribution of food substances in the body can lead to weakened bone structure. Alcohol consumption also creates conditions that adversely affect bone health. The effect of alcoholism on bone metabolism occurs at both the intestinal and cellular levels and impacts the absorption of calcium and its incorporation into bone matrix.

Accidental injury is the leading cause of bone fractures. Falls, motor vehicle crashes, and gunshot wounds are usually accompanied by fractures and other more serious injuries. In addition, risk-taking behaviors, substance abuse, and lower socio-economic status can influence and increase the incidence of fracture injury (Kunkler, 2007).

Treatment

The primary goals of fracture management are to prevent complications while restoring optimum mechanical function with the most favorable cosmetic result. When treating the fracture, the first step involves reduction. This will approximate fragmented bone ends, restore original length, and maintain neurovascular function. Immobilization relieves pain and re-aligns bone ends to allow healing to begin. Immobilization methods include casts, slings, straps, tape, or surgical rods, plates, screws, wires, and pins. Following careful clinical examination, x-rays will verify the fracture line direction, ascertain the amount of displacement, and determine whether management will be by closed or open reduction, internal fixation (ORIF) and/or external fixation.

Closed reduction is the re-alignment of fractured bone ends into anatomical position without surgical intervention. If the fractured bone ends are in proper anatomical position, the non-displaced fracture requires immobilization only with a cast, tape, or sling. When bone ends are displaced, closed reduction using traction and manual manipulation must be done. Depending on the severity of the fracture and the pain involved, closed reduction can be performed in the emergency room with sedation or local anesthesia, or in the operating room under general anesthesia.

If closed reduction is unsuccessful or inappropriate for the fracture type, open reduction and internal fixation (ORIF) and/or external fixation is indicated. In the operating room, the fracture is visualized through an incision. Fragmented bone ends are approximated and stabilized by internal fixation. ORIF is indicated when there is tissue damage with multiple injuries, including injury to nerves and vessels, or when the injury involves a compound, comminuted fracture. If bony defects are extensive, autograft (taken from the patient's own iliac crest or other site) or allograft (taken from another human, usually a cadaver) bone may be used. The bone graft is wired, packed or grafted into the fractured area

Table 6-3
Stages of fracture healing.

Stage	Description	Length
I	Hematoma formation-fracture occurs and hematoma forms at side	1-3 days
II	Fibrocartilage formation-granulation tissue invades the hematoma	3 days-2 weeks
III	Callus formation-granulation tissue matures	2-6 weeks
IV	Ossification-callus bridges the gap between fracture fragments; callus gradually replaced by bone	3 weeks-6 months
V	Consolidation and remodeling-bone reshapes to meet its mechanical requirements	6 weeks-1 year

Adapted from Kunkler, C.E. (2002). Fractures (Chapt. 19). In A.B. Maher, S.W. Salmond, & T.A. Pellino (Eds.), *Orthopaedic nursing* (3rd Ed., pp.609-649). Philadelphia: W.B. Saunders.

Figure 6-1a
Fractures and Fixations

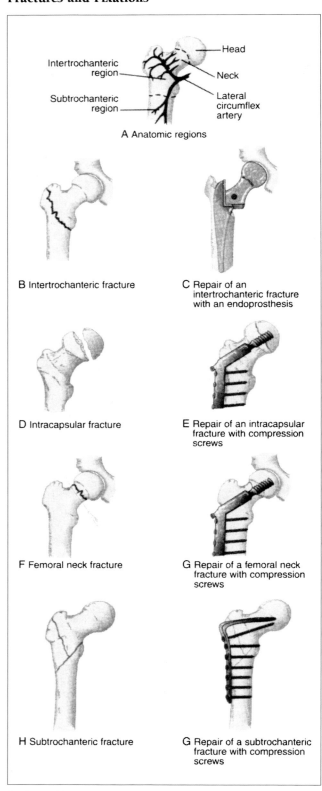

B Intertrochanteric fracture

C Repair of an intertrochanteric fracture with an endoprosthesis

D Intracapsular fracture

E Repair of an intracapsular fracture with compression screws

F Femoral neck fracture

G Repair of a femoral neck fracture with compression screws

H Subtrochanteric fracture

G Repair of a subtrochanteric fracture with compression screws

Reprinted with permission from Black, J.M., & Matassarin-Jacobs, E. (Eds.) (1997). *Medical-surgical nursing: Clinical management for continuity of care* (5th ed., p. 2153). Philadelphia: W.B. Saunders.

Figure 6-1b
Cortical Screws

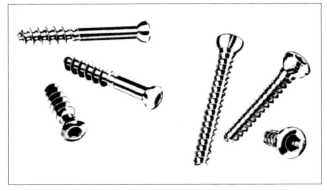

Reprinted with permission from Hilt, N.E. (Eds.) (1984). *Assessment and fracture management of the lower extremities.* Pitman, NJ: National Association of Orthopaedic Nurses. Courtesy of Zimmer, Inc.

Figure 6-1c
Bone Plates

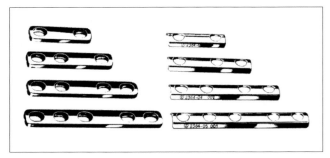

Reprinted with permission from Hilt, N.E. (Eds.) (1984). *Assessment and fracture management of the lower extremities.* Pitman, NJ: National Association of Orthopaedic Nurses. Courtesy of Zimmer, Inc.

Figure 6-1d
Compression Plating with Screws

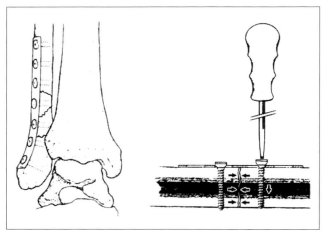

Reprinted with permission from Hilt, N.E. (Eds.) (1984). *Assessment and fracture management of the lower extremities.* Pitman, NJ: National Association of Orthopaedic Nurses. Courtesy of Zimmer, Inc.

to restore shape, fill gaps, add stability, or stimulate bone growth (Morris & Levin, 2007; Murray, 2009).

Internal fixation using devices such as surgical plates, screws, K-wires, pins, and rods (see Figures 6-1a, b, c, and d) usually follows open reduction (Kunkler, 2007). In long bone fractures, intramedullary (IM) rods are commonly inserted percutaneously through the medullary canal to bridge the fracture site. In this way, fixation is accomplished without exposing the fracture. Attaching plates to long bones with screws may also internally fixate limb fractures. Fractures of the patella, ankle, wrist, and elbow are usually repaired using K-wires, pins, and screws. Advantages of internal fixation include early ambulation, shorter hospitalization, and restoration of the bone's anatomical shape.

When fractures are severely comminuted or accompanied by extensive soft tissue wounds, external fixation is the treatment of choice. This method maintains alignment of fractured pelvic or long bones, allowing full access to wounds for assessment, treatment, and early mobilization. External fixation is discussed in more detail later in this chapter.

Bone Healing

Ideal bony union through reconstruction of new bone is achieved by early reduction, adequate immobilization, and sufficient blood supply to the healing bone. Factors influencing the rate at which healing occurs include the individual's age and nutritional status, location and severity of the fracture(s), and other associated injuries. It is important to understand that nicotine, a potent vasoconstrictor, reduces blood flow to a newly formed callus, impairing healing after a fracture. Nonsteroidal anti-inflammatory drugs (NSAIDs) can also diminish bone formation, healing and remodeling (Dahners & Mullis, 2004).

Fracture healing is a process occurring in five stages that do not occur independently, but rather in an overlapping manner (Kunkler, 2007). After the fracture is reduced and immobilized, the body's own internal repair mechanisms become active and initiate healing. See Table 6-3 for a description of the stages of fracture healing.

Occasionally, delayed or non-union of a fracture may occur. This is defined as a fracture that has not healed for 6-8 months after injury. Potential causes of non-union include multiple fracture fragments or extensive bone loss, infection, insufficient blood supply, or uncontrolled, repetitive stress on the fracture. Physical examination may show tenderness with palpation or bone motion at the fracture site and is confirmed by serial X-rays or CT scanning. Interventions to promote healing include electrical stimulation through low-intensity ultrasound, internal or external stimulation, or bone grafting (Morris & Levin, 2007; Murray, 2009).

Pelvis Fractures

The pelvis is made up of three bony structures: the ilium, ichium, and the pubis, forming a ring with the sacrum and coccyx. This anatomy provides great strength to the pelvis. The acetabulum is also part of the pelvis structure. Fracture of the pelvic ring requires a significant force or blunt trauma.

Common mechanisms of injury include motor vehicle accidents, particularly side impact crashes, persons who are hit by a motor vehicle, motorcycle accidents, falls, and crush injury (Kobziff, 2006). A fracture of the pelvis is often accompanied by other injuries including abdominal, thoracic, soft tissue, genitourinary, and head injury. In the United States, pelvic fractures represent 3% of all fractures. Males sustain more high-energy pelvis fractures such as motor

Figure 6-2
Pelvis Fractures

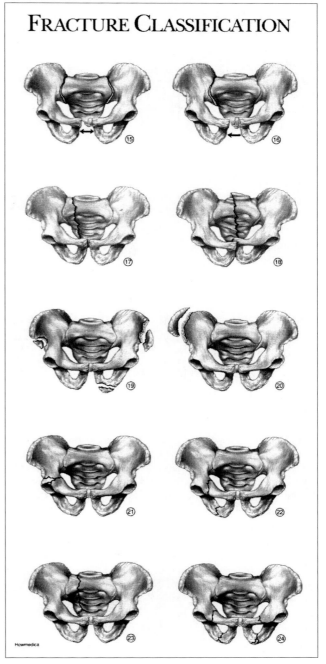

Courtesy of Stryker Orthopaedics.

Table 6-4
Classification Schemes for Pelvic Fractures

Tile's classification[10]	Young and Burgess classification[29]
Type A, Stable A1, Without involvement of pelvic ring A2, With involvement of pelvic ring	**Lateral compression (LC)** I, Sacral compression on side of impact II, Iliac wing fracture on side of impact III, LCI or LCII injury on side of impact with contralteral open-book injury
Type B, Rotationally unstable B1, Open book B2, Ipsilateral lateral compression B3, Contralateral compression	**Anterior posterior compression (APC)** I, Slight widening of pubic symphysis or anterior part of sacroiliac joint with intact anterior and posterior sacroiliac ligaments II, Widened anterior part of sacroiliac joint with disrupted anterior and intact posterior sacroiliac ligaments III, Complete disruption of sacroiliac joint
Type C, Rotationally and vertically unstable C1, Rotationally and vertically unstable C2, Bilateral C3, With associated acetabular fracture	**Vertical shear (VS)** Vertical displacement anteriorly and posteriorly **Combined mechanism (CM)** Combination of other injury patterns

Reprinted with permission of American Association of Critical Care Nurses conveyed through Copyright Clearance Center, Inc.
Frakes, M.A., & Evans, T. (2004). Major pelvic fractures. *Critical Care Nurse, 24*(2), 99-107.

vehicle accidents, while women sustain more low-energy pelvis fractures such as falls (Mechem, 2008). Figure 6-2 represents various types of pelvis fractures.

Patient Assessment

The patient with a pelvis fracture presents in the Emergency Department after stabilization of the fracture and transport from the scene of injury. Relevant medical history and the mechanism of injury should be established. The priority in the management of pelvis fracture is to prevent and control bleeding and hemorrhage. Major blood vessels in the pelvic region include the common iliac and femoral arteries, and the femoral and greater saphenous veins. However, approximately 90% of blood loss can occur from venous bleeding from the bony fracture site (Frakes & Evans, 2004). Large volume blood loss can occur in fractures of the pelvis, making assessment for hypovolemia and hemorrhage important. Initially, the patient examination includes the abdomen, pelvis, back, perineum and upper legs to assess for lacerations, abrasions, open fracture wounds, swelling and bruising, and location of pain. Severe back pain may indicate hemorrhage into the retroperitoneal space. The presence of hematuria and possibility of pregnancy must be determined. Rectal digital examination is performed to evaluate the presence of blood in the rectal vault, assess for an intact rectal wall, palpate the prostate gland, and determine sensation and tone in the rectum. Vaginal examination is important to rule out the possibility of open fracture and determine if the vaginal wall is intact (Kneale, 2005; Smith, 2005). Inspection of the pelvis is done to assess for rotation of the iliac crests, as this indicates serious fracture. Manipulation of the pelvis can be done to determine stability of the pelvic ring. This must be gentle to avoid further injury or stimulate hemorrhage. Neurovascular assessment of the lower extremities is done to determine presence of circulation, sensation, strength, and deep tendon reflexes (Kobziff, 2006).

Radiologic Assessment

To fully assess pelvic fractures, anteroposterior pelvic radiographic images will be utilized. CT scanning allows for visualization of more difficult areas such as the sacrum, sacroiliac joint, posterior arch, and the acetabulum and may facilitate visualization of retroperitoneal hematoma (Frakes & Evans, 2004). A pelvic fracture may be stable or unstable related to where in the pelvic ring the fracture is located and the number of fractures present.

Classification of Pelvic Fractures

Several classification systems for describing the bony injury to the pelvis are available. Most frequently, the Tile classification and the Young and Burgess classification are used. These two systems are compared in Table 6-4.

Fracture Stabilization

Emergent care involves stabilizing the pelvis to manage hemorrhage and reduce long-term effects of a pelvic ring fracture. Stable fractures may be managed using traction and a pelvic sling. Unstable fractures require external and/or internal fixation.

External Fixation

Anterior external fixation can be achieved with the application of a simple frame with two to three pins in each iliac crest. This is particularly useful in "open book" and other unstable fractures. Stabilization with external fixation allows clot formation to control hemorrhage. Early stabilization also reduces the risks of long-term pain and reduced mobility that often follows traumatic pelvis fractures (Frakes & Evans, 2004; Kneale, 2005; Kobziff, 2006).

Internal Fixation

Once the patient is hemodynamically stable, internal fixation may follow in 48-72 hours. Internal fixation provides more stable fracture reduction and helps with early mobilization. Some patients may have a combination of external and internal fixation. This approach helps in stabilizing both anterior and posterior fracture sites (Kneale, 2005).

Orthopaedic nurses need to be vigilant when caring for patients with pelvic fractures, always assessing for additional injury. Recovery from severe pelvic fractures requires long-term rehabilitation and can result in persistent pain and problems with mobility. Nursing management of patients with traumatic injury will be discussed later in this chapter.

Bullet, Blast, Penetrating and Crush Injuries

Bullet Injury

In recent years, it has been reported that gunshots have caused over 30,000 fatal injuries and approximately 100,000 non-fatal injuries in the United States and the numbers continue to rise (National Center for Health Statistics, 2006). Gunshot wounds can be categorized related to velocity. For example, hand-gun bullets are considered to cause low-velocity wounds, and rifle bullets cause high-velocity wounds. Low-velocity injury includes laceration and crushing of tissues which come in immediate contact with the bullet. The entry wound is usually smaller than the exit wound. Low-velocity projectiles may not travel all the way through the body or body part and therefore may be retained. High-velocity bullets often pass completely through the body or body part leaving entry and exit wounds. This projectile causes laceration and crushing of tissues and damage to other structures along the trajectory path. The trajectory cavity will contain bacteria and debris sucked in at the point of entrance, resulting in greater damage to tissue along the missile tract (Bartlett, Helfet, Hausman, & Strauss, 2000). Bullet wounds can result in damage to soft tissue, major organs, bony tissue with fracture, and damage to blood vessels and/or nerves.

Blast Injury

Blast injuries result when an explosive is detonated. While few terrorist attacks have occurred in the United States, those experienced to date involved an explosive device or explosion. In recent military campaigns, blast injuries to the extremities are most commonly seen. The effects of blast injury escalate related to how close the person is to the explosion, and whether the explosion occurs inside or outside of a building. Explosive devices may be loaded with metallic objects that become missiles and cause penetrating injury to soft and bony tissue. Bombs detonated inside a building or vehicle propel fragments that cause penetrating or blunt force injury to persons in the proximity of the explosion (Covy, 2002; Wallace, 2006; Weil, Mosheiff, & Liebergall, 2006). The explosion of a bomb creates a blast wave that includes a shock wave of pressure, followed by a blast wind. Blast injuries are described in Table 6-5.

The types of injuries the orthopaedic nurse expects to see from a blast include traumatic amputation of a limb, concussion, gross wound contamination, compartment syndrome, crush syndrome with resultant rhabdomyolysis and acute renal failure, severe burns, or ear and eye injury. Blast injuries result in high mortality.

Penetrating Injury

Penetrating injuries result when a foreign object is forced through the dermis and into underlying tissues, crushing and tearing the structures. Penetrating injuries can be caused by a bullet from a firearm, and flying debris from a blast. Stab wounds caused by knives, sharp objects, and impalement on objects are also considered penetrating wounds. These types of wounds usually result in tissue contamination with high risk of infection. Impaled objects are usually left in the wound until they can be removed surgically to control potential hemorrhage (Mamaril, Childs, & Sortman, 2007).

Crush Injury

Crush injury involves compression of upper or lower extremities or any part of the body that causes fracture, hemorrhage, edema of muscle tissue, and neurologic compromise. The lower extremity is involved in 74% of crush injuries, upper extremity in 10% of injuries, and the trunk in 9% of injuries (Centers for Disease Control and Prevention, 2008). Crush injury is potentially life-threatening and causes systemic complications including ischemia of the muscle tissue, followed by necrosis. Sudden release of the crushed body part results in reperfusion syndrome and release of myoglobin into circulation. Myoglobin obstructs the renal tubules resulting in acute renal failure. Compartment syndrome can occur. Care of the patient with compartment syndrome is discussed in Chapter 8, *Complications Associated with Orthopaedic Conditions and Surgeries*.

Amputation

Amputation is the removal of a part or all of a limb. Amputations may be done electively by surgical removal or traumatically as a result of an accident. In the United States, approximately 1.7 million persons live with limb loss. The number of amputees continues to increase related to the injuries seen in current military campaigns related to bomb and mine blasts. The need for amputation is precipitated by vascular disease, trauma, cancer and congenital anomalies. The primary cause of amputation is vascular disease.

Table 6-5
Phases of Blast Injury

Blast Phase	Mechanism of Injury
Primary Blast	Over pressurization force impacts the body causing tympanic membrane rupture, lung damage, hollow organ damage and air embolism
Secondary Blast	Projectiles and flying debris cause penetrating and blunt trauma
Tertiary Blast	Structural collapse causes crush injury or entrapment; persons are thrown into fixed objects by the blast wind
Quaternary Blast	All other injuries as a result of the blast: burns, smoke inhalation, exposure and inhalation of toxic substances such as dust containing asbestos and exacerabation of other illnesses

Adapted from DePalma, R.G., Burris, D.G., Champion, H.R., & Hodgson, M.J. (2005). Blast injuries. *The New England Journal of Medicine, 352*(13), 1335-1342.

Figure 6-3a
Levels of Amputation: Upper Extremity

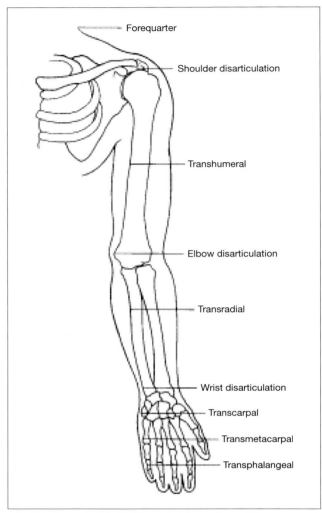

Reprinted with permission from Braddom, R.L. (1996). Forging the physiatric future. *Physical Medicine and Rehabilitation, 77*(11), 4.

Ninety-seven percent of amputations are related to vascular disease and involve the lower extremity, with the remaining 3% involving the upper extremity. Traumatic amputation is the second leading cause of amputation, with 68% involving the upper extremity and 32% the lower extremity. Males are at significantly higher risk of traumatic amputation than females (National Limb Loss Information Center, 2008).

Traumatic amputations often result from accidents with tools such as lawn mowers, snow blowers, and power tools such as saws. Motor vehicle and industrial accidents can be causes of upper and lower extremity amputation. Amputation is considered one of the signature injuries of the war in Iraq. Blast injury from improvised explosive devices (IEDs) used in roadside bombs and suicide bombings account for approximately 70% of the injuries seen in Iraq (Lehman, 2008). Severe injuries that include crushing of tissues often results in blood vessel and nerve damage and leads to

amputation as a way to preserve function in the residual limb. The ability to salvage limbs that have been severely damaged has increased. Some body parts can be reattached or replanted to preserve function, particularly in the hand.

Upper Extremity Amputation

Several levels of amputation can be observed as a result of injury to the upper extremity (see Figure 6-3a). Amputation at the shoulder, or neck of the humerus, is usually the result of severe trauma. Amputations that occur between the axillary fold and the distal supracondyles are referred to as above-the-elbow (AE). Elbow disarticulation is removal of the distal portion of the arm at the level of the humeral condyles. Elbow disarticulation may provide better prosthesis utilization than AE amputation. Below the elbow (BE) amputation, through the forearm, allows the patient to be fitted with a very functional prosthesis if they desire. Amputation through the wrist that preserves the radioulnar joint allows for the continued ability to pronate and supinate and increases the degree of function in the residual limb. Amputation of fingers is common in home, work, and industrial environments. Salvage of the injured finger or fingers is important to preserve the function of the hand. The loss of the thumb is most difficult as this leads to severe deficiencies in ability of the patient to grasp, hold, pick-up or carry items in the

Figure 6-3b
Levels of Amputation: Lower Extremity

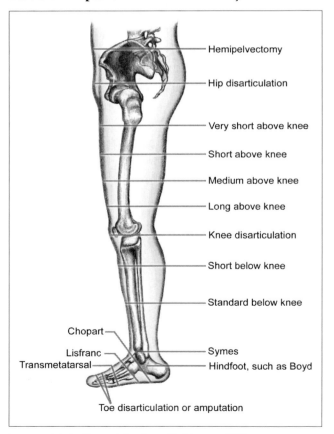

Image reprinted with permission from eMedicine.com, 2010.

hand. If at all possible after a traumatic injury, the thumb should be reconstructed (Schoen, 2000; Williamson, 2002). Upper limb amputations are often more incapacitating because of the loss of the ability to complete many activities of daily living such as eating, dressing, bathing, and driving a car. Amputation results in changes in body image and the adjustments related to loss of a body part.

Lower Extremity Amputation

Hip disarticulation, above-the-knee (AK), and below-the-knee (BK) amputations are often seen in traumatic injuries in the lower extremity. Motor vehicle accidents, blast, and crush injuries are causes of lower extremity amputation. A higher level of function may be offered to the person when the hip and knee joint can be preserved post-amputation. Ankle amputation at the level of the distal tibia and fibula is referred to as a Syme amputation. Amputation through the foot or forefoot can cause considerable gait disturbance and make rapid walking difficult. An injury in this area of the foot may result in further amputation at the ankle or below the knee to provide a more functional residual limb. Amputation of one or more toes may not change a normal walking gait but can decrease the ability to walk rapidly or run. Loss of toes, particularly the great toe, can result in a limping gait due to the loss of push-off that is provided by the great toe (Schoen, 2000; Williamson, 2002). Figure 6-3b shows levels of lower limb amputation.

Residual Limb Care

In the immediate postoperative period, the upper extremity residual limb may be elevated to reduce edema. The lower extremity residual limb should remain extended and not be elevated to prevent hip and knee flexion contracture. To help decrease edema, elastic bandage wraps, shrinker socks or stockings, or rigid dressings may be used.

Phantom Limb Pain

It is common for the patient to report sensation and persistent pain in the missing limb immediately after surgery and even long past the loss of the limb. This painful sensation is referred to as phantom limb pain. While this can happen with any amputation, it is more common after surgical amputation of a chronically painful limb than in traumatic injury or amputation. It is important for the nurse to recognize that this pain is real and must be treated. Phantom limb pain may not be relieved by opioid analgesic medications. Other medications such as beta-blocking agents, antiepileptic drugs, and antispasmodics may be more effective in managing phantom limb pain (Baower & Reuter, 2009).

Promoting Mobility

The orthopaedic nurse should collaborate with the physical therapist and occupational therapist to design a patient exercise program and plan for assistance with activities of daily living. Use of assistive devices will be included in the therapy. Physical therapists use rigid dressings and shrinker socks to decrease edema and shape the residual limb to prepare for fitting of a prosthesis. A prosthetist will assist the patient to be fitted with an appropriate prosthesis.

Body Image and Lifestyle Adaptation

The patient who loses a body part may experience body image changes that include feelings of inadequacy. Finding a mentor who has also experienced loss of a body part can help. The remaining portion of the limb is referred to as the residual limb, as the use of the word "stump" can evoke thoughts of uselessness. A patient may seem to be adjusting well during the hospitalization period but may have difficulty coping once they are discharged and the difficulties of functioning with limb loss become apparent. It is important to refer the patient to support groups that may be available in the community.

Nursing Considerations in Care of the Trauma Patient

When a patient with a traumatic injury presents to the Emergency Department they must be assessed in a systematic way. Following stabilization of the patient's condition, preparations for operative fixation of fractures, wound debridement and exploration, and repair of other injuries may occur. Postoperative care includes ongoing nursing diligence in assessment for bleeding and hemodynamic stability. Nursing assessment of neurologic and neurovascular status is essential. Careful pain assessment is important as changes in pain levels can signal a complication. Careful nursing management of external fixation, wounds and dressings, drains, and other equipment and devices can decrease the risks of complications during the recovery phase. See Table 6-6 for a list of common nursing diagnoses pertaining to the patient who has sustained a traumatic injury.

Careful management of potential complications in the postoperative and recovery phases will decrease the risks to the patient for further dysfunction and potential disability. The orthopaedic nurse must be ever watchful when caring for persons who have experienced musculoskeletal trauma.

Table 6-6
Nursing Diagnoses for the Patient with Traumatic Injury

- Impaired Comfort, Acute Pain related to physical injury; phantom limb pain
- Impaired Physical Mobility related to musculoskeletal impairment
- Impaired Skin Integrity related to crush injury; tissue loss or damage
- Self-care Deficit related to bathing/hygiene, grooming/dressing
- Imbalanced Nutrition: Less Than Body Requirements related to increased metabolic processes
- Grieving related to loss of function or independence secondary to trauma
- Ineffective Coping related to changes in body integrity secondary to loss of limb, trauma
- Disturbed Body Image related to changes in appearance, loss of limb, loss of body function
- Hopelessness related to impaired ability to cope secondary to impaired functional abilities

Table 6-7
Classification of Major Types of Traction

Traction	Type	Term	Duration	Other
Cervical				
Skin traction	Skin	Short-term	Intermittent	
Skeletal traction	Skeletal	Short-term or long-term	Continuous	
Halo traction	Skeletal		Continuous	Traction via halo vest
Upper Extremity				
Side-arm traction	Skin or skeletal		Continuous	Vertical suspension to forearm
Overhead/90-90			Continuous	Vertical traction to humerus; horizontal suspension to forearm
Dunlop	Skin	Short-term	Continuous	
Pelvic				
Pelvic belt	Skin	Short-term	Intermittent	
Pelvic sling	Skin	Long-term	Continuous	
Lower Extremity				
Bryant	Skin	Long-term	Continuous	Bilateral; vertical suspension
Buck	Skin	Short-term	Continuous	Unilateral or bilateral
Russell	Skin	Usually short-term	Continuous	Balanced suspension
Lower extremity 90-90	Skin or skeletal		Continuous	Suspension; unilateral (children) or bilateral (adults)
Skeletal traction with balanced suspension	Skeletal	Long-term	Continuous	Usually unilateral

Adapted from *An Introduction to Orthopaedic Nursing* (2004). In C. Mosher (Ed.), (3rd ed., p. 76). Chicago, IL: National Association of Orthopaedic Nurses.

Understanding actions to take early in the patient's episode of care will assist in providing excellent outcomes in the recovery and rehabilitation phases.

Care of Patients in Traction, Casts, or External Fixation Devices

Therapeutic modalities have been used for centuries to immobilize an injured part of the musculoskeletal system to provide treatment and healing. Immobilization secures the affected area to prevent injury, provide alignment, promote healing, and reduce pain. Forms of immobilization include traction, casts, and external fixators. The principles used for the care and management of patients with immobilization devices are fundamental for the provision of standard orthopaedic nursing practice.

Traction

Traction is defined as the application of a pulling force to an injured or diseased part of the body or an extremity while countertraction pulls in the opposite direction (Kunkler, 2007). The pulling force of traction is typically achieved through the application of weights but may also be done manually. Countertraction is generally provided by the patient's body.

The goal of traction is to exert a pulling force on an extremity or body part to immobilize, realign, or prevent spasm. The purposes of traction are:

- To reduce, realign, and promote healing of fractures, dislocations, and subluxations.

- To decrease muscle spasms associated with fractures, low back pain, or cervical whiplash.

- To correct, lessen, or prevent deformities or contractures.

- To provide immobilization to prevent soft tissue damage.

- To promote rest of a diseased, injured, or painful joint.

- To expand a joint space during arthroscopic or joint reconstruction surgery.

Traction is not used as frequently today due to the advances in instrumentation for fracture repairs and new methods of trauma management. Improved femoral and acetabular prostheses, along with femoral shaft instrumentation, have decreased the need for skeletal traction. Skeletal traction is generally used for patients with multiple trauma who are not candidates for immediate surgical repair of their orthopaedic injuries. Patients with abdominal or thoracic injuries may require traction stabilization of fractures prior to surgical intervention. In addition, the use of external fixators has reduced the need for traction in patients with significant fracture displacement and soft tissue injury. Buck's traction may be used preoperatively with hip fracture patients to reduce spasm and decrease pain. Individuals with unstable cervical spine injuries may be treated with cervical skeletal traction, but will most likely have surgical intervention or a halo vest applied. Because of the advantages of early mobilization and the increased costs of lengthened hospital stays, traditional traction management is reserved for patients whose outcomes would be less successful with other interventions.

Classifications

Manual traction uses the hands to exert a pulling force on the extremity or part that requires immobilization or

Figure 6-4
Bed Frame with a Telescoping Bar

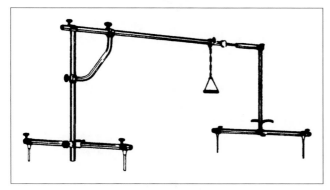

Reprinted with permission from the *Traction Handbook* (2000). Warsaw, IN. Zimmer, p. 13.

Figure 6-5
Cross Clamp

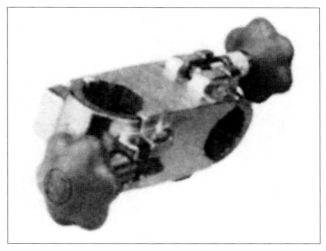

Reprinted with permission from the *Traction Handbook* (2000). Warsaw, IN. Zimmer, p. 69.

Figure 6-6
Single Camp Bar

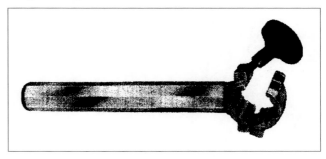

Reprinted with permission from the *Traction Handbook* (2000). Warsaw, IN. Zimmer, p. 70.

realignment. The use of manual traction is usually reserved for very stable fractures prior to splinting or casting, application of skin or skeletal traction, or surgical reduction (Zimmer Orthopaedic Surgical Products, Inc., 2009). This type of traction can be used as a temporary measure in an emergency when traction ropes break, pins loosen in an extremity or halo vest, or in a first aid situation.

Skin traction is the application of a pulling force applied directly to the skin using foam splints or boots, traction strips, or slings. It is used as a temporary measure when only a moderate amount of longitudinal force (5-7 pounds) is required for a relatively short period of time. In adults, skin traction is often used prior to surgical reduction or skeletal traction, or to reduce spasms in an extremity with a fracture. There is high risk for skin irritation and breakdown with this type of traction; therefore, the apparatus must be removed frequently to monitor the skin condition. Another disadvantage of skin traction is its ineffectiveness in controlling limb rotation (Zimmer Orthopaedic Surgical Products, Inc., 2009). It is difficult to consistently maintain the pulling force of skin traction. The skin traction apparatus requires frequent assessment to make sure it is smooth and securely applied to the largest possible surface area. Buck's traction is a commonly used form of skin traction.

Skeletal traction applies force directly to the bone and allows the use of 20-30 pounds of force for up to 4 months (Zimmer Orthopaedic Surgical Products, Inc., 2009). Skeletal traction requires the use of Steinman pins or Kirschner wires in long bones and tongs for cervical traction. A spreader bar attaches to the pins or wires to transmit the force to the bone. Skeletal traction is most beneficial for unstable fractures, severely displaced fractures, or those where muscle pull must be overcome to maintain alignment, such as with femoral fractures. It is most often used with balanced suspension, where the suspension is provided by means of a rope and free hanging weights at the other end of the limb to provide balance.

In addition, traction can be classified according to the type of pulling force or mechanism applied. Traction can be static (continuous) or dynamic (intermittent). It can also be running (straight) or balanced suspension. Table 6-7 summarizes the classifications of the major types of traction.

Mechanics of Traction

It is helpful for the nurse to be knowledgeable about basic equipment used in an overbed frame or traction framework. Most facilities use a basic straight frame (see Figure 6-4), consisting of a telescoping overhead bar with two vertical bars attached to two plain bars, which fit into IV pole holders at the head and foot of the bed. Figure 6-5 illustrates the double cross clamp used to connect two traction bars together on the basic frame. Some facilities may use a 4-poster or Balkan frame, which provides greater stability. The Balkan Frame is especially useful with obese patients.

The basic frame is extended with additional plain bars (see Figure 6-6) that vary from 5-36 inches. These bars are used to attach the pulleys and weights. Pulleys are attached via single cross clamps or can be built into the traction bars.

Figure 6-7
How to Tie a Slip Knot

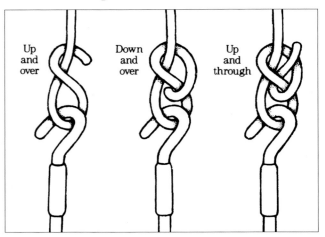

Reprinted with permission from the *Traction Handbook* (2000). Warsaw, IN. Zimmer, p. 10.

Other necessary pieces of traction equipment include traction cord, weights, slings, spreader bars, and foot plates.

Nurses caring for orthopaedic patients should be aware of several general precautions regarding the assembly of traction equipment. These precautions are as follows:

- Single or double clamps must be positioned so that the knobs are on the top of the horizontal bars.

- The flat surface must be on top for all horizontal bars and on the side for upright bars to assure maximum stability.

- Traction should be set up with the bed in the lowest position and the patient centered in the bed.

- Weights should never hang over the patient's body.

- Pulleys may be lubricated with silicone spray prior to set up but never after the traction is set up unless the physician is present. This can alter the pulling force of the traction.

- Never reuse traction cord.

- Slipknots are used to tie traction and should be secured with adhesive tape (see Figure 6-7).

- A quick visual inspection of traction should be done by all nursing staff entering the patient's room (Zimmer Orthopaedic Surgical Products, Inc., 2009).

Immobility and the associated risks are an important consideration with the patient in traction. Specialty beds can be used with traction to aid in lowering the risk of skin breakdown or respiratory complications. Equipment can be applied to low air loss beds, but the nurse must be aware of the slippery surface of the mattress and the potential for malalignment. Appropriate safety must be maintained and the patient positioned to prevent skin shearing. Traction can be attached to specialty beds for the bariatric population; however, extra reinforcement may be indicated.

Principles of Traction

The following principles should be incorporated into the care and management of all patients with traction:

- Always maintain the prescribed line of pull. Any disruption in the line of pull, including changing pulleys or raising/lowering bars, can alter the alignment and cause pain and spasm.

- Always maintain continuous pull unless the traction is ordered as intermittent. Never remove traction without a physician's order. Buck's traction would be an exception in order to provide skin care.

- Prevent friction that will interfere with the line of pull. This includes weights that touch the floor, knots that rest on the pulleys, and plates against the foot of the bed, linen, or traction ropes.

- Identify and maintain countertraction. The patient's body usually provides the countertraction. If the patient slides down in bed, the countertraction is lost. Countertraction can be difficult with the elderly patient in Buck's traction who may be too underweight to provide the necessary countertraction. Keeping the bed as flat as tolerated, considering the patient's physical condition, will help maintain the patient's position. Elevating the foot of the bed can also prevent the patient from sliding downward.

- Never add or remove weights without a physician's order.

Cervical Traction

Cervical skin traction is used for minor injuries such as sprains, whiplash, cervical myositis, and subluxation or dislocation. It is generally used short-term due to the potential for skin irritation. Cervical traction is applied with the bed flat and may be set up with the standard overhead frame. The components of cervical skin traction include the chin strap and the spreader bar with weights attached. Cervical traction is less commonly used than in the past and is usually accomplished with collars and braces.

Nursing care of the patient in cervical traction includes an assessment of the fit of the head halter and the direction of pull of the cervical weights. Paresthesias of the face and jaw may occur if the halter is not applied correctly. Jaw pain may develop if weights are too heavy and should be reported to the physician immediately. In addition, a careful skin assessment is necessary to monitor the chin, ears, mandible, and occiput for pressure areas. Diet modifications may be required due to difficulty chewing and swallowing. In order to establish eye contact with the patient, the nurse must stand close to the bed.

Cervical skeletal traction is achieved through the use of Crutchfield, Vinke, or Gardner-Wells tongs inserted directly into the skull and attached to weights. This type of traction stabilizes the vertebrae, reducing the possibility of spinal cord damage or further injury (Zimmer Orthopaedic Surgical Products, Inc., 2009). Constant traction must be maintained. If a pin loosens, the physician must be notified immediately. The nurse must maintain manual traction if there is disruption of the skeletal traction. Sandbags or cervical collars may be

Figure 6-8
Buck's Traction

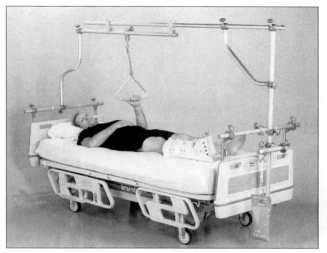

Reprinted with permission from the *Traction Handbook* (2000). Warsaw, IN. Zimmer, p. 29.

Figure 6-9
Russell Traction

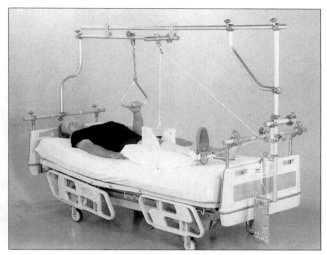

Reprinted with permission from the *Traction Handbook* (2000). Warsaw, IN. Zimmer, p. 33.

helpful to maintain cervical alignment. Because of the extreme immobility of patients in cervical traction, turning frames and specialty rotating beds may be used. Skin assessment is a priority as pressure points and skin breakdown can quickly develop. Assessing key pressure points is necessary every 2 to 4 hours. Pin sites are assessed at least each shift for signs of inflammation or infection. Pin site care is discussed later in the chapter under "External Fixation."

Upper Extremity Traction

There are two major types of upper extremity traction: side arm traction and overhead (or 90-90) traction. Both types of traction can be applied by the skin or skeletal method, and the nursing care is similar for both. Upper extremity traction is used to stabilize fractures or dislocations of the elbow, humerus, or shoulder. Traction is applied to the humerus, with the forearm in balanced suspension (Zimmer Orthopaedic Surgical Products, Inc., 2009). Side arm traction is generally used to immobilize fractures or dislocations of the humerus or shoulder. Overhead or 90-90 traction is a continuous suspension traction that is used to treat supracondylar fractures of the elbow, humerus, or shoulder.

Patients with upper extremity traction are maintained in the supine position. A trapeze will aid in self-care and enable the patient to assist in repositioning. Countertraction beyond the patient's body weight may be necessary to maintain upper extremity traction. Options include folded blankets placed under the mattress and frame on the affected side of the bed, shock blocks, or a vest restraint to maintain the patient's position.

Frequent back care is necessary to prevent skin breakdown. The traction strips and ace bandages must be carefully applied and checked to avoid wraps that overlap, are too tight, or cut into the elbow or wrist. Bandages must be applied evenly, as tight wrappings at the proximal end of the

arm will cause swelling (Zimmer Orthopaedic Surgical Products, Inc., 2009). Active and passive exercises of the wrist and fingers will help maintain joint mobility and circulation. The elevated position of the hand may cause it to feel cold, even though circulation is adequate.

Lower Extremity Traction

Lower extremity traction is used to treat fractures or injuries of the hip, femur, knee, or lower leg. Skin or skeletal traction may be used depending on the injury and treatment goals. Types of lower extremity traction include Buck's, Russell, skeletal balanced suspension, and the Bohler-Braun frame.

Buck's Traction

Buck's traction is a continuous longitudinal skin traction (see Figure 6-8) sometimes used for preoperative fractured hip immobilization (Perry & Potter, 2009). Buck's traction can also be used to immobilize femur or pelvic fractures, prevent hip flexion contractures, and reduce muscle spasms postoperatively. Skin traction is applied with a foam boot that is connected by rope and pulley to a 5-7 pound weight. Countertraction is provided by the patient's body. Additional countertraction may be gained by elevating the foot of the bed.

Skin assessment and care is a major nursing measure for patients in Buck's traction. The skin should be carefully assessed for abrasions, vascular insufficiency, and edema. Since the majority of patients in Buck's traction are elderly, the potential for skin breakdown is greatly increased. Elevating the heels off of the bed with a pillow or rolled towel or blanket will help relieve pressure in this area. Care must also be taken so that the boot is not too tight across the dorsum of the foot and anterior leg or calf. In addition, pressure on the peroneal nerve must be prevented to avoid foot drop. Intermittent pneumatic or sequential compression devices should not be applied under the Buck's traction boot.

Figure 6-10
Skeletal Balanced Suspension Traction

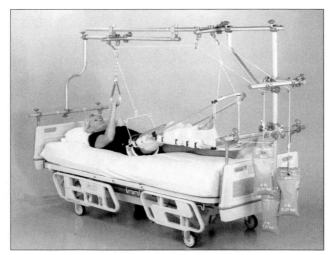

Reprinted with permission from the *Traction Handbook* (2000). Warsaw, IN. Zimmer, p. 37.

Russell Traction

Russell traction (see Figure 6-9) is continuous balanced suspension skin traction, used to treat femoral and hip fractures and certain knee injuries. The traction set-up uses a sling under the knee with a continuous rope that goes through four pulleys to the weight. Due to the pulley system, the pulling force on the foot is double the weight applied. Countertraction is applied with physician order and can be achieved by elevating the foot of the bed or gatching the knee (Perry & Potter, 2009).

Nursing care of the patient in Russell traction requires careful review of the position of the sling, since an alteration can change the direction of pull. Using a skin marker to make a line on the thigh at both the proximal and distal edges of the sling will help keep alignment intact. A trapeze is useful for bed mobility, and passive and active exercises are encouraged.

Skeletal Balanced Suspension Traction

Skeletal balanced suspension traction is indicated for treating fractures of the femoral shaft, hip, or lower leg (see Figure 6-10). Patients with skeletal balanced suspension traction often have multiple injuries from motor vehicle accidents or major trauma. The advantage of balanced suspension traction is increased bed mobility for the patient. Long-term use of skeletal balanced suspension traction is less common than in the past. Current surgical interventions to treat traumatic injuries are more frequently used, and traction may be applied only long enough to stabilize other injuries.

Skeletal balanced suspension traction is achieved through the insertion of a Steinman pin or Kirschner wire into the distal femur. The pin or wire is attached to a traction bow and connected to ropes, pulleys, and weights. A Thomas or Brady leg splint is used to elevate and support the thigh and upper leg. The ischial ring is padded for comfort and

suspended with pulleys and weights. The Pearson attachment is a padded metal frame that supports the lower leg. A footplate is attached to prevent foot drop. The distal end of the Pearson attachment is connected to the distal end of the Thomas splint with traction rope. Countertraction, provided through weights, generally equals the amount of weight suspending the leg (Perry & Potter, 2009).

Maintaining traction alignment and patient positioning are two key measures in the nursing care of the patient in balanced suspension traction. Traction alignment should be checked by all members of the nursing team with each entrance into the patient's room. The full or half ring at the proximal end of the Thomas splint should be padded with sheepskin to promote comfort and changed in case of soiling. The Thomas splint must be positioned so to avoid pressure on the groin. The affected leg should not rotate externally, as this alters the pull of traction and places pressure on the peroneal nerve. Slings on the Pearson attachment should be placed so that the heel and Achilles tendon do not carry the weight of the lower leg (Zimmer Orthopaedic Surgical Products, Inc., 2009). The head of the bed can be raised slightly for comfort, but for at least an hour of each shift, the bed should be flat to promote hip extension.

Ongoing nursing assessments include a thorough evaluation of the patient's skin and neurovascular status of the affected extremity. Pin site care must be maintained and is discussed later in "External Fixation." Patients should be instructed to perform active plantar and dorsiflexion of the foot to help prevent foot drop. Initially, the patient will experience much discomfort and will be reluctant to move. However, with time and encouragement, the patient will increase bed mobility.

Bohler-Braun Frame

The Bohler-Braun frame is used with comminuted or unstable fractures of the femur or tibia, or open fractures with extreme soft tissue damage. The metal frame that elevates and supports the thigh and calf can be used with skin or skeletal traction.

Care must be taken to assure that the proximal end of the Bohler-Braun frame does not press into the perineum. The entire frame must be padded with sheepskin or felt. Padding should not press on the popliteal space, Achilles tendon, or heel. The patient's skin should be assessed frequently

Casts

A cast is a temporary, circumferential, rigid device used to immobilize an extremity. Casts have been used for years to aid in the healing of fractures. Materials have evolved from starched cloth strips, to Plaster of Paris, to current synthetic materials. The cast usually covers the fractured area as well as the joints above and below the injury to provide immobilization of the injured site for alignment and healing.

If an injured extremity is edematous, a splint may be applied prior to casting. A splint is not circumferential, however, the same precautions apply for patient care as those for casting. A splint is usually a temporary measure and is replaced by a cast when appropriate.

The primary purpose of a cast is for immobilization, generally of a fracture. Casting maintains alignment, supports and protects the bone to promote healing, and may allow for early weight bearing. Other indications for cast application include postoperative application to provide additional support, serial casting to prevent or correct deformities, post-injury with severe sprains or strains to decrease pain, and post-amputation to shrink and mold the residual limb. The advantages of using a cast for treatment are the relative ease of application, minimal care requirements, decreased need for hospitalization, and increased patient mobility (Kunkler, 2007).

Casts changes are based on the nature of the injury and condition of underlying tissues. Casts are usually changed every 2 to 4 weeks to inspect the skin and incision line, if applicable, and reassess fracture healing and alignment. In addition, the cast is changed if it becomes too loose or too tight; the patient complains of pain; it becomes excessively wet, soiled, or damaged; or if a foreign object is placed in the cast. X-rays are initially obtained every 1-2 weeks to assess position, alignment, and healing of the fracture and then at the time of cast removal.

Casting Materials

Casting tapes used today are either natural or synthetic. The type of material used will vary based on physician preference, indications for the cast, and number of potential cast changes. A hybrid cast may also be applied, using plaster under fiberglass material.

Plaster of Paris incorporated into a bandage roll is a natural casting material that has been used for years. Some physicians still prefer it for its moldability, and use it especially for severely displaced fractures or when multiple cast changes are anticipated. Plaster casts require longer drying time, must be handled with the palms of the hands when wet, placed on a soft surface when wet to prevent indentations, and repositioned to promote drying and prevent heat entrapment. Plaster casts are heavier than synthetic casts and lose their integrity if exposed to water.

Synthetic cast materials are used more frequently because they are strong and durable, lightweight, and harden and dry almost immediately. These qualities facilitate rapid ambulation following casting. The most common synthetic casting material is fiberglass, but polyester/cotton knit tape impregnated with a resin or a latex free polymer may also be used (Kunkler, 2007). Synthetic casts are often used for nondisplaced fractures, closed fractures, or in a well-healing fracture following several cast changes.

Types of Casts

Casts can be grouped into extremity casts and body casts. The upper extremity can be casted with a short- or long-arm cast, or a cylinder, hanging, or thumb spica cast. In the lower extremity, short- and long-leg casts as well as cylinder or abduction boots can be used.

Body casts encompass not only the affected limb, but also a portion of the torso. Types of body casts include a hip spica, spinal body vest, and airplane or shoulder spica casts.

Since these casts are very restrictive, they are generally not used unless other measures are unable to provide the necessary immobilization.

Cast Application

Supplies required for cast application include the appropriate cast material, gloves, stockinette, cast padding, moisture barrier liner, and tepid water. Casting material is supplied in rolls and is dipped in water to apply. Gloves are worn during application to maintain universal precautions and protect the applicator's skin from irritation from the casting materials.

The casting process begins by positioning the extremity in alignment. Since this may be painful for the patient, pain medication should be administered if necessary. Clean dressings should be applied to an incision if present. A stockinette is applied to the extremity and should be at least 2 inches longer on each end than the fitted cast, in order to fold over the edge of the cast for a smooth finish. The stockinette must be applied smoothly, as wrinkles can cause pressure and skin breakdown. Cast padding is then applied with special attention to bony prominences or incision sites. The casting tape is applied from the distal to the proximal end of the extremity. Each turn overlaps the previous one by half the width. In small areas, it may be necessary to tuck the casting material for a good fit. Molding the cast after each roll provides for good conformity. The stockinette is folded back onto itself on both ends, and a final roll of cast tape is applied. Fiberglass casts should be assessed for rough or sharp edges that may need to be petalled or shaped.

Cast Splitting or Windowing

Since casts are circumferential immobilizers, they can cause pressure or edema. Edema may also be present due to injury. Casts may need to be split or bivalved to relieve the resultant pressure. Indications for cast splitting include increasing pain, pressure or swelling in the extremity, signs of neurovascular compromise such as decreased circulation or loss of sensation or function, or compartment syndrome.

A cast is windowed by cutting out a specific area to permit inspection of the patient's skin, an incision, or a wound, or to relieve pressure. If there is soft tissue damage, the window facilitates frequent wound assessments and dressing changes. The window piece should be saved as it is often reinserted. Both cast splitting and windowing are done using the cast saw.

Cast Removal

The cast is removed using a cast saw with a vibrating blade rather than a spinning blade. The vibration decreases the chance of cutting the patient during use, but the noise can be frightening if the patient is not warned. In addition, the vibration causes increased warmth of the blade and may also cause discomfort to an injured area or incision. The extremity must be supported while removing the cast as well as afterward. The patient's skin must be washed gently, and lotion should be applied. Dead skin is typical following cast removal and should be allowed to slough off naturally.

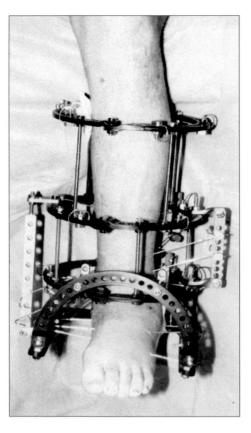

**Figure 6-11
Smith &
Nephew
Ilizarov
Circular
Fixator**

Reprinted with
permission from
*An Introduction to
Orthopaedic
Nursing* (2004).
In C. Mosher (Ed.),
(3rd ed., p. 83).
Chicago, IL:
National
Association of
Orthopaedic
Nurses.

Complications

Complications associated with cast application include compartment syndrome, neurovascular compromise, and skin breakdown. See Chapter 8, *Complications Associated with Orthopaedic Conditions and Surgeries*, for further discussion of complications.

Cast syndrome or superior mesenteric artery syndrome may occur in patients with body casts, due to compression of the duodenum, aorta, and vertebral column (Sprague, 1998). The compression can cause partial or complete obstruction of the duodenum or superior mesenteric artery. The nurse should ensure that the abdominal window is adequate in the cast, auscultate bowel sounds, and palpate the abdomen. Symptoms of cast syndrome include prolonged nausea, abdominal pressure and pain, and persistent and projectile vomiting. Symptoms can develop days or weeks after cast application. The physician should be notified immediately to develop a plan of care, which may include avoiding oral intake, instituting intravenous fluids, and introducing nasogastric tube suctioning. If symptoms are not relieved, cast removal may be necessary.

Nursing Considerations

Nurses must complete routine neurovascular assessments on all patients with casts (see Chapter 1, *Musculoskeletal Anatomy and Neurovascular Assessment*). The patient should be questioned regarding pain, pressure, numbness, or tingling. The nurse should also monitor for symptoms of compartment syndrome.

Patient education is an important aspect related to cast management. Elevation of the involved extremity will help to reduce swelling. The patient may shower if the cast is covered with a commercial shower guard or large plastic bag to seal the cast. Nothing should be put inside the cast, as this may cause skin irritation or damage. The patient should be instructed to self-monitor for signs of infection if an incision is present by noting increased pain, swelling, drainage, or foul odor from the cast.

The goal for the patient with impaired mobility is the ability to safely ambulate with the appropriate assistive device. Collaboration with physical therapy is essential to instruct the patient in the use of an assistive device for ambulation. Discussion of safety considerations for home, work, or school should take place.

External Fixation

External fixation is a method of immobilization that employs percutaneous pins or wires in bone that are attached to a rigid external frame (Kunkler, 2007). Fixators, classified according to the design of the components, can be unilateral, bilateral, triangular, or circular (see Figures 6-11and 6-12) and made of aluminum, titanium, graphite, or nylon. The pins are either transfixing or half pins that go partially into the bone (Redemann, 2002).

Indications and Advantages

External fixators are most commonly used to treat complicated, open fractures with segmental loss of bone and severe soft tissue damage. Fixators can also be used to improve alignment and stability in extremely unstable fractures. The surgical plan for nonunions, malunions, joint arthodesis, and simple fractures can also incorporate the use of an external fixator. The circular frame is often used for bone tissue distraction and lengthening for the treatment of a congenital defect or traumatic injury (Redemann, 2002).

A key advantage of external fixation is access to the injured site for primary and secondary procedures related to vascular and soft tissue injuries, while rigid stability of fractures is maintained. Skeletal stability with rigid fixation allows bone

Figure 6-12
EBI Dynafix External Fixator

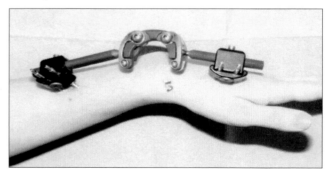

Reprinted with permission from *An Introduction to Orthopaedic Nursing* (2004). In C. Mosher (Ed.), (3rd ed., p. 83). Chicago, IL: National Association of Orthopaedic Nurses.

healing to occur. The external fixator maintains bone and muscle bulk with the percutaneous approach and can also enhance potential early mobilization.

Complications

While external fixators provide many advantages, complications can occur with their use (Lucas & Davis, 2005). The most common complications are pin tract infections, loss of alignment, joint stiffness or contractures, and delayed healing or nonunion. Instability of the fixator frame or loose wires can cause complications postoperatively.

Pin tract inflammation and infection in a patient with external fixation can be extremely damaging to the healing process and can occur even when specific protocols are followed. The nurse must monitor pin sites for signs of infection such as redness, warmth, swelling at the site; white, yellow, or green drainage or odor at the pin site; and fever. Clear fluid drainage from pin sites is expected within 48-72 hours after insertion. Pin site care should be completed at least every 8 hours or more often as needed in the first 48-72 hours after insertion when drainage is heaviest. After this initial period, pin site care can be done daily as long as the pin remains stable in the bone. Chlorhexidine 2mg/mL solution may be the most effective cleansing agent for pin sites (Holmes & Brown, 2005). Betadine solution, betadine ointment, alcohol, and peroxide should be avoided as these agents can cause tissue damage, loosening of pins, and deterioration of the pin itself (Holmes & Brown, 2005). The patient and family must be taught to continue pin site care at home after discharge. The ability to shower and get the pin sites wet is determined by the orthopaedic surgeon.

Nursing Considerations

The nurse must perform a thorough neurovascular assessment of the affected extremity. If the fixation device is used for distraction and lengthening, it is important to immediately identify neurovascular compromise that can occur due to rapid distraction or incorrect alignment. Observation of pin sites must occur with each patient assessment. The patient must adhere to specific activity and weight bearing orders. The fixator device should not be used to lift the extremity, as this can put inappropriate pressure on bars and pins and alter alignment. Educating the patient and family is critical, as care of the external fixator will be primarily managed at home (Kunkler, 2007). A specific plan of care for limb lengthening must be communicated, and the patient and family must clearly understand and demonstrate the correct procedure.

Traction, casts, and external fixation are methods used to immobilize and treat fractures and joint injuries, some of which can include soft tissue damage as well. Individualized patient assessment, combined with appropriate nursing interventions, can lead to the desired outcomes.

Psychosocial Impact of Trauma

No matter the cause, the trauma victim experiences a disruption in his/her life. The trauma precipitates a crisis for both the patient and family which can surface at anytime throughout the continuum of care. The patient and family will have a need for open communication and information, compassion and compassionate care, and the maintenance of hope. Responses to the traumatic event will be based on an individual's perception of the event, support systems, and previous coping skills. During the recovery period, the patient may exhibit withdrawal, depression, and avoidance of eye contact; denial of injury or emotions; make excessive demands; be overly compliant or non-compliant with the shared plan of care and instructions; be unable to problem solve or identify resources; become easily frustrated; express negativity; or exhibit self-destructive behaviors (Martinez, 2009). The nurse can intervene with the patient by establishing a trusting relationship; identifying and contacting family and agency supports; clarifying misconceptions, explaining procedures; structuring the environment; allowing choices; and setting limits and time frames. It is important for the nurse to give realistic information to the patient and family without extinguishing hope.

Families also benefit by having a healthcare team member as a liaison during the recovery process to update them regarding the patient's condition and explain care interventions. The nurse can learn valuable information about the traumatic event from the family that can help influence the patient's care. Families must be periodically updated about the patient's condition. Self-care for the family must be encouraged to enhance their ability to be supportive to the patient during the recovery process. Throughout the hospitalization of the patient, the nurse advocates for both the patient and family by making referrals to psychiatric clinicians, social workers, clergy and spiritual advisors, physical, occupational and alternative therapists, and outside agencies and resources to help patients and their families cope with the crisis and to promote the most functional and positive outcomes.

References

American Academy of Orthopaedic Surgeons (2007). *Stress Fractures.* Retrieved February 18, 2010, from http://orthoinfo.aaos.org/topic. cfm?topic=A00112

American Academy of Orthopaedic Surgeons (2007). *Hip Dislocation.* Retrieved February 19, 2010, from http://orthoinfo.aaos.org/topic. cfm?topic=A00352

Bartlett, C.S., Helfet, D.L., Hausman, M.R., & Strauss, E. (2000). *Journal of the American Academy of Orthopaedic Surgeons, 8*(1), 21-36.

Bauer, T.C., & Reuter, J.T. (2009). Analgesia, Sedation, and Neuromuscular Blockade in the Trauma Patient. In K. McQuillan, M. Makic, & E. Whalen, (Eds.), *Trauma nursing: From resuscitation through rehabilitation* (4th ed., p. 407). St. Louis: W.B. Saunders.

Black, J.M. (1997). Nursing care of clients with musculoskeletal trauma or overuse. In J.M. Black & E. Matassarin-Jacobs (Eds.), *Medical – surgical nursing: Clinical management for continuity of care* (5th ed., pp. 2129-2170). Philadelphia: W. B. Saunders.

Bongiovanni, M.S., Bradley, S.L., & Kelley, D.M. (2005). Orthopedic trauma critical care nursing issues. *Critical Care Quarterly 28*(1), 60-71.

Carpenito-Moyet, L.J. (2008). *Nursing diagnosis: Application to clinical practice* (12th ed.). Philadelphia: Lippincott, Williams, & Wilken.

Centers for Disease Control and Prevention. *Blast injuries: Essential facts.* Retrieved May 30, 2009, from http://emergency.cdc.gov/masscasualties/blastessentials.asp

Centers for Disease Control and Prevention. *National vital statistics reports.* Retrieved June 6, 2009, from http://www.cdc.gov/nchs/nvss.htm

Covey, D.C. (2002). Blast and fragment injuries of the musculoskeletal system. *Journal of Bone and Joint Surgery, 84,* 1221-1234.

Dahners, L., & Mullis, B. (2004). Effects of nonsteroidal anti-inflammatory drugs on bone formation and soft-tissue healing. *Journal of the American Academy of Orthopaedic Surgeons, 12*(3), 139-143.

DePalma, R.G., Burris, D.G., Champion, H.R., & Hodgson, M.J. (2005). Blast injuries. *The New England Journal of Medicine, 352*(13), 1335-1342.

Frakes, M.A., & Evans, T. (2004). Major pelvic fractures. *Critical Care Nurse, 24*(2), 18-30.

Hilt, N. (Ed.). (1984). *Assessment and fracture management of the lower extremities* (p. 56, 57). Pittman, NJ: National Association of Orthopaedic Nurses.

Holmes, S.B, & Brown, S.J. (2005). Skeletal pin site care: National Association of Orthopaedic Nurses guidelines for orthopaedic nursing. *Orthopaedic Nursing, 24*(2), 99-107.

Kneale, J.D. (2005). Care of the patient with a pelvic injury. In J. Kneale, & P. Davis (Eds.), *Orthopaedic and trauma nursing* (2nd ed., pp. 450-469). St. Louis: Elsevier.

Kobziff, L. (2006). Traumatic pelvic fractures. *Orthopaedic Nursing, 25*(4), 235-241.

Kunkler, C.E. (2007). Therapeutic modalities. In National Association of Orthopaedic Nursing, *NAON Core curriculum for orthopaedic nursing* (6th ed., pp. 227-256). Chicago, IL: National Association of Orthopaedic Nurses.

Lehman, C. (2008). Mechanisms of injury in wartime. *Rehabilitation Nursing, 33*(5),192-205.

Lucas, B., & Davis, P.S. (2005). Why restricting movement is important. In J. Kneale, & P. Davis (Eds.), *Orthopaedic and trauma nursing,* (2nd ed., pp. 130-132). St. Louis: Elsevier.

Mamaril, M.E., Childs, S.G., & Sortman, S. (2007). Care of the orthopaedic trauma patient. *Journal of Anesthesia Nursing, 22*(3), 184-194.

Martinez, R. (2009). Psychological impact of trauma. In K. McQuillan, M. Makic, & E. Whalen (Eds.), *Trauma nursing: From resuscitation through rehabilitation* (4th ed., pp.422-446). St. Louis: W.B. Saunders.

Mayo Clinic (2008). *Dislocation.* Retrieved February 19, 2010, from http://mayoclinic.com/health/dislocation/DS00239

Mechem, C.C. (2008). *Pelvic fracture.* Retrieved May 30, 2009, from http://emedicine.medscape.com/article/825869-print

Morris, N., & Levin, B. (2007). Complications. In *Core curriculum for orthopaedic nursing.* (6th ed., pp. 395-431). Chicago, IL: National Association of Orthopaedic Nurses.

Murray, C.A. (2009). Care of patients with musculoskeletal trauma. In D.D. Ignatavicius, & M.L. Workman, *Medical surgical nursing: Patient centered collaborative care* (6th ed., pp. 1178-1211). St. Louis: W.B. Saunders.

National Center for Health Statistics. *NCHS data on injuries.* Retrieved June 3, 2009, from http://www.cdc.gov/nchs.injury.htm

National Limb Loss Information Center (2008). *Amputation statistics by cause.* Retrieved May 30, 2009, from http://www.amputeecoalition.org/fact_sheet/amp_stats_cause.html

Redemann, S. (2002). Modalities for immobilization. In A.B. Maher, S.W. Salmond, & T.A. Pellino (Eds.), *Orthopaedic nursing* (3rd ed., pp. 302-323). Philadelphia: W.B. Saunders.

Nelson, F., & Blauvelt, C. (2007). *A manual of orthopaedic terminology.* (7th ed.). Philadelphia: Mosby.

Perry, A.G., & Potter, P.A. (2009). *Clinical nursing skills and techniques.* (7th ed). Philadelphia: Mosby.

Petersen, V. *Trauma tertiary surveys.* Retrieved June 17, 2009, from http://www.trauma.org/archive/nurse/tertiarysurvey.html

Schoen, D.C. (2000). Care of the patient with amputation. In D.C. Schoen, *Adult orthopaedic nursing* (pp. 445-465). Philadelphia: Lippincott.

Smith, B. (2005). *How to manage that pelvic fracture.* Retrieved May 30, 2009, from http://rn.modernmedicine.com/rnweb/article

Sprague, J. (1998). Cast syndrome. *Orthopaedic Nursing, 17*(4), 12-16.

Taber, C. (2005). *Taber's cyclopedic medical dictionary,* (20th ed.). Philadelphia: F.A. Davis.

Wallace, G.L. (2006). Blast injury basics: A guide for the medical speech-language pathologist. *The ASHA Leader, 11*(9), 26-28.

Weigelt, J., Brasel, K., & Klein, J. (2009) Mechanism of Injury. In K. McQuillan, M. Makic, & E. Whalen (Eds.) *Trauma nursing: From resuscitation through rehabilitation* (4th ed., pp.178-199). St. Louis: W.B. Saunders.

Weil, Y.A., Mosheiff, R., & Liebergall, M. (2006). Blast and penetrating injuries to the extremities. *Journal of the American Academy of Orthopaedic Surgeons, 14*(10), 136-139.

Williamson, V. (2002). Amputation. In A.B. Maher, S.W. Salmond, & T.A. Pellino, (Eds.), *Orthopaedic nursing* (3rd ed., pp. 650-673). Philadelphia: W.B. Saunders.

Zimmer Orthopaedic Surgical Products, Inc. (2009). *The Traction Handbook.* Warsaw, IN: Author.

Chapter 7

Pain Management

Cathy D. Trame, MS, RN, CNS, BC

Objectives

- Identify five variables that influence patient pain assessment.

- Describe the pathology of three orthopaedic pain sources.

- Compare treatment strategies for the management of chronic orthopaedic pain versus postoperative orthopaedic pain.

Key Terms

Acute pain: pain of short duration that resolves in the expected amount of time after injury or surgery.

Addiction: craving for a substance to achieve a euphoric effect.

Adjuvants: medicines or therapies that potentiate the primary medicine or therapy.

Chronic pain: pain of longer duration that does not resolve in the expected amount of time after injury or surgery.

Complex Regional Pain Syndrome (CRPS): CRPS Type I is pain extending beyond the initial peripheral nerve injury and out of proportion to the expected amount of pain; CRPS Type II is pain following a peripheral nerve pathway and out of proportion to the expected amount of pain.

Dependence: physiologic response to a drug that will cause adverse symptoms if the drug is abruptly stopped.

Neuropathic: abnormal pain pathway that is related to one or more nerves.

Nociceptive: normal pain pathway of peripheral nerve receptors.

Pseudoaddiction: behavior that appears to be addiction but develops due to under-treated pain and resolves once the pain is relieved.

Radicular/Radiculopathy: nerve root compression resulting in nerve dysfunction evidenced by changes in sensory, motor, and reflex function.

Somatic: pain arising from skin, muscle, tendons, joints, bone, or viscera.

Tolerance: increasing amounts of a drug are required to achieve the same effect.

Visceral: pain arising from organs.

Orthopaedic injuries, disease processes, and surgeries will induce acute pain and potentially chronic pain. It is estimated that 76.5 million Americans (26%) have chronic pain (American Pain Foundation (APF), 2009). Unfortunately, 40% of chronic pain patients do not have adequate pain relief (Heit & Gilson, 2008). Common causes of chronic pain are often orthopaedic in nature such as low back pain and arthritis. Demographic changes in our society are increasing the risk for developing chronic pain. In the United States, obesity affects 33.3% American males, 35.3% females, and 16.3% children (Swartz, Mobley, & Felix, 2009; National Center for Health Statistics, 2007). According to the UN Population Division statistics (2006), the increase in probable lifespan for women in developing countries exceeds 80 years. The combination of excess stress on the musculoskeletal system due to body weight and surviving to an older age potentiates the likelihood of orthopaedic-related pain.

Acute pain induced by trauma or surgery can be enormously debilitating and lead to chronic pain. Total knee arthroplasty is known to be one of the most painful surgeries performed (American Academy of Orthopaedic Surgeons (AAOS), 2007). Other causes of orthopaedic pain may include pressure on a nerve, within a compartment, tissue extravasation secondary to inflammation and swelling, or muscular pain secondary to manipulation and stretching. Researchers at University of Washington found that 62.7% of patients with a major trauma injury one year ago still experienced injury-related pain (Barclay & Lie, 2008). The wide variety of sources of orthopaedic-related pain can make diagnosis and treatment complex. The challenge for the nurse is to accurately treat the source of pain while aggressively managing the symptom of pain.

Pain Assessment

A thorough pain assessment can often provide characteristic clues to the origin of the painful process. Discovery of the source allows the nurse to succinctly identify the appropriate treatment. A standardized approach to conducting the assessment will yield valuable information to formulate a plan of care.

The patient's report of pain is to be believed; that is, McCaffery recognized as early as 1968 that "pain is what the experiencing person says it is and it exists when the person says it does". Utilizing a standardized scale that the patient selects allows the nurse to evaluate whether the patient perceives that the pain is worsening or improving. Once the patient selects a scale, the same scale should be utilized in future pain assessments. Patients should be asked to determine their pain goal; that is, at what level the pain would be tolerable for them. The health care provider can then work toward an acceptable level for the patient. The goal should be documented and visible to all health care providers.

Pain Scales

The most commonly used pain scale is the Numerical Rating Scale (Figure 7-1). The scale is known to be reliable and valid for assessing pain in persons able to understand the concept that "0" is no pain and "10" is the worst pain imaginable. Multiple researchers have documented that even cognitively impaired persons can often reliably report pain using this scale (Puntillo et al., 2009). The Numerical Rating Scale can vary in increments up to the most severe pain being "100," and be horizontally or vertically placed. There is mounting evidence that a vertical scale is easier for geriatric patients to interpret due to the visual association between a rising temperature on a thermometer and increasing levels of pain (Gagliese, Weizblit, Ellis, & Chan, 2005).

The Visual Analog Scale is simply a visual continuum of pain along a line. The patient may be asked to mark a point on the scale that best reflects the severity of their pain.

Figure 7-1
Numerical Rating Scale – Wong Baker Faces Scale

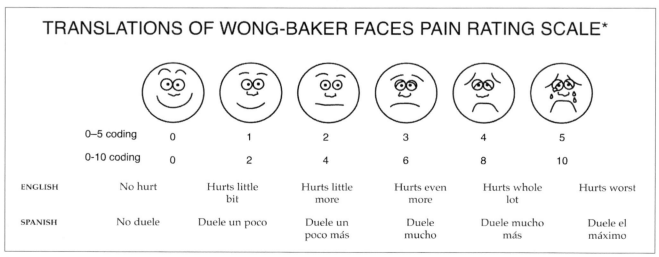

Reprinted with permission from Wong, D.L., Hockenberry-Eaton, M., Wilson, D., Winkelstein, M.L., & Schwartz, P. (2001) P. Wong's Essentials of pediatric nursing (6th ed., p. 1301). St. Louis: Mosby. Copyrighted by Mosby, Inc. Reprinted by permission.

Table 7-1
Selected quality of life indicators that influence chronic pain or chronic illness.

Physical/functional Well Being	Emotional Well-Being	Social Well-Being	Spiritual Well-Being
Age	Distress/stressors	Family role	
Health status	Consequences of pain	Relationships (family, friends, significant others)	Religion
Nutritional status	Self-esteem	Participation in leisure activities	
Independence	Coping methods	Community Support	
Pain/consequences of pain	Anxiety	Employment status	Spiritual beliefs
Access to health care services	Depression	Ethnicity/culture	Values/ethics
Quality of sleep		Socio/economic status	
Energy level		Social isolation	
Sexual functioning		Sexuality	
Exercise		Education level	
Physical Mobility			
Education level			

Chart content developed by Cheryl Rawe, RNC, BA, 2003.

Young children, neonates, and comatose patients cannot reliably use the Numerical Rating Scale or Visual Analog Scale without the cognitive ability to understand numeric or proportional increases and decreases.

The Faces scale (Figure 7-1) may be appropriate for illiterate persons, children, or anyone who prefers the scale. Wong and Baker originally created this scale with numbers 0-5 (Wong, Hockenberry-Eaton, Winkelstein, & Schwartz, 2001), but over the years, some researchers have superimposed a 0-10 scale with proven reliability (Herr et.al., 2006). Patients who have difficulty using scales may be able to gauge pain by "mild, moderate, or severe." If patients seem functionally better, but continue to report a consistent number, they may be able to report a percentage of pain improvement since the previous assessment or treatment.

The dilemma over selection of a behavioral pain scale for adults has not been resolved. Evaluation of behaviors of nonverbal, comatose, demented, or cognitively impaired persons are not consistent, thereby making assignment of numbers unreliable. The only reliable indicator exhibited when studying a variety of non-verbal causes, is a change from baseline behavior (Herr et al., 2006). Caregivers and/or family members familiar with the patient can give the best clues to changes from baseline behavior and should be contacted.

Factors Influencing Pain Assessment

A thorough pain history should include:

- **Pain frequency and duration**—how often the pain occurs, if the pain comes and goes, and how long the pain has been present, precipitating factors in the past;

- **Pharmacologic and non-pharmacologic treatments in the past**—effectiveness and response, most recent regimen including herbal medicines and over-the-counter medicines;

- **History of substance abuse and/or opioid tolerance**—recency, type, amount and frequency of consumption of substance;

- **Coping ability**—support systems, history of psychiatric disorders, family attitudes and involvement;

- **Expressions of pain**—words used (children and geriatric patients may use terminology other than "pain"), past behaviors during painful episodes.

The longer the patient has experienced the pain, the more difficult the pain is to treat, secondary to development of abnormal neural pathways (Bushnell & Basbaum, 2008). Complicating factors such as emotional pain or a substance abuse history must be acknowledged and treated along with the pain. Nursing assessment should include a complete history to report to the physician, as pain is influenced by multiple factors. A thorough evaluation of functionality with acute pain and chronic pain should influence treatment decisions. If the patient has chronic pain, overall quality of life may be affected and should be assessed (Table 7-1).

Description

The minimum inpatient pain assessment must at least include description, location, duration, frequency, and reassessment after intervention (The Joint Commission (TJC), 2008). Documentation tools that trigger these basic assessment requirements provide a helpful structure (Figure 7-2). Additionally, reported factors that improve or worsen pain help steer treatment regimens. For instance, activity-related pain should be managed with short, quick-acting medications versus long-acting medications. Specific word descriptors such as "sharp, dull, aching, or crushing", along with pain location and radiation, provide important clues for identifying the pain source. Treatment may be modified based on the descriptors documented and reported

Figure 7-2
Pain Assessment/Comfort Management Flowsheet

PAIN ASSESSMENT / COMFORT MANAGEMENT

Pain Score: 0=No Pain 1=Mild Pain 5=Moderate Pain 10=Severe Pain N=Nonverbal
Non-Verbals: Cr=Crying S=Sweating G=Grimacing R/A=Restless/Agitation SL=Sleeping R=Resting C=Calm NC=New onset confusion O=Other
Pain Characteristic: T=Throbbing S=Sharp C=Cramping D=Dull B=Burning A=Aching P=Pressure R=Radiates O=Other
Pain Frequency: B=Brief I=Intermittent C=Constant
Sedation Scale: 1=Wide awake 2=Drowsy 3=Sleeping but easily arousable 4=Difficult to arouse or weak 5=Unarousable or paralyzed
Respiratory Quality: S=Shallow E=Even U=Unlabored L=Labored V=Vent D=Deep
Relief Measures: M=Medicate P=Positioned H=Heat C=Cold A/E=Activity/Exercise Ma=Massage D=Diversion T=TENS O=Other
Plan/Comments: R=Resting M=Monitor Re=Re-medicate N=Notify physician O=Other E=Effective Ø=No interventions required

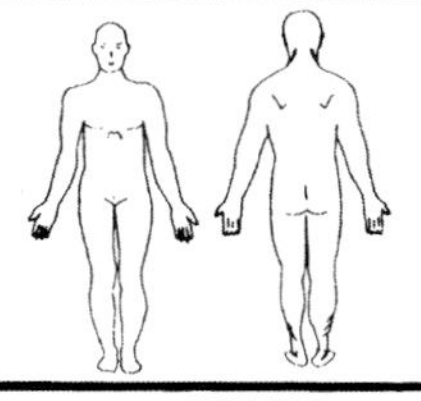

Number Pain Sites 1, 2, 3

Pain Goal: | Pain Scale — numbers / faces / colors — use the same scale each time | RESPONSE

Date Time	Pain Score	Pain Location (Body Map)	Pain Characteristic/ Non-verbals	Pain Frequency	Medication Administered	Dose	Route	Sedation Score	Resp Rate & Quality	Relief Measures / Comments	Initials	Time	Pain Score	Sedation Score	Plan / Comments	Initials
					SEE MAR											
					SEE MAR											

Reprinted with permission and developed by Miami Valley Hospital Pain Performance Team facilitated by Carol Roberts, RN, BSN, 2001.

by the nurse. A concise pain location report may trigger the physician to order further diagnostic tests.

Cultural Factors

Cultural factors may influence how the patient responds to and reports pain, while the health care providers may harbor their own cultural biases. "Cultural" may be used to describe ethnic background or geographical upbringing, as well as familial cultural influences. Briggs & Martin (2008) noted that under-reporting, over-reporting, enhanced emotional and behavioral responses, or subdued emotional and behavioral responses may all be learned behaviors related to life history and/or cultural influences. Health care practitioners are influenced by educational level, personal experiences, and past pain education, thus forming subjective opinions about the patient's report of pain (Idvall, Berg, Unosson, & Brudin, 2005; Sloman, Rosen, Rom, & Shir, 2005). In response, pain may be under-treated or over-treated.

Assessment, often complicated by a variety of factors, is not as simple as a number. All of the variables discussed must be considered to formulate a comprehensive plan of care. It may be advisable to enlist the help of a pain specialist or psychologist when the assessment reveals a complicated picture. The nurse may act as facilitator to obtain additional consultations by providing a comprehensive assessment for the physician.

Pain Origins

Knowledge regarding normal and abnormal pain pathways provides needed information to steer treatment choices. Orthopaedic injuries involve a wide variety of painful processes. Normal nociceptive transmission may be somatic or visceral. Somatic pain describes pain arising from skin, muscle, bone, tendon, or tissue. A somatic pain process is always present with an orthopaedic injury. Visceral pain is pain arising from organs. Visceral pain would only be associated with orthopaedic pain if extensive inflammation, swelling, or structural deformity from bone disease or injury compromises an organ in the immediate vicinity.

Abnormal pain processing involves neuropathic pain, which may be peripheral or central in nature. Peripheral neuropathic pain may arise from a single injured nerve (mononeuropathy) or from multiple nerves (polyneuropathy). Orthopaedic injuries more likely include single nerves in close proximity to injured bone. The polyneuropathies typically stem from disease processes such as diabetic neuropathy or vascular disease.

Central neuropathy is pain mediated from the central nervous system as in spinal cord or brain injury. Since spinal cord injury often results from trauma, orthopaedic injuries may occur simultaneously. Injuries or diseases affecting bone in the back may compress the spinal cord or the nerves branching off the cord at the bony outlets, causing severe neuropathic pain. An example of brain-induced neuropathy would be extremity pain related to stroke, tumor, or aneurysm. Complex Regional Pain Syndrome (CRPS) Types I and II are abnormal developments of chronic pain related to an acute injury of a nerve or nerve bundle, typically of an extremity (previously termed Reflux Sympathetic Dystrophy or "RSD"). Mild pressure sensations and temperature changes are abnormally read as painful by the patient. CRPS can be extremely difficult to treat and require invasive interventions such as nerve blocks and/or brain surgery.

Neuropathic pain is much more difficult to treat than nociceptive pain. Adjuvant medicines, in addition to opioids, are typically required to alleviate symptoms associated with neuropathy. Opioid and non-steroidal anti-inflammatory drugs (NSAIDs) are usually effective for nociceptive pain but do not comprehensively treat neuropathic pain. The following section will discuss pharmacologic options preferred for specific types of pain.

Pharmacologic Management

The goal of pharmacologic management of acute and chronic pain should be improvement in function and quality of life. Complete pain relief should never be assured or expected, and may not be realistic in all situations. Although the goal is to provide the most optimum pain relief possible, complicating neuropathic pain or intolerable side effects from analgesic medications may prevent complete relief. Multidisciplinary management in conjunction with medication should ideally restore the person to an acceptable level of activity with attention to quality of life. Limitations in activity due to medications or intolerable side effects of medications should be addressed by dose reduction, change to another similar medication, or additional pharmacologic management specific to the symptom experienced. Constipation, a common side effect with opioids and complicated by immobility from orthopaedic injuries, should be addressed prophylactically with a fiber-rich diet, increased fluids, and bowel stimulants as needed. Over-sedation with opioids may impede rehabilitation; therefore, adjuvant medications and non-pharmacologic means should always be included in the treatment regimen. Nursing reports of observable side effects will assist the physician to determine needed medication adjustments.

Opioids

Opioids are the mainstay for the short-term management of moderate to severe pain. Although most types of pain respond to opioids, up to 38% of patients do not respond, even with aggressive titration (Becker, Sjorgen, Bech, Olsen, & Eriksen, 2000). Awareness of the "Clinical Guidelines for Chronic Opioid Therapy in Patients with Noncancer Pain" is important when a patient needs to be maintained on opioids for a chronic condition (American Pain Society (APS)/American Academy of Pain Medicine (AAPM), 2009).

Adjuvant medication along with opioids has been repeatedly shown to reduce overall opioid consumption and side effects (APS, 2008). Despite the controversial use of opioids for chronic pain, 21 organizations have issued a joint consensus statement in support of opioid use for chronic non-malignant pain (APF, 2009). The American Geriatric Society's (AGS) guideline on the pharmacologic management of persistent pain in older adults (2009), the APS guidelines for the use of opioids for the treatment of chronic pain (2009), and even the U.S. Drug Enforcement Agency (Controlled Substances Act, 2009) have issued statements in support of prudent use of opioids in chronic non-malignant pain that does not respond to other medications or modalities, or when the risk of side effects from non-steroidal drugs outweighs the benefits.

The "gold standard" for the treatment of moderate to severe acute pain is morphine. Efficacious analgesia combined with cost-effectiveness make morphine a commonly used opioid. Other common opioids for moderate to severe pain are hydromorphone (Dilaudid®) and fentanyl. Hydromorphone is indicated for use in renally-compromised patients because it has minimal metabolites to accumulate thereby causing fewer side effects (APS, 2008). Meperidine (Demerol®) is rarely indicated for extended use due to its neurotoxic metabolite, normeperidine, the accumulation of which, with repeated doses, may induce seizures. Due to the poor analgesic effect and risks associated with meperidine, usage has gradually declined over the past 20 years and is not recommended (APS, 2008). The short half-life of fentanyl allows the drug to be started and stopped for short-term use or for intermittent patient evaluation. These properties make fentanyl the opioid of choice for procedural pain or for use in the intensive care unit (Rawe et al., 2009).

Long-acting opioids may be useful when the patient has established opiate tolerance, a recent history of drug abuse, or around-the-clock pain. The extended release action may better cover baseline analgesic requirements in combination with short-acting opioids. If the patient has no established baseline opiate tolerance, long-acting agents may be dangerous and should be titrated slowly upward, based on the usage of breakthrough opiates. An equianalgesic dosing chart should be used to more accurately predict the dosage the patient may be able to tolerate (see Table 7-2). Because effects of different opioids can be unpredictable, even within the same class, a dose reduction of one-third to one-half the previous 24-hour dose total is recommended when switching opioids (Katzung, 2007). The nurse should watch for signs of oversedation when a new or different opioid is being trialed. Since there are at least 7 known mu-receptor sub-types, opiate rotation may be beneficial for improved analgesic effect with a resulting reduction in side effects (DuPen, Shen, & Ersek, 2007).

Patient controlled analgesia (PCA) is a common form of pain management for conscious trauma patients or postoperative patients. Although PCA has been shown to improve patient satisfaction in past studies, pain is not optimally controlled when the patient falls asleep and gets behind on the analgesic. Larijani and colleagues (2005) found that 75% of postoperative patients reported moderate to severe pain at rest with standard doses of PCA. If around-the-clock pain is anticipated, a long-acting opioid or low dose continuous PCA opioid infusion should be considered for the night of surgery. Breakthrough immediate-release opioid dosing should be calculated at 5% to 15% of the total 24-hour dose (Tennant, Liu, & Hermann, 2002; Brookhoff, 2000). Short-acting agents are particularly useful for activity-related pain. See the "Dosing" section for further discussion of dosing.

Non-Steroidal Anti-Inflammatory Drugs (NSAIDs), Aspirin, and Acetaminophen (Tylenol®)

Simple analgesics such as NSAIDs, aspirin (ASA), or acetaminophen are often effective for musculoskeletal pain or somatic pain (Table 7-3). Short-term therapy, especially with inflammatory processes, can effectively be managed with over-the-counter NSAIDs in therapeutic prescriptive doses. NSAIDs and ASA must be used with caution due to the increased risks associated with gastrointestinal irritation (GI), bleeding, and renal toxicity. The risks associated with side effects exclude the use of more than one NSAID at a time, and NSAIDs should be consumed at the lowest possible dose to achieve analgesia. Maximum effects of NSAIDs will be reached at maximum doses, and escalation will not improve analgesia.

Concerns regarding contraindications and side effects of NSAIDs and ASA must be weighed in relation to low dose opioid use when analgesics are to be rendered on a long-term basis. Adjuvant use of these medicines when pain is more severe has consistently exhibited a reduction in opioid use and should be included in the medication regimen unless contraindicated (APS, 2008). Since NSAIDs are effective for all types of pain, the nurse should ask the physician to consider a NSAID unless contraindicated. Gastrointestinal

Table 7-2
Equianalgesic Dosing Chart

Opioid Agonist Available dosage forms	Approximate equianalgesic dose[1]		Recommended starting dose for moderate to severe pain (adults and children ≥50 kg body weight)[2]	
	Oral	**Parenteral**	**Oral**	**Parenteral**
Morphine A wide variety of dosage forms are available including 15 mg, 30 mg tablets; 10 mg, 20 mg, suppositories; 10 mg/ 5 ml, 20 mg/ml oral liquid; 4 mg, 8 mg, 10 mg, 15 mg syringes; PCA	30 mg q 3-4 hrs (around the clock dosing) 60 mg q 3-4 hrs (single or intermittent dosing)	10 mg q 3-4 hrs	15-30 mg q 3-4 hrs	10 mg q 3-4 hrs
MS Contin (Morphine, *controlled release*) 15 mg, 30 mg, 60 mg, 100 mg, 200 mg tablets	90-120 mg q 12 hrs	Not available	15-30 mg q 12 hrs	Not available
Kadian (Morphine, *sustained release*) 20 mg, 30 mg, 50 mg, 60 mg, 100 mg capsules with sustained release pellets	180-240 mg once daily	Not available	N/A – patients are usually converted from another dosage form	Not available
Codeine 15 mg, 30 mg, 60 mg tablets; 30 mg, 60 mg syringes	180-200 mg q 3-4 hrs	130 mg q 3-4 hrs	60 mg q 3-4 hrs[3]	60 mg q 2 hrs[3] (IM/SQ)
Fentanyl Transdermal 12.5 mcg/hr, 25 mcg/hr, 50 mcg/hr, 75 mcg/hr, 100 mcg/hr patch	25 mcg/hr transdermal fentanyl = 12 mg/day parenteral morphine = 36 mg/day oral morphine. Most patients are adequately maintained with q 72 hour Fentanyl[4]		Not appropriate for acute pain. Doses greater than 25 mcg/hr should not be used for initiation of Fentanyl patch therapy in non-opioid-tolerant patients.[4]	
Dilaudid (Hydromorphone) 2 mg, 4 mg, 8 mg tablets 5 mg/5ml oral liquid 3 mg suppository 2 mg/ml, 10 mg/ml and injection	7.5 mg q 3-4hrs	1.5 mg q 3-4 hrs	6 mg q 3-4 hr	1.5 mg q 3-4 hrs
Hydrocodone (in Lortab, Vicodin) Only in combination; see table 2	30 mg q 3-4 hrs	Not available	10 mg q 3-4 hrs	Not available
Levo-Dromoran (Levorphanol) 2 mg tablet	4 mg q 6-8 hrs	2 mg q 6-8 hrs	4 mg q 6-8 hrs	2 mg q 6-8 hrs
Demerol (Meperidine) 50 mg, 100 mg tablet 50 mg/5 ml oral liquid; 25 mg, 50 mg, 75 mg, 100 mg syringes; PCA	300 mg q 3-4 hrs	100 mg q 3 hrs	Not recommended	100 mg q 3 hrs[5]
Methadone (Dolophine) 5 mg, 10 mg tablets 10 mg/ml, 5 mg/5ml, 10 mg/5ml oral liquid; 10 mg/ml injection	10 mg q 6-8 hrs	5 mg q 6-8 hrs	5 mg q 6-8 hrs	2.5 mg q 6-8 hrs
Roxicodone (Oxycodone, also in Percocet, others) 5 mg, 15 mg 30 mg tablet 5 mg/5 ml. 20 mg/ml oral liquid	30 mg q 3-4 hrs	Not available	10 mg q 3-4 hrs	Not available
OxyContin (Oxycodone, controlled release) 10 mg, 20 mg, 40 mg, 80 mg, 160 mg tablet	60 mg q 12 hrs	Not available	10 mg q 12 hrs	Not available
Centrally acting NON–OPIOID – this is NOT an opioid and does not have cross tolerance				
Tramadol (Ultram) 50 mg tablet		Not available	50 mg q 6 hrs	Not available

[1] Published tables vary in the suggested doses that are equianalgesic to morphine. Clinical response is the criterion that must be applied for each patient; titration to clinical responses is necessary. Because there is a not complete cross-tolerance among these drugs, it is usually necessary to use a lower than equianalgesic dose when changing drugs and to re-titrate to response.

[2] Recommended doses do not apply for adult patients with body weight less than 50 kg. Recommended doses do not apply to patients with renal or hepatic insufficiency or other conditions affecting drug metabolism and kinetics.

[3] Codeine doses > 65mg often are not appropriate because of diminishing incremental analgesia with increasing nausea, constipation, and other side effects

[4] Because of the increase in serum fentanyl concentration over the first 24 hours following initial system application, the initial evaluation of the maximum analgesic of Duragesic cannot be made before 24 hours of wearing. The initial Duragesic dosage may be increased after 3 days. During the initial application of Duragesic, patients should use short-acting analgesics as needed until analgesic efficacy with Duragesic is attained. Thereafter, some patients still may require periodic supplemental doses of other short-acting analgesics for "breakthrough" pain.

[5] Meperidine therapy should be limited to short term therapy of 48 - 72 hours.

Chart content developed by Sandra P. Dean, Pharm. D., 2003; updated 2009 by Cathy Trame, MS, CNS.

Table 7.3
Non-steroidal Anti-inflammatory Drugs

	Usual Adult Dose (for adults and children ≥ 50kg body weight)	Dosage Forms Available
Acetaminophen (Tylenol, others)[1]	650 mg q 4-6 hrs	325 mg, 500 mg , 650 mg tablets 60 mg, 160 mg chewable tablets 120 mg, 650 mg suppository 650 mg/25 ml & 160 mg/5 ml elixir
Aspirin	650 mg q 4-6 hrs	325 mg tablet 300 mg & 600 mg suppository 325 mg enteric coated tablet
Diclofenac (Voltaren)	100 – 200 mg /day in divided doses bid, tid or qid	25 mg, 50 mg, 75 mg tablets 100 mg XR tablet (for once daily dosing)
Diflunisal (Dolobid)	500-1500 mg daily in 2-3 divided doses	250 mg, 500 mg tablets
Etodolac (Lodine)	200-400 mg q 6-8 hrs	200 mg, 300 mg capsules
Fenoprofen (Nalfon)	200-600 mg every 4-6 hours; max 3200 mg/day	200 mg, 300 mg capsules; 600 mg tablets
Ibuprofen (Motrin, Advil, others)	400-600 mg q 6 hrs or 800 mg tid	200 mg, 400 mg, 600 mg, 800 mg tablets 100 mg/5ml oral suspension
Indomethacin (Indocin)	25-50 mg tid	25 mg, 50 mg capsules 75 mg SR capsule 50 mg suppository
Ketoprofen (Orudis, Oruvail)	12.5-75 mg/dose every 4-6 hrs; max 300 mg/day Extended release: 100- 200 mg qd	12.5 mg tablets 25 mg, 50 mg, 75 mg capsules 100 mg, 150 mg, 200 mg extended release capsules
Ketorolac (Toradol)	Injection: 15 mg IV or 30 mg IM single dose : 15 mg IV/IM q 6 hrs; maximum of 20 doses or 5 days. Oral – Only for continuation of IV/IM therapy: 10 mg q 4-6 hrs; max of 40mg/day. **Total ketorolac therapy should not exceed 5 days.**[2]	15mg, 30 mg, 60 mg injection; 10 mg tablet
Nambumetone (Relafen)	1000-2000 mg qd as single dose or divided doses given bid	500 mg tablet
Naproxen (Naprosyn)	250-275 mg q 6-8 hrs	250 mg, 375 mg, 500 mg tablets
Oxaprozin (Daypro)	600-1200 mg qd; max 1800 mg /day	600 mg tablets and caplets
Piroxicam (Feldene)	20 mg qd	10 mg capsule
Sulindac (Clinoril)	150-200 mg bid	150 mg, 200 mg tablets
Trilisate[3]	1000-1500 mg bid to tid	500 mg, 750 mg tablets
Selective COX-2 Inhibitor		
Celecoxib (Celebrex)	200-400 mg daily in 1-2 divided doses	100 mg, 200 mg, 400 mg capsules

[1] Acetaminophen lacks the peripheral anti-inflammatory and antiplatelet activities of the NSAIDS.

[2] Patients ≥ 65 yrs old, with renal impairment, or weighing <50kg require doses of ONE-HALF the normal dose, maximum 60mg/day.

[3] May have minimal platelet activity.

Chart content developed by Sandra P. Dean, Pharm. D., 2003; updated 2009 by Cathy Trame, MS, CNS.

irritation can be reduced by using a COX-2 inhibitor versus a NSAID. Alternatively, a NSAID could be used in combination with misoprostol (Cytotec®), an H2 antagonist such as ranitidine (Zantac®), or a proton pump inhibitor such as lansoprazole (Prevacid®) (Katzung, 2007). The cost of using COX-2 inhibitors versus gastrointestinal (GI) protectants along with an over-the-counter NSAID are comparable.

Acetaminophen up to 4000 mg (4 grams) per day, the maximum daily dose, is recommended for first-line treatment for osteoarthritis and mild chronic pain. The Federal Drug Administration (FDA) recommends that persons who consume more than 2 ounces of alcohol per day should reduce the 24-hour limit of acetaminophen to 2.5 grams per day due to risk of liver toxicity. Persons with known liver disease should avoid the use of acetaminophen. The dosage should be divided into 500 - 1000 mg, 4 times per day. If the pain is moderate to severe, acetaminophen is rarely effective or appropriate as a single analgesic. Combination analgesics containing acetaminophen and an opioid will have dose limits secondary to the acetaminophen 4-gram-per-day maximum (see Table 7-4). For example, the maximum amount of acetaminophen/propoxyphene (Darvocet N-100®) is six tablets per day, 650 mg of acetaminophen per tablet, which would total 3900 mg of acetaminophen. The nurse should counsel the patient about acetaminophen limits as well as con-commitant alcohol use, as patients often take additional acetaminophen or consume alcohol and do not realize the dangers.

The use of NSAIDs or COX-2 inhibitors has been controversial due to past publications revealing interference with bone healing. A study of 288 patients who underwent spinal fusion did not fuse adequately when ketorolac was used postoperatively (Glassman et al., 1998). Inhibition of fusion was amplified as volume and dose of ketorolac was increased. Another study of rabbits undergoing spinal fusion compared celecoxib (Celebrex®) and indomethacin (Indocin®) with controls and found indomethacin significantly interfered with fusion (Long, Lewis, Kuklo, Zhu, & Riew, 2002), while celecoxib did not interfere. A third study with mice revealed interference in healing of bone fractures with administration of COX-2 inhibitors (Simon, Manigrasso, & O'Connor, 2002). Another study concluded that in human subjects following spinal fusion, short term use of ketorolac (Toradol®) 0.5 mg/kg not more than 15 mg times 6 doses, did not inhibit fusion and did reduce morphine consumption (Munro et.al., 2002). Finally, Sucato and associates (2008), found no interference with bone fusion when ketorolac was administered after spinal fusion for idiopathic scoliosis. Conclusively, when fracture healing or bone fusion is the desired outcome, NSAIDs and COX-2 inhibitors should be used sparingly for short periods of time, pending further refutive research. Table 7-3 lists suggested dosing of various NSAIDs.

Topical NSAIDs have been introduced that act locally at the site of the pain versus systemically. The advantage of the topical agents is the reduced and nearly eliminated risk of GI adverse effects. Trial of a topical NSAID is worthwhile in lieu of the systemic effects of alternative medicines. Two of the preparations currently available are: Flector® patch 1.3% dosed every 12 hours (contains diclofenac) or Voltaren® (diclofenac) gel 2-4 grams dosed up to 4 times daily. Caution must still be exercised if the patient has had an acute myocardial infarction or has congestive heart failure (PDR, 2008).

Muscle Relaxants

The addition of muscle relaxants for spasm, often associated with bone injury, can greatly reduce or eliminate the need for opioids. The spasm stimulates production of lactic acid, which is known to trigger the nociceptive pathway (Katzung, 2007). Failure to control spasm may complicate and slow rehabilitation after an orthopaedic injury. A variety of skeletal muscle relaxants are available for short term use following acute injury. Individual response and side effects (typically sedation) should dictate which agent achieves the best outcome for the patient. A long-acting muscle relaxant with once daily dosing is now available (Amrix®), which does help minimize the sedation associated with these drugs. The nurse should prompt the physician to consider a muscle relaxant in addition to an opioid to achieve optimal analgesia.

Steroids

Steroids have been effective in reducing inflammation by interfering with the arachidonic acid cascade and blocking nociceptive input (Katzung, 2007). Administration with invasive techniques such as regional or local blocks may be preferred for site-specific pain versus oral administration that increases systemic side effects. Steroids may be indicated for rheumatologic conditions, chronic back or neck pain with radiculopathy, and inoperable tumors or inflammatory conditions (particularly involving the joint) of varied etiologies. Contraindications for steroids include diabetes, depression, or psychosis (Katzung, 2007). Multiple side effects of steroids, particularly with long term use include, but are not limited to, GI disturbance, psychological effects, cushionoid effects, hypertension, hyperglycemia, fluid retention, osteoporosis, compression fractures, myopathy, skin rashes, and thinning of connective and subcutaneous tissues (Katzung, 2007).

Local Anesthetics

Long- or short-acting local anesthetics may be utilized for neuropathic syndromes to interfere with the sodium ion channels, thereby dulling pain sensation. The most common use of local anesthetics in the orthopaedic population is via nerve block administration during the intraoperative phase (see "Invasive Therapies"). Topical application with a 5% Lidoderm® (lidocaine) patch, to a contained painful area (not open wound) can be analgesic with minimal systemic absorption. Patch application may pre-empt the need for more invasive management with local anesthetics, resulting in a significant risk reduction to the patient. The Lidoderm® patch is currently being researched for osteoarthritic back and knee pain following anecdotal reports of patient improvement with application, however there are still no controlled, randomized trials available for review in orthopaedic populations. Local anesthetics may be injected locally for myofascial pain or near nerve roots or nerve root bundles to calm the neuropathic sensation and/or numb the area. Oral forms of local anesthetics are rarely employed for orthopaedic injuries or surgeries due to the risk of cardiotoxicity.

Anticonvulsants and Antidepressants

Adjuvant medication is often helpful for neuropathic pain. Logically, the lowest possible dose should be used to minimize short- and long-term side effects. Side effects of antidepressants can be minimized by using the class of secondary amine tricyclics or SNRI's (serotonin norepinephrine re-uptake inhibitors) (APS, 2008). All persons with neuropathic pain (burning, searing, or electric-like) should be trialed on a tricyclic antidepressant or anticonvulsant as a first line adjuvant. If greater than 50% reduction in pain is achieved, patient function improves, and side effects are tolerable, the therapy should be continued long-term (Holmquist, 2001). Adjuvants for neuropathic pain may be effective as singular analgesics but should be prescribed in combination with opioids when pain continues to impair function and is intolerable to the individual. Anticonvulsants block neuropathic pain by inhibiting the ion channels that stimulate the nerve, while antidepressants suppress neuropathic pain by inhibiting

Table 7-4
Opioid Acetaminophen Combinations and Tablet Limits/24 Hours

	Content per tablet, capsule or 5 ml	Daily limit[1]	Usual adult dose
Tylenol w/Codeine #2	Acetaminophen 300 mg Codeine 15 mg	13 tablets	1-2 tablets q 4 hrs
Tylenol w/Codeine #3	Acetaminophen 300 mg Codeine 30 mg	13 tablets	1-2 tablets q 4 hrs
Tylenol w/Codeine #4	Acetaminophen 300 mg Codeine 60 mg	13 tablets	1-2 tablets q 4 hrs
Tylenol w/Codeine Elixir	Acetaminophen 120 mg Codeine 12 mg (12.5 ml = one Tylenol #3 tablet)	167 ml (13 doses of 12.5 ml)	12.5 ml q 4 hrs
Lortab 5; Vicodin	Acetaminophen 500 mg Hydrocodone 5 mg	8 tablets	1-2 tabs q 4-6 hrs; max of 8 tabs/day
Lortab 7.5 mg tab	Acetaminophen 500 mg Hydrocodone 7.5 mg	8 tablets	1 tab q 4-6 hrs
Vicodin ES	Acetaminophen 750 mg Hydrocodone 7.5 mg	5 tablets	1 tab q 4-6 hrs; up to 5/day
Vicodin HP	Acetaminophen 660 mg Hydrocodone 10 mg	6 tablets	1 tab q 4-6 hrs
Lortab Elixir	Acetaminophen 167 mg Hydrocodone 2.5 mg (15 ml = Lortab 7.5)	120 ml (8 doses of 15 ml)	15 ml q 4-6 hrs
Darvocet-N-50	Acetaminophen 325 mg Propoxyphene Napsylate 50 mg[2]	12 tablets	2 tab q 4-6 hrs
Darvocet-N-100	Acetaminophen 650 mg Propoxyphene Napsylate 100 mg[5]	6 tablets	1 tab q 4-6 hrs
Wygesic	Acetaminophen 650 mg Propoxyphene 65 mg[5]	6 tablets	1 tab q 4-6 hrs
Percocet 5/325	Acetaminophen 325 mg Oxycodone 5 mg	12 tablets	1-2 tabs q 4-6 hrs
Percocet 7.5/500	Acetaminophen 500 mg Oxycodone 7.5 mg	8 tablets	1 q 4-6 hrs
Percocet 10/650	Acetaminophen 650 mg Oxycodone 10 mg	6 tablets	1 tab q 4-6 hrs
Tylox	Acetaminophen 500 mg Oxycodone 5 mg	8 tablets	1 tab q 4-6 hrs
Ultracet	Acetaminophen 325 mg Tramadol 37.5 mg	12 tablets	1-2 tabs q 4-6 hrs

Note: There are a variety of products which contain a combination of acetaminophen and an opioid. Clinicians should be aware of the acetaminophen content of these products. To avoid acetaminophen toxicity, in patients requiring additional pain relief consideration should be given to switching to a product with a higher proportion of opioid:acetaminophen rather than additional doses of lower proportion product.

[1] Published tables vary in the suggested doses that are equianalgesic to morphine. Clinical response is the criterion that must be applied for each patient; titration to clinical responses is necessary. Because there is a not complete cross-tolerance among these drugs, it is usually necessary to use a lower than equianalgesic dose when changing drugs and to re-titrate to response.

[2] Recommended doses do not apply for adult patients with body weight less than 50 kg. Recommended doses do not apply to patients with renal or hepatic insufficiency or other conditions affecting drug metabolism and kinetics.

[3] Codeine doses > 65mg often are not appropriate because of diminishing incremental analgesia with increasing nausea, constipation, and other side effects

[4] Because of the increase in serum fentanyl concentration over the first 24 hours following initial system application, the initial evaluation of the maximum analgesic of Duragesic cannot be made before 24 hours of wearing. The initial Duragesic dosage may be increased after 3 days. During the initial application of Duragesic, patients should use short-acting analgesics as needed until analgesic efficacy with Duragesic is attained.. Thereafter, some patients still may require periodic supplemental doses of other short-acting analgesics for "breakthrough" pain.

[5] Meperidine therapy should be limited to short term therapy of 48 – 72 hours.

Chart content developed by Sandra P. Dean, Pharm. D., 2003; updated 2009 by Cathy Trame, MS, CNS.

serotonin re-uptake, thereby allowing more available serotonin to neuromodulate the pain (Katzung, 2007). Examples of chronic neuropathic pain related to orthopaedic injury or disease are post-amputation pain, myelopathic or radicular pain from spinal stenosis, arachnoiditis or fibrosis, or complex regional pain syndromes. If the patient reports "burning, shooting, or electric-like pain," the pain is likely neuropathic. The nurse should describe the patient's pain utilizing these descriptors to prompt the physician to order appropriate adjuvants for treating neuropathic pain.

Glucosamine

Glucosamine, considered an herbal biological agent, deserves recognition as a proven adjuvant for reduction in weight-bearing joint pain (APS, 2002). Glucosamine is thought to stimulate the production of cartilage matrix and act as a chondroprotective agent with antioxidant activity. The APS guidelines for the management of pain in osteoarthritis (OA) recommend the use of 1500 mg of glucosamine per day for joint pain associated with OA. Some glucosamine preparations may be combined with chondroitin 4-sulfate, thought to provide some anti-inflammatory effects and stimulate cartilage production. There are a limited number of small studies on chondroitin 4-sulfate, demonstrating improvement in pain and function for joint pain associated with osteoarthritis (APS, 2002).

Other

Bone pain may arise from a variety of sources. Identifying and aggressively managing the source of the pain obviously will reduce the need to manage the symptom of pain. Pharmacologic or non-pharmacologic management should ideally target the source of the pain. Radiation therapy, chemotherapy, or surgery may be the most effective treatment to manage pain associated with tumor, bone deformity, or secondary neural compression. Management of infectious processes such as diskitis or septic arthritis may be targeted with antibiotics. Fractures may be stabilized with splints, casts, cement (as in vertebroplasty or kyphoplasty), or other orthotics, affording drastic reductions in the amount of pain experienced. Additionally, biophosphonates inhibit osteoclast activity, providing analgesic relief when calcium leaks from the bone (APS, 2008). Primary management of the pain source, with secondary management of the pain symptom, will produce the best outcome.

Route of Administration

The oral route of drug administration is the least invasive and should be utilized whenever possible (APS, 2008). When the oral route is contraindicated, subcutaneous or intravenous routes may be utilized for opioid administration. The intramuscular route of administration should be avoided if possible, as it does not provide reliable absorption, increases the risk for abscess, and is more painful (APS, 2008). As soon as the patient tolerates oral intake, the nurse should ask for transition to oral analgesics by notifying the physician.

Nerve blocks with local anesthetic can also be utilized for short-term management of trauma or surgery pain but may be under-utilized if there isn't a "pain service" available to follow up with the patients regarding efficacy and side effects (Sharrock, 2002). Localized nerve blocks such as femoral nerve block and sciatic nerve block for total knee replacement have increased in popularity due to the greatly reduced opioid intake and improved pain control. The epidural or intraspinal route of drug administration may sometimes be preferred for painful surgeries or trauma. Total hip, fractured ribs, or traumatic amputations—typically extremely painful—can be well-controlled with opioid and/or local anesthetic infusions into the epidural or intraspinal space (Klasen et al., 2005). Based on the American Society of Regional Anesthesia (ASRA) consensus statement (2002), a one-time epidural/intrathecal bolus dose of opioid may provide short-term postoperative pain management if a continuous infusion is contraindicated. Before inserting or removing an epidural catheter, make sure the patient is not on an anticoagulant, due to the risk of formation of an epidural hematoma. Check with the physician regarding the ASRA guidelines for use of anticogulants with neuraxial analgesia prior to catheter insertion or removal.

Dosing

Analgesia should be dosed based on the patient's report of pain, pain goal, pain frequency, and previous response to a defined dose of medication. The nurse should review the previous efficacy of the dose and any side effects before determining the next dose to be administered. If the last dose was ineffective, inadequate, or did not mediate the pain for the expected time frame, the nurse should contact the physician to adjust the dose or dose interval.

Frequency refers to how long the pain stays: does it come and go or stay all the time? Does something specific aggravate the pain that could be pre-treated? Answers to these questions guide medication dosing. If the patient reports pain around-the-clock (ATC) or always present, a long-acting analgesic is preferred; however, a short-acting analgesic on a scheduled basis may be more cost-effective. The disadvantages of repetitive dosing of short-acting agents are nurse inconvenience, interruption of the patient's sleep, and increased nausea. A conversion to long-acting oral or transdermal opioids can be used when baseline opiate tolerance has been established. NSAIDs or acetaminophen can be given ATC in place of opioids when pain is less severe, or in addition to opioids, to reduce overall opioid consumption. The nurse should inform the physician when pain is consistently present so ATC dosing can be ordered. Pain exacerbated by activity such as physical therapy or ambulation can be pre-treated with short-acting agents. Treatment with prn medication to assure pre-treatment for painful activities is an important nursing intervention. Intravenous patient controlled analgesia (PCA) or patient controlled epidural analgesia (PCEA) can be utilized for short-term management until the patient can tolerate oral medication (APS, 2008).

Pre-treatment of surgical pain has been termed "pre-emptive." Conflicting research regarding the efficacy of various modalities has made pre-emptive treatment controversial to operationalize. The studies that have shown efficacy in decreasing pain scores postoperatively have typically employed multi-modal analgesia—combinations of 2 or more analgesics—all with pharmacologic actions at varying levels of the nociceptive pathway. A study of patients with knee surgery by Menigaux, Adam, Guignard, Sessler, and Chauvin (2005) concluded that preoperative gabapentin (Neurontin®) reduced anxiety and improved functional recovery. Gabapentin given 2 hours preoperatively reduced morphine consumption and pain scores following brachial plexus injury, and after lower extremity orthopaedic surgery (Prabhaker, Arora, Bithal, Rath, & Dash, 2007; Montazeri, Kashefi, & Honarmand,

2007). Several NMDA (N-methyl D-aspartate) antagonists given pre-emptively have reduced opioid consumption and pain scores following acute trauma and following lumbar disk surgery (Galinski et al., 2007; Aveline, Hetet, Vautier, Gautier, & Bonnet, 2006).

Most of the pre-emptive research that has been done with NSAID's or COX-2 inhibitors has revealed significant pain reduction and less postoperative opioid consumption. Due to the large body of research on this class of drugs, pre-emptive administration should be considered for orthopaedic surgery. One study demonstrated significant opioid sparing and improved pain scores and active range of motion (ROM) when patients having total knee arthroplasty received 400 mg celecoxib 1 hour prior to surgery and 200 mg celecoxib every 12 hours for five days postoperatively (Huang et.al., 2008). Other studies on COX-2 inhibitors not currently available in the U.S. have repeatedly shown reduced opioid use and decreased pain scores postoperatively (Riest et al., 2008; Petkas et al., 2007; Takada et al., 2007; Toivonen, Pitko, & Rosenberg, 2007; Tuzuner, Ucok, Kucukyavuz, Alkis, & Alanoglu, 2007; & Yamashita et al., 2006).

Invasive Therapies

Epidural steroid with or without local anesthetic can decrease inflammation of nerve roots off of the spinal column, as in back pain or neck pain with radiculopathy. Complex regional pain syndrome (CRPS) may be unresponsive to traditional, non-invasive pain management regimens. The epidural route may be chosen to interrupt or "break the cycle" of neuropathy. Epidurals may be utilized intraoperatively or postoperatively for pain control for a variety of orthopaedic surgeries including knee arthroplasty, ilizarov bone stabilization, hip arthroplasty, or leg amputation. A variety of other nerve blocks with local anesthetic can be performed to specifically target the surgical area. Femoral nerve blocks for knee surgery or axillary nerve blocks for upper extremity surgery are examples. Nerve blocks of all types are useful for decreasing analgesic use and providing optimum pain control in the early postoperative phase. Continuous femoral nerve blocks (CFNB) were found to be preferred by patients over continuous epidural infusions (CEI) in postoperative total knee arthroplasy (Sundarathiti, 2009). Although pain control was superior with the epidural infusions, patient satisfaction was higher in the CFNB group and the patients experienced less side effects. Other studies with continuous femoral nerve block have been shown to provide superior analgesia after total joint replacement as compared to IV analgesia or single shot nerve blocks (DeRuyter, et al., 2006; Duarte, Fallis, Slonowsky, Kwarteng, & Yeung, 2006; Salinas, Liu, & Mulroy, 2006). A combination of CFNB along with sciatic block, in total knee replacements, improved pain control postoperatively by adding analgesic coverage to the posterior portion of the knee (Pham Dang et al., 2005).

Intra-articular blocks are quite common for relieving all types of joint irritation. Steroids are often used to relieve inflammation in the joint and thereby delay or prevent surgery (Neustadt & Altman, 2007). Hyaluronic acid has

Figure 7-3
Implantable Pump

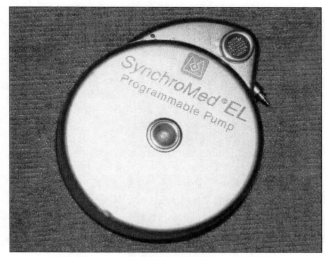

Photography by Sandra P. Dean, PharmD, 2003.

Figure 7-4
Implantable Spinal Cord Stimulator

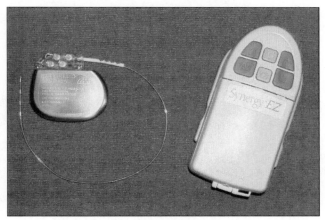

Photography by Sandra P. Dean, PharmD, 2003.

also shown promise for reducing mild to moderate knee pain when patients have osteoarthritis (Dagenais, 2006; Petrella & Petrella, 2006). Local anesthetic infusions into the joint intra-operatively and postoperatively have been shown to decrease general anesthetic requirements and and/or improve postoperative function and recovery (Charalambous, Tryfonidis, Alvi, Kumar, & Hirst, 2006). Unfortunately, the literature is not consistently conclusive regarding the reduction of pain scores when local anesthetic is used intra-articularly.

Myoneural nerve blocks, often termed "trigger points," can relieve muscular pain by injection of local anesthetic, steroid medication, and/or a dry needle (Elliott, et al., 2002). Bone disease or injury may trigger myofascial pain or may be a direct result of injury incurred at the time of the orthopaedic injury. Chronic myofascial pain is most likely to develop after a trauma, thereby making aggressive pain treatment paramount in the acute phase (Bushnell & Basbaum, 2008).

Implantable devices may serve as a last resort for unmanageable chronic pain or intolerance to side effects of medications. Implanted pumps with drug reservoirs release medication through a catheter into the intraspinal or epidural space (Figure 7-3). The dorsal column stimulator or spinal cord stimulator (SCS) is another implantable device (Figure 7-4). Generator leads provide stimulation to the area of the spinal cord from which the pain originates. The signal creates a vibration sensation that replaces the pain and triggers the body's production of endogenous opioid (endorphins). A SCS is most often used to treat chronic back pain.

Guidelines for Pain Management in Osteoarthritis, Rheumatoid Arthritis, and Juvenile Chronic Arthritis

The American Pain Society (APS, 2002) published comprehensive guidelines for the management of osteoarthritis and rheumatoid arthritis. Table 7-5 summarizes pharmacologic and non-pharmacologic management of the diseases and related symptoms.

A practice guideline, Diagnosis and Treatment of Low Back Pain: A Joint Clinical Practice Guideline (Chou et al., 2007),

has been published to help direct the care that primary care providers utilize to diagnose and treat low back pain. These guidelines may be accessed on the American Pain Society website at ampainsoc.org.

Non-Pharmacologic Pain Management

Rehabilitation of the orthopaedic patient involves active participation in pain-relieving strategies. From injury to preoperative, postoperative and recovery phases, non-medicinal treatment can enhance healing and improve functionality (Kolasinski, 2007). Exercise, weight loss, occupational therapy, and physical therapy affect acute outcomes, as well as functional outcomes associated with chronic pain (Stitik & Hochberg, 2007; Ellison, Finley, & Paice, 2002). Although there are some conflicting research outcomes regarding complementary therapies, individual patient benefits versus risks should ultimately determine choices (Table 7-6).

Patient Education

A multitude of studies done on the relationship of preoperative pain education and patient satisfaction with postoperative pain management have consistently demonstrated that education related to pain management will positively influence patient satisfaction and in some studies, decrease pain scores (Niemi-Murola et al., 2007; Oshodi, 2007; Walker, 2007). One of the most important

Table 7-5

Osteoarthritis/ Rheumatoid Arthritis Summary of Guidelines from American Pain Society, (2002)

Degree of Pain	Osteoarthritis	Rheumatoid Arthritis
Mild pain	**Pharmacologic** Acetaminophen up to 4 gm/24 hrs. **Non-pharmacologic** Patient education Cognitive-behavioral strategies Weight loss Exercise 30 minutes most days of week. Physical/occupational therapy Assistive devices Massage	**Pharmacologic** Disease modifying drugs Sulfasalazine Acetaminophen up to 4 gm/24hrs. **Non-pharmacologic** Patient education Cognitive-behavioral strategies Weight loss Exercise 30 minutes most days of week. Physical/occupational therapy Assistive devices
Moderate to severe pain	**Pharmacologic** COX-2 selective NSAID's Non-selective NSAID's +misoprostol Glucosamine Tramadol Neuropathic agents if indicated Intra-articular hyaluronic acid Glucocorticoid injection Opioids Experimental medications **Non-pharmacologic** Continue interventions as with mild pain Consider surgery	**Pharmacologic** Sulfasalazine Methotrexate Leflunomide Biologic therapy COX-2 selective NSAID's Non-selective NSAID's +misoprostol Tricyclic antidepressants Intra-articular hyaluronic acid Topical agents Glucocorticoid injection Opioids Oral glucocorticoids Experimental drugs **Non-pharmacologic** Continue interventions as with mild pain Consider surgery

Chart content developed by Cathy Trame, RN, MS, CNS.

Table 7-6
Non-pharmacologic Pain Management

Modality	Uses (rule-out danger to spinal cord, nerve roots)	Expected Outcomes
Exercise and physical therapy	Orthopaedic injuries Arthritis Radicular pain Spinal stenosis Rotator cuff tears Snapping hip Thoracic outlet syndrome Post Total joint replacement Post Bone stabilization	Improved range of motion. Decreased joint stress and shock. Reduction of pain, emotional stress, depression, and hopelessness.
Thermal treatment – Heat (Deep heat via US may worsen pain in arthritic hips and knees, minimal low back pain relief)	Muscular pain and stiffness.	Improved strength and function. Reduction in stiffness. Reduction of pain and spasm.
Thermal treatment – Cold	Any inflammatory process. Incisional pain.	Reduction of inflammation. Reduction of pain and spasm.
Massage	Muscular pain and stiffness. Contraindicated for bleeding risk, spread of infection, or clot dislodgment.	Reduction of pain and spasm. Stress relief. Improved sleep.
Acupuncture	Rheumatologic disorders. Osteoarthritis. Low back pain. Carpal tunnel syndrome.	Reduction of pain with decreased analgesic use.
Relaxation and Imagery	Low back pain (chronic). Cancer pain. Rheumatoid arthritis (short term).	Diminished stress response. Reduction of pain. Reduction of tight muscles. Reduction in anxiety.
TENS	Low back pain (chronic). CRPS. Orthopaedic surgery.	Reduction of pain.
Electromagnetic Therapy	Osteoarthritic knees. Other joint pain. (No impact on neurogenic pain.)	Reduction of pain.
Therapeutic touch	None proven.	
Weight loss.	Any bone or muscle pain exacerbated by weight bearing.	Reduction of pain.

Chart content developed by Cathy Trame, RN, MS, CNS, 2003.

interventions for patients with chronic conditions such as osteoarthritis is education (Stitik & Hochberg, 2007). Classes, written information, internet education, and care provider discussions have a major impact on patient outcomes and their importance should not be underestimated.

Exercise and Physical Therapy

The benefits of exercise and physical therapy to the patient include improved range of motion, decreased joint stress and joint shock, and reduction of pain. An exercise program should be devised with a professional so that painful conditions are improved rather than exacerbated (Stitik & Hochberg, 2007; Ellison, Finley, & Paice, 2002). If pain is not adequately managed with pharmacotherapy, an exercise program may be avoided or refused by the patient. Practitioners have a responsibility to make sure that pain does not interfere

with the patient's rehabilitation (TJC, 2008). Exercise programs should be encouraged and maintained on a long-term basis. Ultimately, the patient's level of function is expected to improve through exercise, thereby reducing emotional distress, depression, and hopelessness.

Physical therapy has been shown to provide enormous benefits for all types of orthopaedic injuries and diseases including arthritis, radiculopathies from neck or back injuries, spinal stenosis, rotator cuff tears, snapping hip, thoracic outlet syndrome, and post-recovery from total joint replacements or bone stabilization. The physical therapy program should be started after dangerous pathology is excluded and pain control is optimized. Short-term physical therapy for the acute rehabilitation phase should be followed with education regarding long-term maintenance and prophylaxis (Stitik & Hochberg, 2007). Weight loss should be encouraged to reduce the amount of stress on the frame and joints of the body.

Thermal Treatment

Heat application, combined with active exercise with range of motion and strengthening, enhances pain relief. Improvements in strength, function, and stiffness are additional benefits (APS, 2002). Short-term pain relief can be achieved with heat by reducing spasm, increasing relaxation, and improving flexibility. Heat should be reserved for chronic pain versus an acute orthopaedic injury or disease flare with swelling, as heat will induce increased inflammation along with enhanced fluid collection. The resulting increase in swelling and localized congestion may actually worsen the pain (Stitik & Hochberg, 2007). Deep heat via ultrasound may actually worsen pain in arthritic knees and hips (APS, 2002), while providing minimal or no pain relief for chronic low back pain (Acute Low Back Problems Guideline Panel, 1994).

Cold application reduces local inflammation and provides a local anesthetic effect, thereby reducing pain and spasm. Direct application of ice to an incision can enhance analgesic medications by providing local numbing and reducing swelling.

Massage

The stimulation of specific nerve fibers by manipulation of muscles and tissues may block nociceptive impulses from the brain. More intense massage may trigger the release of endogenous opioids, thus mediating the pain signal. Other benefits of massage such as anxiety reduction, stress relief, and improved sleep can all influence pain levels. Contraindications for massage include bleeding risks, spread of infection, and risks of clot dislodgment. After screening for potential risks, massage should be considered as a beneficial adjuvant to medical management in all types of musculoskeletal disorders (Cochrane Reviews, 2009).

Acupuncture

The use of acupuncture has been shown to offer benefits for rheumatologic disorders by reducing pain scores and decreasing analgesic use in some studies, however functionality has not been consistently affected (Kolasinski, 2007). The theory behind acupuncture is that, in the healthy individual, there is normal energy flow through the body called "Qi." When Qi is disrupted, abnormal pathophysiology occurs. Acupuncture is thought to restore the flow of Qi and can be performed with dry needles or with lidocaine.

Osteoarthritis, low back pain, and carpal tunnel syndrome are other conditions that have benefited from acupuncture. Patients with significant degenerative bone changes do not respond to acupuncture as well as others (Elliott et al., 2002; Freedman, 2002).

Relaxation and Imagery

Muscular relaxation, imagery, or distraction techniques can effectively diminish the stress response. These techniques become more effective when practiced over time by training the body's neuromodulation system to respond to learned cues. Release of endorphins and added stimulation to neural circuits reduces the intensity of the pain signal (Bushnell & Basbaum, 2008). There are numerous relaxation and imagery techniques available that can contribute to a relaxed state.

Deep breathing exercises, such as slow inhalation with pursed lip exhalation or progressive muscle relaxation with purposeful release of individual tense muscles, are two of the most commonly practiced techniques. These exercises are easy to teach and practice at the bedside. Effective imagery requires the individual to be able to remove himself from the present. Imagining, on a regular basis, a substance dissolving an object that represents the pain can provide effective pain control. Autogenic relaxation combines mental and physical stimuli along with passive concentration. Reductions in anxiety and pain have provided some benefit for low back pain and cancer-related pain. Muscle relaxation training for individuals with rheumatoid arthritis provided short-term improvements in function (6 months) but no long-term improvement after 12 months (APS, 2002). Since anxiety was associated with greater pain, worse function, and more use of resources in the first year after TKA, relaxation techniques may be of benefit to patients experiencing anxiety (Brander, Gondek, Martin, & Stulberg, 2007).

Transcutaneous Electrical Nerve Stimulation (TENS)

TENS therapy, typically initiated by a physical therapist, provides stimulation to peripheral nerves that transmit a vibration signal to the brain. Evidence suggests that the distraction effect of tying up neural circuits, an endorphin effect from the nerve stimulation, and a placebo effect all contribute to improved analgesia from the TENS unit. TENS units improved visual analog pain scores with decreased analgesic use for chronic back pain in elderly patients (Grant, Bishop-Miller, Winchester, & Faulkner, 1999). TENS has also been shown to decrease analgesic use in patients with complex regional pain syndrome (Greene, 2001). A 2009 Cochrane review showed that TENS provided analgesic relief as compared to placebo in patients with osteoarthritic knees (Osiri et al., 2009), and for the treatment of rheumatoid arthritis in the hand (Brosseau et al., 2009).

Orthopaedic surgery is just one type of surgery that has been shown to benefit from TENS application postoperatively, although it is rarely used (Acute Pain Management Guideline Panel, 1992). The use of TENS should be considered and trialed as an adjuvant treatment for all types of orthopaedic pain since there are virtually no side effects associated with this therapy.

Magnetic Therapy

Electromagnetic therapy is thought to influence the relationship between the atoms in the body with the external environment (Jacobson, Gorman, Yamanashi, Saxena, & Clayton, 2001). Because of this magnetic interaction between atoms, biological systems can be altered. Jacobson, et al. (2001) have demonstrated a significant reduction in pain associated with osteoarthritic knees by exposing the knees to low-amplitude magnetic fields. A 49% reduction in pain scores was achieved after 2 weeks of electromagnetic therapy (176 patients were randomized into a placebo or treatment group). Magnetic therapy has only shown benefits for joint pain and has little impact on neurogenic pain (Jenkner, 2002). Modest improvements in pain were noted in two studies related to osteoarthritis (Hulme, Welch, deBie, Judd, & Tugwell, 2009). Exciting research will unveil future applications for magnetic therapy but more research is urgently needed. The topical application of therapeutic magnets has not conclusively been proven effective for pain relief; however, minimal risk is involved with a trial of this modality.

Other

Multiple other modalities could be discussed; however, little conclusive research is available related to quality outcomes for orthopaedic patients. As a general rule, if a complementary therapy is perceived to be helpful to the patient and does not cause harm, it should be employed.

Pain and Addiction

The use of opioids for pain control is influenced by practitioners' and patients' fears of addiction. Patients may restrict their own opioid use based on personal fears or fear of being judged by friends or family members. The question naturally arises: do clinicians create addiction by prescribing opioids for pain control? Statistically, opioid addiction rarely occurs related to the use of medicines to treat pain. In a landmark study by Porter & Jick (1980), the incidence of potential addiction related to an acute pain episode in a hospital was 4 in 12,000 patients, or a mere 0.03%. Other studies related to prescribing opioids for chronic malignant or non-malignant pain over extended periods of time, indicate addiction rates that are higher than with acute treatment, so treatment and outcomes should be monitored. The American Society of the Interventional Pain Physicians (ASIPP) produced an extensive guideline in 2008 for the use of opioids in the management of chronic non-cancer pain (Trescot et al., 2008). The guideline provides useful information for structuring a treatment plan for the patient that is on opioids for an extended period beyond the acute phase of recovery. The concept of true addiction is often poorly defined and misconstrued by the public. Tolerance, physical dependence, and addiction are frequently erroneously used interchangeably, creating confusion for patients and health care workers. Consequently, people with severe pain problems may be under-treated related to addictive labels.

The American Academy of Pain Medicine (AAPM), American Pain Society (APS), and the American Society of Addiction Medicine (ASAM) jointly issued a consensus paper in 2001 that clearly defined the differences among addiction, tolerance, and physical dependence (American Pain Foundation, 2001). Addiction is defined as "a primary chronic, neurobiologic disease, with genetic, psychosocial, and environmental factors influencing its development and manifestations. It is characterized by behaviors that include one or more of the following: impaired control over drug use, compulsive use, continued use despite harm, and

craving" (AAPM, APS, & ASAM Consensus Statement published by American Pain Foundation, 2001). Even the most astute practitioner may have difficulty discriminating addictive behaviors from behaviors manifested as a result of poor pain management. These behaviors, labeled as "pseudoaddiction", escalate when painful conditions are under-treated. The victim may develop cunning or creative ways to attempt self-treatment or exhibit dramatic outbursts to convince health care practitioners that their pain is real. Clock-watching, hoarding opioids during periods of remission to be used for painful exacerbations, aggressive complaining about symptoms, or even openly acquiring drugs from additional medical sources may occur.

Physical dependence often develops in patients taking opioids for an extended period. Dependence is more common than tolerance. Dependence is "a state of adaptation that is manifested by a drug class specific withdrawal syndrome that can be produced by abrupt cessation, rapid dose reduction, decreasing blood level of the drug, and/or administration of an antagonist" (AAPM, APS, & ASAM Consensus Statement published by American Pain Foundation, 2001). Patients may shamefully describe themselves as addicted because they have attempted to reduce or stop their opioids and experienced withdrawal symptoms.

"Tolerance is a state of adaptation in which exposure to a drug induces changes that result in a diminution of one or more of the drug's effects over time" (AAPM, APS, & ASAM Consensus Statement published by American Pain Foundation, 2001). Since cross-tolerance among opioids in the same class is not universal, opioid rotation is recommended to maintain the lowest possible analgesic requirement while minimizing side effects.

Treatment of acute pain is typically less complex than chronic pain because the duration of pain is shorter, predictable, and follows a typical course of improvement. Baseline requirements of long-acting opioids to replace existing opioid usage and/or illicit drug use are necessary to adequately manage the additional acute needs. Management of the acute situation includes immediate bolusing to meet increased opioid requirements with titration to level of comfort. Although patient controlled analgesia (PCA) may be controversial due to self-controlled dosing, PCA usage may actually be preferential because dosing is not reliant on potentially judgmental caregiver decision-making. The intravenous route characteristically induces a "rush" or euphoric effect and should be discontinued as soon as oral opioids are tolerated. When indicated, regional analgesia such as nerve blocks or epidural analgesia should be employed to reduce opioid requirements during the acute phase. Continuous epidural or local anesthetic infusions postoperatively may eliminate the need for intravenous opioids.

Advancement to less potent oral analgesics can be employed when the epidural or local infusion is discontinued. The media has widely publicized that long-acting oral preparations of opioids, when improperly crushed and injected, could be considered to be highly addictive and widely abused. When opioids need to be used, the patient's preferred drug of abuse should be avoided, and a single opioid agent should be utilized whenever possible. Around-the-clock dosing should be employed on a scheduled basis at a specific time; for example 8:00 a.m., 2:00 p.m., and 9:00 p.m. Current technology, which is FDA approved in the U.S., provides a long-acting oral opioid packaged in a liposome that will release an antagonist if crushed, thus negating the euphoric effects of the drug. This technology will continue to be employed with new long-acting analgesics.

Adjuvant medications, as with any pain management regimen, should be maximized to decrease or eliminate opioid requirements. General principles of adjuvant use for pain management, as outlined by the American Pain Society (2008), should be instituted. Use of around-the-clock non-steroidal anti-inflammatory drugs (NSAIDs) should be employed except when contraindicated. Alternative substitution with acetaminophen to a maximum of 4 grams per day should be prescribed when NSAIDs are not feasible. Specific adjuvants for neuropathic pain, such as anticonvulsants and tricylic antidepressants or SNRI's, should be employed around-the-clock for chronic syndromes. In addition to other adjuvants, muscle relaxants should be utilized to reduce painful spasms that exacerbate the pain reaction.

Certainly, a multidisciplinary approach with a team including psychiatry, psychology, addictionology, and pain management specialists, will illicit ideal outcomes for patient management. The treatment plan should be formulated with the patient, and agreed upon, preferably with obtainment of the patient's signature. In essence, the patient is entering into a contractual agreement with the care provider. A copy of the written plan should be provided to the patient. For an acute pain situation, specific parameters regarding length of opioid use, taper, and anticipated time of discontinuance should be discussed. If treatment is for a chronic pain problem, specifics about the use of one prescribing physician for opioids, rules regarding lost prescriptions, random urine screening, and parameters for relapse should be discussed and included in the plan. Frequent office visits to the opioid prescriber should be scheduled, with a one-week supply of opioid ordered at a time to reduce the risk of potential overuse or overdose in the known addict.

Non-pharmacologic adjuvants such as physical therapy, transcutaneous electrical stimulation (TENS), heat, ice, relaxation, imagery, massage, and acupuncture should be offered when appropriate for either acute or chronic pain. Other therapies for chronic back pain such as dorsal column stimulators may be effective for some patients. Documentation of pain treatment with opioids should include a complete description of the characteristics of the pain with measurable scoring, frequency of the pain (often tracked with a diary for chronic pain), amount of analgesic being used, functionality including activities of daily living, work, leisure, and sleep habits, and any evidence of relapse or opioid misuse. Guidelines for treatment and follow-up should be based on "Clinical Guidelines for Chronic Opioid Therapy in Patients with Noncancer Pain" (APS/AAPM, 2009). Documentation serves to protect the nurse and/or physician in the event a regulatory agency would investigate,

while maximizing the patient's pain management from a global perspective.

Structured detoxification after acute recovery, as well as rehabilitation, may be indicated. Support groups that offer psychological support and enhance coping ability are an important part of the recovery process for the addict. Relapse is very common and considered a normal part of addiction recovery. Controlling risks of relapse such as increased stress, negativity, money accessibility, free time, and poor support mechanisms will reduce the most common triggers of relapse.

Geriatric Considerations

Assessment of pain in the geriatric patient can be challenging. Elderly patients may view pain as a personal weakness, a punishment, or an impending disease, and may be reluctant to report it. Pain can be viewed as a segway to loss of independence. Many elderly also fear addiction to pain medications (Barkin, Barkin, & Barkin, 2007). Terms used by elderly to describe pain may be different than those used by younger individuals, such as "sore", "achy", or "stiff". Presence of pain in the elderly may also be complicated by depression and isolation (Barba, Tesh, & Kohlenberg, 2007). All of these influences impact the degree of pain, and how and when the patient may report pain.

Medication management may be challenging as well. Geriatric patients experience a decline in renal clearance and liver metabolism as a normal part of aging. The inability to effectively clear metabolites of the opioids makes this population more vulnerable to confusion, opioid oversedation, and respiratory depression. Ideally, non-opioid medications, non-pharmacologic interventions, and nerve blocks should be used whenever possible in order to minimize the opioid requirement for the older adult. Medication selection should cause the least amount of central nervous system depression possible.

The American Geriatric Society (AGS) issued a statement in May 2009 indicating that for patients aged 75 or older, "NSAID's and COX-2 Inhibitors should be used rarely since the risks related to hypertension, heart failure, and renal failure outweigh benefits. Opioid therapy should be considered if the elderly patient has moderate to severe pain, or a diminished quality of life" (AGS, 2009). As with all medications, the benefits must outweigh the risks. When opioids need to be employed, one should start low and go slow until the patient's tolerance is determined.

Certain opioids should be avoided in the older adult related to reduced creatinine clearance. These include propoxyphene (Darvocet®) and meperidine (Demerol®) (Barkin et al., 2007). Both of these drugs have metabolites that accumulate and cause neurotoxicity. Metabolites of propoxyphene can also cause cardiac dysrhythmias and pulmonary edema. As with all patients, particularly the elderly, methadone should only be used by practitioners familiar with prescribing the drug.

Many adjuvant medications used to treat neuropathic pain such as anticonvulsants, tricyclic antidepressants, serotonin norepinephrine re-uptake inhibitors (SNRI's), and local anesthetic patches, can be cost-prohibitive for someone on a fixed income with limited prescription coverage. Long-acting opioid agents tend to be more costly than short-acting agents. It is important to determine the patient's ability to pay for their prescriptions and work with the physician to make sure the medications are affordable for the patient.

Constipation is a major concern when patients lack mobility. In the geriatric patient, the risk of constipation is complicated by age and pain medications. Bowel prophylaxis with a stool softener, coupled with a stimulant, should be employed on a scheduled basis a minimum of twice daily. The bowel regimen should be continued as long as the patient requires opioids and/or is immobile.

Summary

Orthopaedic pain involves multiple facets of care. Immediate treatment of the source of pain through stabilization, disease management and/or surgery, in conjunction with aggressive pain management, provides the best outcome for the patient. There is mounting evidence that chronic pain can be prevented by the implementation of multi-modal analgesic strategies as early as possible in the acute phase (Bushnell & Basbaum, 2008). Pain should not be allowed to interfere with active rehabilitation or quality of life. The nurse can be the patient's advocate to promote a comfortable and functional recovery.

References

Acute Low Back Problems Guideline Panel (1994). *Acute low back problems in adults.* AHCPR Pub. No. 95-0642. Rockville, MD: Agency for Health Care Policy and Research.

Acute Pain Management Guideline Panel (1992). *Acute pain management: Operative or medical procedures and trauma.* AHCPR Pub. No.92-0032. Rockville, MD: Agency for Health Care Policy and Research.

American Academy of Orthopaedic Surgeons (2007). *Total knee replacement.* Retrieved August 18, 2009, from http://orthoinfo.aaos.org/

American Geriatric Society (2009). *Pharmacological management of persistent pain in older persons.* Retrieved August 18, 2009, from http://www.americangeriatrics.org/education/final_recommendations.pdf

American Pain Foundation (2001). Addiction, physical dependence, tolerance. Confused? *The Pain Connection,* Spring, 2001, p.1, 4.

American Pain Foundation (2009). *Chronic pain and opioid treatment.* Retrieved August 18, 2009, from http://www.painfoundation.org/Publications/OpioidTherapy.pdf

American Pain Foundation (2009). *Pain facts and figures.* Retrieved August 18, 2009, from http://www.painfoundation.org/page/asp?file=Newsroom/PainFacts.htm

American Pain Society (2002). *Guideline for the management of pain in osteoarthritis, rheumatoid arthritis, and juvenile chronic arthritis.* Glenview, IL: American Pain Society.

American Pain Society (2008). *Principles of analgesic use in the treatment of acute and cancer pain* (6th ed.). Glenview, IL: Amertican Pain Society.

American Pain Society/American Academy of Pain Medicine (2009). *The use of opioids for the treatment of chronic pain.* A consensus statement from the American Academy of Pain Medicine and the American Pain Society. Retrieved August 18, 2009, from http://www.ampainsoc.org/advocacy/opioids.htm

American Society of Regional Anesthesia (2002). *Neuraxial anesthesia and anticoagulation. Consensus statements.* Chicago, IL: American Society of Regional Anesthesia.

Aveline, C., Hetet, H., Vautier, P., Gautier, J., & Bonnet, F. (2006). Preoperative ketamine and morphine for postoperative pain control after lumbar disk surgery. *European Journal of Pain, 10*(7), 653-658.

Barba, B., Tesh, A., & Kohlenberg, E. (2007). Recognize the many facets of gerontological nursing. *Nursing Management, 38*(1), 35-41.

Barclay, L., & Lie, D. (2008). Patients may need better pain interventions after traumatic injury. *Archives of Surgery, 143*(3), 282-287.

Barkin, R., Barkin, S., & Barkin, D. (2007). Pharmacotherapeutic management of pain with a focus directed at the geriatric patient. *Rheumatic Disease Clinics of North America, 33,* 1-31.

Becker, N., Sjorgen, P., Bech, P., Olsen, A., & Eriksen, J. (2000). Treatment outcomes of chronic non-malignant pain patients managed in a Danish multidisciplinary pain center compared to general practice. A randomized controlled trial. *Pain, 84*(1), 203-211.

Brander, V., Gondek, S., Martin, E., & Stulberg, S. (2007). Pain and depression influence outcome 5 years after knee replacement surgery. *Clinical Orthopaedics and Related Research, 464,* 21-26.

Briggs, K., & Martin, F. (2008). Target processing is facilitated by motivationally relevant cues. *Biological Psychology 78*(1), 29-42.

Brookoff, D. (2000). Chronic pain: 1. A new disease. *Hospital Practice, 35*(7), 45-59.

Brosseau, L., Yonge, K., Welch, V., Marchand, S., Judd, M., Wells, G., … Tugwell, P. (2009). *Transcutaneous electrical nerve stimulation (TENS) for the treatment of rheumatoid arthritis in the hand.* Retrieved August 18, 2009, from http://www.cochrane.org/reviews/en/ab004377.html

Bushnell, M., & Basbaum, A. (2008). The senses: A comprehensive reference. *Pain, 5.* Philadelphia: Elsevier.

Charalambous, C., Tryfonidis, M., Alvi, F., Kumar, R., & Hirst, P. (2006). Purely intra-articular versus general anesthesia for proposed arthroscopic partial meniscectomy of the knee: A randomized controlled trial. *Arthroscopy, 22*(9), 972.

Chou, R., Qaseem, A., Snow, V., Casey, D., Cross, T., Shekelle, P., … Owens, D. (2007). Diagnosis and treatment of low back pain: A joint clinical practice guideline from the American College of Physicians and the American Pain Society. *Annals of Internal Medicine, 147*(7), 478-91.

Cochrane Reviews (2009). *Massage.* Retrieved August 18, 2009, from www.cochrane.org/reviews/en/index_list_m.html

Dagenais, S. (2006). Intra-articular hyaluronic acid (viscosupplementation) for knee osteoarthritis. *Issues in Emergency Health Technology, 94,* 1-4.

DeRuyter, M., Brueilly, K., Harrison, B., Greengrass, R., Putzke, J., & Brodersen, M. (2006). A pilot study on continuous femoral perineural catheter for analgesia after total knee arthroplasty. *The Journal of Arthroplasty, 21*(8), 1111-1117.

DuPen, A., Shen, D., & Ersek, M. (2007). Mechanisms of opioid-induced tolerance and hyperalgesia. *Pain Management Nursing, 8*(3), 113-121.

Duarte, V., Fallis, W., Slonowsky, D., Kwarteng, K., & Yeung, C. (2006). Effectiveness of femoral nerve blockade for pain control after total knee arthroplasy. *Journal of PeriAnesthesia Nursing, 21*(5), 311-316.

Elliott, J., Knox, K., Renaud, E., St.Marie, B., Sharoff, L., Swift, M., … Vanni, L. (2002). Chronic pain management. In B. St.Marie (Ed.), *Core curriculum for pain management nursing* (pp. 273-347). New York: W.B. Saunders.

Ellison, N., Finley, R., & Paice, J. (2002). Achieving pain relief in osteoarthritis. Dannemiller Memorial Educational *Foundation Pain Report, 1*(4), 6-7.

Freedman, J. (2002). An audit of 500 acupuncture patients in general practice. *Acupuncture Medicine, 20*(1), 30-34.

Gagliese, L., Weizblit, N., Ellis, W., & Chan, V. (2005). The measurement of postoperative pain: A comparison of intensity scales in younger and older surgical patients. *Pain, 117*(3), 412-420.

Galinski, M., Dolveck, F., Combes, X., Limoges, V., Smail, N., Pommier, V., ...Adnet, F. (2007). Management of severe acute pain in emergency settings: Ketamine reduces morphine consumption. *American Journal of Emergency Medicine, 25*(4), 385-390.

Glassman, S., Rose, S., Dimar, J, Puno, R., Campbell, M., & Johnson, J. (1998). The effect of postoperative nonsteroidal anti-inflammatory drug administration on spinal fusion. *Spine, 23*(7), 834-838.

Grant, D., Bishop-Miller, J., Winchester, M., & Faulkner, S. (1999). A randomized comparative trial of acupuncture versus transcutaneous electrical nerve stimulation for chronic back pain in elderly. *Pain, 82*(1), 9-13.

Greene, W. (Ed.) (2001). Reflex sympathetic dystrophy and complex regional pain syndromes. In *Essentials of musculoskeletal care* (2nd ed., pp. 65-68). Rosemont, IL: American Academy of Orthopaedic Surgeons.

Heit, H., & Gilson, A. (2008). DEA: Revisited. *Pain Medicine, 9*(7), 924-926.

Herr, K., Coyne, P., Key, T., Manworren, R., McCaffery, M., Merkel, S., ...& Wild, L. (2006). Pain assessment in the nonverbal patient: Position statement with clinical practice recommendations. *Pain Management Nursing, 7*(2), 44-52.

Holmquist, G. (2001). Drug decisions for patients with chronic non-cancer pain syndromes. *Drug Benefit Trends*, May 2001, 1-12.

Huang,Y., Wang, C.M., Wang, C.T., Lin, W., Horng, L., & Jiang, C. (2008). Perioperative celecoxib administration for pain management after total knee arthroplasty –A randomized, controlled study. *BMC Musculoskeletal Disorders, 3*(9), 77.

Hulme, J., Welch, V., deBie, R., Judd, M., & Tugwell, P. (2009). *Electromagnetic fields for the treatment of osteoarthritis.* Retrieved August 18, 2009, from http://www.cochrane.org/reviews/en/ab003523.html

Idvall, E., Berg, K., Unosson, M., & Brudin, L. (2005). Differences between nurse and patient assessments on postoperative pain management in two hospitals. *Journal of Evaluation in Clinical Practice, 11*(5), 444-451.

Jacobson, J., Gorman, R., Yamanashi, W., Saxena, B., & Clayton, L. (2001). Low amplitude, extremely low frequency magnetic fields for the treatment of osteoarthritic knees: A double blind clinical study. *Alternative Therapies, 7*(5), 54-65.

Jenkner, F. (2002). A global view of evolving pain treatment modalities. *Practice Pain Management, 2*(4), 29-33.

Katzung, B. (Ed.) (2007). Basic and clinical pharmacology (10th ed.). New York: McGraw-Hill.

Klasen, J., Haas, M., Graf, S., Harbach, H., Quinzio, L., Jürgensen, I., ... Hempelmann, G. (2005). Impact on postoperative pain of long-lasting pre-emptive epidural analgesia before total hip replacement: A prospective, randomized, double-blind study. *Anaesthesia, 60*(2), 118-123.

Kolasinski, S. (2007). Complementary and alternative medicine. In Moskowitz, R., Altman, R., Hochberg, M., Buckwalter, J., & Goldberg, V. (Eds.), *Osteoarthritis: Diagnosis and medical-surgical management* (4th ed., pp.303-311). Philadelphia: Lippincott, Williams, & Wilkins.

Larijani, G., Sharaf, I., Warshal, D., Marr, A., Gratz, I., & Goldberg, M. (2005). Pain evaluation in patients receiving intravenous patient-controlled analgesia after surgery. *Pharmacotherapy, 25*(9), 1168-1173.

Long, J., Lewis, S., Kuklo, T., Zhu, Y., & Riew, K. (2002). The effect of cyclooxygenase-2 inhibitors on spinal fusion. *The Journal of Bone and Joint Surgery, 84-A*(10), 1763-1768.

McCaffery, M. (1968). *Nursing practice theories related to cognition, bodily pain, and man-environment interactions.* Los Angeles: UCLA Students Store.

Ménigaux, C., Adam, F., Guignard, B., Sessler, D., & Chauvin, M. (2005). Preoperative gabapentin decreases anxiety and improves early functional recovery from knee surgery. *Anesthesia and Analgesia, 100*(5), 1394-1399.

Montazeri, K., Kashefi, P., & Honarmand, A. (2007). Pre-emptive gabapentin significantly reduces postoperative pain and morphine demand following lower extremity orthopaedic surgery. *Singapore Medical Journal, 48*(8), 748-751.

Munro, H., Walton, S., Malviya, S., Merkel, S., Voepel-Lewis, T., Loder, R., ...Farley, F. (2002). Low dose ketorolac improves analgesia and reduces morphine requirements following posterior spinal fusion in adolescents. *Canadian Journal of Anaesthesia, 49*(5), 461-466.

National Center for Health Statistics (2007). *Center for Disease Control.* Retrieved August 18, 2009, from http://www.cdc.gov/obesity/data/index.html

Neustadt, D., & Altman, R. (2007). Intra-articular therapy. In R. Moskowitz, R. Altman, M. Hochberg, J. Buckwalter, & V. Goldberg (Eds.), *Osteoarthritis. Diagnosis and medical/surgical management* (4th ed., pp. 287-301). Philadelphia: Lippincott, Williams, & Wilkins.

Niemi-Murola, L., Poyhia, R., Onkinen, K., Rhen, B., Makela, A., & Niemi, T. (2007). Patient satisfaction with postoperative pain management – Effect of preoperative factors. *Pain Management Nursing, 8*(3), 122-129.

Oshodi, T. (2007). The impact of preoperative education on postoperative pain. Part 1. *British Journal of Nursing, 16*(12), 706-710.

Oshodi, T. (2007). The impact of preoperative education on postoperative pain. Part 2. *British Journal of Nursing, 16*(13), 790-797.

Osiri, M., Welch, V., Brosseau, L., Shea, B., McGowan, J., Tugwell, P., ... Wells, G. (2009). *Transcutaneous electrical nerve stimulation for knee osteoarthritis.* Retrieved August 18, 2009, from http://www.cochrane.org/reviews/en/ab002823.html

Petkas, Z., Sener, M., Bayram, B., Eroglu, T., Bozdogan, N., Donmez, A., ...Uckan, S. (2007). A comparison of preemptive analgesic efficacy of diflunisal and lornoxicam for postoperative pain management: A prospective, randomized, single-blind, crossover study. *International Journal of Oral and Maxillofacial Surgery, 36*(2), 123-127.

Petrella, R., & Petrella, M. (2006). A prospective, randomized, double-blind, placebo controlled study to evaluate the efficacy of intraarticular hyaluronic acid for osteoarthritis of the knee. *Journal of Rheumatology, 33*(5), 951-956.

Pham Dang, C., Gautheron, E., Guilley, J., Fernandez, M., Waast, D., Volteau, C., ...Pinaud, M. (2005). The value of adding sciatic block to continuous femoral block for analgesia after total knee replacement. *Regional Anesthesia and Pain Medicine, 30*(2), 128-133.

Physicians' Desk Reference 2009 (2008). (63rd ed.). Montvale, NJ: Medical Economics.

Porter, J., & Jick, H. (1980). Addiction rare in patients treated with narcotics. *New England Journal of Medicine, 302*(2), 123.

Prabhakar, H., Arora, R., Bithal, P., Rath, G., & Dash, H. (2007). The analgesic effects of preemptive gabapentin in patients undergoing surgery for brachial plexus injury – A preliminary study. *Journal of Neurosurgical Anesthesiologists, 19*(4), 235-238.

Puntillo, K., Pasero, C., Li, D., Mularski, R., Grap, M., Erstad, B., ... Sessler, C. (2009). Evaluation of pain in ICU patients. *Chest, 135*(4), 1069-1074.

Rawe, C., Trame, C., Moddeman, G., O'Malley, P., Biteman, K., Dalton, T., ...Walker, S. (2009). Management of procedural pain: Empowering nurses to care for patients through clinical nurse specialist consultation and intervention. *Clinical Nurse Specialist, 23*(3), 131-137.

Riest, G., Peters, J., Weiss, M., Dreyer, S., Klassen, P., Stegen, B., ... Eikermann, M. (2008). Preventive effects of preoperative parecoxib on post-discectomy pain. *British Journal of Anesthesia, 100*(2), 256-262.

Salinas, F., Liu, S., & Mulroy, M. (2006). The effect of single-injection femoral nerve block versus continuous femoral nerve block after total knee arthroplasty on hospital length of stay and long-term functional recovery within an established clinical pathway. *Anesthesia and Analgesia, 102*, 1234-1239.

Sharrock, N. (2002). Postoperative pain management. In G. Scuderi, & A. Tria, (Eds.), Surgical techniques in total knee arthroplasty (pp.680-86). New York: Springer-Verlag.

Simon, A., Manigrasso, M., & O'Connor, J.P. (2002). Cyclo-oxygenase 2 function is essential for bone fracture healing. *Journal of Bone and Mineral Research, 17*(6), 963-975.

Sloman, R., Rosen, G., Rom, M., & Shir, Y. (2005). Nurses' assessment of pain in surgical patients. *Journal of Advanced Nursing, 52*(2), 125-132.

Stitik, T., & Hochberg, M. (2007). Baseline program. In R. Moskowitz, R. Altman, M. Hochberg, J. Buckwalter, & V. Goldberg (Eds.), Osteoarthritis. Diagnosis and medical/surgical management (4th ed., pp. 257-65). Philadelphia: Lippincott, Williams, & Wilkins.

Sucato, D., Lovejoy, J., Agrawal, S., Elerson, E., Nelson, T., & McClung, A. (2008). Postoperative ketorolac does not predispose to pseudoarthrosis following posterior spinal fusion and instrumentation for adolescent idiopathic scoliosis. *Spine, 33*(10), 1119-1124.

Sundarathiti, P. (2009). A comparison of continuous femoral nerve block and continuous epidural infusion in postoperative analgesia and knee rehabilitation after total knee arthroplasty. *Journal of the Medical Association of Thailand, 92*(3), 328-334.

Swartz, D., Mobley, E., & Felix, E. (2009). Bile reflux after Roux-en-Y gastric bypass: An unrecognized cause of postoperative pain. *Surgery for Obesity and Related Diseases, 5*, 27-30.

Takada, M., Fukusaki, M., Terao, Y., Yamashita, K., Inadomi, C., Takada, M., ...Sumikawa, K. (2007). *Journal of Clinical Anesthesia, 19*(2), 97-100.

Tennant, F., Liu, J., & Hermann, L. (2002). Intractable pain. *Practical Pain Management, 2*(3), 8-11.

The Joint Commission (TJC) (2008). *The 2009 comprehensive accreditation manual for hospitals: The official handbook.* Oakbrook Terrace, IL: The Joint Commission.

Toivonene, J., Pitko, V., & Rosenberg, P. (2007). Etoricoxib pre-medication combined with intra-operative subacromial block for pain after arthroscopic acromioplasty. *Acta Anaesthesiology Scandanavica, 51*(3), 316-321.

Trescot, A., Helm, S., Hansen, H., Benyamin, R., Glaser, S., Adlaka, R., ...Manchikanti, L. (2008). Opioids in the management of chronic non-cancer pain: An update of American Society of the Interventional Pain Physicians' Guidelines. *Pain Physician, 11*, S5-S62.

Tuzuner, A., Ucok, C., Kucukyavuz, Z., Alkis, N., & Alanoglu, Z. (2007). Preoperative diclofenac sodium and tramadol for pain relief after bimaxillary osteotomy. *Journal of Oral and Maxillofacial Surgery, 65*(12), 2453-2458.

U.S. Drug Enforcement Agency (2009). *Drug abuse prevention and control.* In U.S. Drug Enforcement Administration, Food and drugs. Retrieved August 18, 2009, from http://www.usdoj.gov/dea/pubs/csa.html

United Nations Population Division, DESA (2006). *World population aging 1950-2050. Demographic determinants of population aging.* Retrieved August 18, 2009, from http://www.un.org/esa/population/publications/worldageing19502050/index.htm

Walker, J. (2007). What is the effect of preoperative information on patient satisfaction? *British Journal of Nursing, 16*(1), 27-32.

Wong, D. L., Hockenberry-Eaton, M., Wilson, D., Winkelstein, M. L. & Schwartz, P. (2001). *Wong's essentials of pediatric nursing* (p. 1301). St. Louis: Mosby.

Yamashita, K., Fukusaki, M., Ando, Y., Fujinaga, A., Tanabe, T., Terao, Y., & Sumikawa, K. (2006). Preoperative administration of intravenous flurbiprofen axetil reduces postoperative pain for spinal fusion surgery. *Journal of Anesthesia, 21*(2), 294.

Complications Associated With Orthopaedic Conditions and Surgeries

Nancy Morris, PhD, APRN

Objectives

- Identify risk factors for select complications associated with orthopaedic conditions and surgical procedures.

- Initiate interventions to prevent or minimize complications associated with orthopaedic conditions and surgical procedures.

- Provide the education and counseling necessary for the patient and family regarding the prevention and treatment of complications associated with orthopaedic conditions and surgical procedures.

Key Terms

Allogenic blood: blood taken from a different individual than the one receiving it.

Autologous blood: blood donated from the same individual who will be receiving it.

Delirium: a disturbance of consciousness with reduced ability to focus, sustain, or shift attention; a change in cognition (memory deficit, disorientation, language disturbance); or the development of a perceptual disturbance that occurs over a short period of time and tends to fluctuate over the course of the day.

Fasciotomy: incision of the connective sheath that separates or holds together a group of muscles.

Gastrocolic reflex: a sensory stimulus that causes strong peristaltic waves in the colon when food enters the stomach.

Pulse Pressure: the difference between systolic and diastolic blood pressure.

Total knee arthroplasty, laminectomy, open reduction and internal fixation of the distal radius, and tibial rodding are all examples of orthopaedic surgical procedures performed daily with predominantly positive outcomes. Surgical interventions, however, are not without risk. Successful outcomes are a reflection of the knowledge, skill, and collaborative efforts of the entire health care team. Quality perioperative care provided by the health care team with the appropriate equipment and adequate resources is essential to optimal outcomes.

Identification of risk factors and patient characteristics that increase the likelihood of complications after orthopaedic surgery enable the health care team to be proactive rather than reactive. Early identification of risk and timely initiation of interventions will help to prevent and minimize complications. Complications associated with orthopaedic injuries and procedures can be significant such as venous thromboembolic conditions, compartment syndrome, fat embolism syndrome, delirium, hemorrhage, and surgical site infection. Other complications that can occur during the postoperative period include hospital acquired pneumonia, nausea and vomiting, constipation, urinary retention, and impaired skin integrity.

A brief explanation of the pathophysiology and medical management of these complications will lead to a discussion of nursing assessment, interventions, and outcome indicators. The specific complications identified and the associated nursing care apply to most orthopaedic conditions and surgical procedures requiring an overnight hospital stay.

General Risk Factors Related to Surgical Procedures

A thorough assessment will help the nurse with early recognition of potential postoperative complications. Knowledge of specific risk factors will enable the nurse to design a plan of care to prevent or minimize complications and contribute to optimal outcomes after surgery.

In general, increasing age is associated with increased rates of morbidity, functional dependence, and mortality after surgery (Finlayson & Birkmeyer, 2009). This is related to the normal physiologic changes of aging as well as the increasing likelihood of comorbidities. Older adults are thus at increased risk for complications requiring early initiation of preventative strategies and increased attentiveness to the signs and symptoms of the onset of complications.

Comorbidity is also a risk factor for complications after surgery. Pulmonary complications are increased in patients with reactive airway disease, chronic obstructive pulmonary disease, significant kyphosis, and in those who smoke tobacco. Increased risk for poor wound healing, surgical site infections, and impaired skin integrity are seen in patients with diabetes and in immunocompromised, obese, or malnourished patients. Cardiovascular complications are increased in patients with symptomatic or significant arrhythmias, unstable angina, congestive heart failure, severe valvular disease, and in those who have had a myocardial infarction within 30 days (Fleisher et al., 2007). The risk for impaired skin integrity is higher in patients with depression,

impaired nutritional status, and altered sensory perception. Venous thromboembolic events are seen more frequently in patients with malignancy, varicose veins, obesity, congestive heart failure, stroke, deficiencies in the clotting cascade, and pregnancy. Awareness of the risks associated with specific medical conditions prompts the nurse to target interventions and hopefully prevent the occurrence of complications.

Medication use can also influence recovery. Drugs such as warfarin, corticosteroids, and nonsteroidal anti-inflammatory drugs can negatively affect healing, bleeding, and coagulation (Wallvik, Själander, Johansson, Bjuhr, & Jansson, 2007). The risk for a thromboembolic event may be increased in patients who take oral contraceptives or hormone replacement therapy (Lidegaard, Lokkegaard, Svendsen, & Agger, 2009). Postoperative use of opioids increases the likelihood of constipation (Holzer, 2008). Postoperative delirium may be precipitated or aggravated by the use of drugs with anticholinergic effects (Hshieh, Fong, Marcantonio, & Inouye, 2008). A review of all medications that a patient is using is an important aspect in determining the risk for postoperative complications.

The nature and circumstances of an injury itself may be associated with increased risk of infection. Bone displacement, comminution of the bone, multiple bone involvement, vascular injury with compromised perfusion, significant soft tissue injury, an open fracture, and wound contamination all increase the risk of infection. Prolonged time between injury and stabilization of fractured bones not only increases the risk of infection but also increases the risk for soft-tissue injury, vascular compromise, and fat embolism syndrome, especially if the injury involves a long bone.

Patients are at risk for complications beginning at the time of injury or surgery and extending throughout the recovery period. Identification of risk and initiation of appropriate interventions to prevent or minimize complications is an important role for the orthopaedic nurse.

Venous Thromboembolic Conditions

Venous thromboembolic conditions (VTE) of primary concern in the postoperative period include deep vein thrombosis (DVT) and pulmonary embolism (PE). The frequency of these conditions is difficult to assess since many venous thromboses and pulmonary emboli are clinically silent. Diagnostic efforts are also not very sensitive or specific, making definitive diagnosis more difficult. VTEs are the most common life-threatening complications associated with major orthopaedic surgery of the hip and knee. It is important for nurses to be aware of the risk factors for VTE, strategies that can be used to minimize the risk, and early signs and symptoms of VTE so that treatment measures can be instituted in a timely manner when needed.

Pathophysiology

A thrombus is a fibrin clot. Following injury to a blood vessel, prothrombin is converted to thrombin. Thrombin then prompts the conversion of fibrinogen to fibrin, and a fibrin plug forms to reduce the flow of blood from a ruptured vessel (Turkoski, 2000). Clotting rarely occurs when vascular integrity and blood flow are normal. In the 19th century, Rudolph Virchow described a triad of factors—endothial injury, hypercoagulable state, and venous stasis—that affect coagulation within a blood vessel (Carter, 1994). Virchow's triad is thought to upset the normal balance between blood-clotting activators and inhibitors, which typically prevents circulating blood from clotting inappropriately. In particular, venous stasis and either endothelial injury or hypercoagulable states are recognized as major risk factors for thrombus formation.

Mobility is often limited during recovery from orthopaedic surgical procedures. Immobility causes a lack of pumping action in the large muscles of the legs and, subsequently, a decreased venous blood flow. Blood consequently pools in the venous valve cusps of the lower limbs, setting the stage for the formation of a fibrinous group of cells that can develop into a thrombus. Clinical symptoms appear when the thrombus is large enough to block blood flow in one of the large vessels.

Once a thrombus is formed, it may undergo lysis, become organized, persist as an unorganized or partially organized fibrin, or become dislodged and carried in the circulation as an embolus (Barloon, Bergus, & Seabold, 1997). A pulmonary embolus (PE) is a thrombus obstructing a significant portion of the pulmonary arterial bed. For optimal gas exchange to occur within the lungs, ventilation must match perfusion. When an embolus blocks a pulmonary artery or branch, flow distal to the embolus is either partially or totally occluded. The increased pulmonary vascular resistance caused by the PE results in pulmonary hypertension and increased right ventricular workload. All of these pathologic events lead to hypoxia and the clinical manifestations of PE (Tapson & Witty, 1995).

Risk Factors

The primary risk factors for venous thromboembolism are patient-related, procedure-related, and anesthesia-related (see Table 8-1). Many adults undergoing orthopaedic procedures will have one or more of these risk factors, making prevention a primary consideration.

Prevention and Nursing Interventions

The optimal prophylactic regimen for prevention of venous thromboembolism after orthopaedic surgery is controversial, but there is universal consensus that some form of thromboembolic prophylaxis, especially after joint replacements, is important (Geerts et al., 2008). VTE prophylaxis involves the use of nonpharmacologic and pharmacologic regimens. Nonpharmacologic interventions include early ambulation, elastic stockings, intermittent pneumatic compression devices, use of a bone vacuum technique during surgery, and inferior vena caval filters. Pharmacologic methods include low molecular weight heparin (LMWH) (i.e., Lovenox®), warfarin (Coumadin®), fondaparinux (Arixtra®), and vitamin K antagonists (VKA).

Early ambulation should be a routine part of postoperative care for all patients, unless an absolute contraindication exists. Elastic stockings should be applied preoperatively

Table 8-1
Risk Factors for Venous Thromboembolism

Patient Related	■ older age ■ previous thromboembolism ■ malignancy ■ varicose veins ■ obesity ■ trauma ■ congestive heart failure ■ stroke ■ oral contraceptive use ■ pregnancy ■ deficiencies in clotting cascade related to: antithrombin III, protein C, protein S, fibrinogen, or plasminogen ■ postoperative complications: bleeding, MI, pneumonia, UTI
Procedure Related	■ pelvic, hip, or leg surgery ■ repair of fractured pelvis or hip ■ surgery > 30 minutes ■ postoperative immobilization ■ postoperative infection ■ re-operation
Anesthesia Related	■ general anesthesia

Adapted from Gangireddy, C., Rectenwald, J.R., Upchurch, G.R., Wakefield, T.W., Khuri, S., Henderson, W., …Henke, P.K. (2007). Risk factors and clinical impact of postoperative symptomatic venous thromboembolism. *Society for vascular surgery, 45*, 335-342.
and
Katoli, P., Henderson, M.C., & White, R.H. (2003). DVT prophylaxis and anticoagulation in the surgical patient. *The Medical Clinics of North America, 87*, 77-110.

and continued throughout the recovery period as an adjunct to pharmacologic prophylaxis. Graduate elastic compression stockings reduce venous hypertension, decrease edema, and improve microcirculation. Stockings that are too tight will increase venous pressure below the knee and delay venous emptying. Measurement of the circumference and length of each leg is important to assure appropriate fit (Kaboli, Henderson, & White, 2003).

There are two types of intermittent pneumatic compression devices used to prevent VTE (Kaboli et al., 2003). One provides sequential pneumatic compression of the leg, and the other is a "foot-pump" device that compresses the venous plantar plexus of the foot. These work by having a direct effect on pumping venous blood, thereby reducing stasis.

Inferior vena cava filters, which trap emboli and prevent their travel to the pulmonary circulation, are typically only used for previous history of a VTE/PE, absolute contraindication to anticoagulation, or failure of adequate anticoagulation. In most cases, clots trapped by the filter undergo endogenous thrombolysis. The risks of inferior venal caval filters include migration of the filter, recurrent DVT, inferior vena caval thrombosis, and postphlebitic syndrome (Kaboli et al., 2003).

Consensus on the best pharmacologic approach to prevent VTE is evolving. Low molecular weight heparins (LMWH) are recommended for VTE prophylaxis. They have more antifactor X activity than unfractionated heparin and do not prolong the partial thromboplastin time. LMWH requires less frequent dosing and laboratory monitoring, has a lower incidence of heparin-induced thrombocytopenia, and a more predictable dose-response relationship. This leads to reduced protein binding, and carries less risk of osteoporosis than unfractionated heparin (Green, 2003; Turkoski, 2000). Routine laboratory test monitoring is unnecessary when using LMWH because of its predictable pharmacokinetics. The only exceptions are for pregnant patients, those with renal failure, and neonates or other low-weight patients for whom weight-based dosing may not be accurate. For these exceptions, anti-Xa plasma levels are the preferred test for assessing and guiding accurate dosing (Hemker, Dieri, & Beguin, 2005). It is important to periodically measure platelet levels of patients using LMWH to identify the potential of heparin-induced thrombocytopenia. In addition to teaching patients about the need for periodic blood tests, patients and their families must also be taught how to administer the LMWH which is given as a subcutaneous injection.

Warfarin may be used as prophylaxis for VTE for patients undergoing hip and knee arthroplasty although it is no longer recommended as preferred therapy (Geerts et al., 2008). The major advantages of warfarin are its low cost and ability to be given orally. Warfarin, however, requires frequent blood tests to monitor the INR which is used to adjust dosage. The potential risk for bleeding is also a concern with the use of warfarin. Nurses play a large role in educating patients and their families about the potential drug-drug, drug-food, drug-dietary supplements/herbal products, and drug-alcohol interactions with warfarin. Nurses must also counsel patients about safety measures to decrease the likelihood of bleeding such as shaving with an electric razor rather than a blade, and reducing risk of falls which may cause traumatic bleeding.

The Seventh American College of Chest Physicians (ACCP) Consensus Conference on Antithrombotic Therapy provides evidence-based guidelines for the prevention of VTE in surgical patients (Geerts et al., 2008). The evidence suggests that patients undergoing a total hip or knee arthroplasty or surgery for repair of a hip fracture should receive either low molecular weight heparin, fondaparinux (Arixtra®), or a vitamin K antagonist (VKA) with an international normalized ratio target of 2.5 (range 2-3) for 10-35 days for prophylaxis against VTE. Medication prophylaxis should be accompanied by early ambulation and elastic stockings. Intermittent pneumatic compression should also be used for repair of a hip fracture or a total hip arthroplasty. The evidence in inconclusive for use of intermittent pneumatic compression for patients undergoing a total knee arthroplasty (Geerts et al., 2008).

Nurses have a role in establishing and implementing protocols for VTE prophylaxis. Standards of care, care plans, and clinical pathways should incorporate strategies for VTE prevention. Knowledge of risk factors and identification of patients at risk facilitate the nurse's efforts to provide preventive measures. If using anticoagulants, one must balance the bleeding risk against the risk of thromboembolism associated with the operative procedure and postoperative mobility restrictions (Kaboli et al., 2003).

Clinical Manifestations and Assessment

Clinical diagnosis of DVT is fairly nonspecific and often inaccurate, as many individuals may have a DVT without any symptoms. The classical physical findings of DVT relate to inflammation and obstruction, including unilateral swelling of the thigh and/or lower leg, erythema, warmth, and tenderness. The pain may be described as aching, cramping, sharp, dull, severe, or mild. The discomfort may be constant or intermittent and often increases with movement and weight bearing. Homans sign is **not** specific to or sensitive for DVT. Doppler ultrasonagraphy with compression is the imaging study of choice to confirm symptomatic DVT. Ultrasonography has high sensitivity and specificity. It allows for direct imaging of the clot, and is portable (Schellong et al., 2007). The combination of low clinical probablility for a DVT and a normal D-dimer test result has been shown to effectively rule out DVT (ten Cate Hoek, 2005). Ultrasonography is used for those patients with a likely clinical probability of DVT or an abnormal D-dimer test result (Gibson et al., 2009).

Pulmonary emboli also are often undetected or misdiagnosed because of the nonspecificity of PE symptoms. Presenting symptoms of those with suspected PE include dyspnea, tachycardia, and low pulse oximetry (Kim et al., 2008). Chest pain, apprehension, confusion, anxiety, restlessness, cough, hemoptysis, diaphoresis, palpitations, and syncope may also occur. The patient's skin can feel cool or warm and may become cyanotic. Given the vague and unspecific manifestations of both DVT and PE, it is important to consider theses diagnoses when a patient presents with the symptoms described above. Although not definitive, arterial blood gases, chest x-ray, and electrocardiogram may contribute to the diagnostic workup for PE. In the early stages of PE, arterial blood gas (ABG) results may identify a respiratory alkalosis with a decreased pO_2 and a decreased pCO_2. With massive PE, ABGs will show a decreased pO_2 and an increased pCO_2. A chest x-ray is often normal but can be helpful in ruling out other pulmonary perfusion problems. An electrocardiogram should be obtained and evaluated for the presence of an inverted T-wave segment, indicating hypoxemia. D-dimer assays may be obtained. A spiral CT is the gold standard for detection of PE (Kim et al., 2008). Ventilation–perfusion lung scanning (VQ scan) remains an alternative to CT angiography when injection of a contrast dye is a concern. Although a normal scan can rule out the disease, the scan results in false negatives in up to a third of patients with suspected pulmonary embolism, meaning inconclusive findings are frequent (Anderson et al., 2007).

Treatment

Full-dose anticoagulation is the major treatment for DVT and PE. Anticoagulation will prevent the formation of new thrombi and allow dissolution of current thrombi by intrinsic fibrinolytic mechanisms. For patients with objectively confirmed deep vein thrombosis or pulmonary embolism, recommended treatment includes anticoagulant therapy with subcutaneous low-molecular-weight heparin, monitored intravenous or subcutaneous (SC) unfractionated heparin, unmonitored weight-based SC unfractionated heparin, or SC fondaparinux (Kearon et. al., 2008). If a PE is confirmed, oxygen and respiratory support should be initiated. If an oral anticoagulant is going to be taken for several months, it is important that the patient understands the purpose of the medication, food and drug interactions, the need for blood tests, untoward side effects, and precautions that accompany oral anticoagulant use.

Compartment Syndrome

Compartment syndrome, a potentially limb-threatening complication, can be prevented if recognized and treated early. There are four main compartments in the lower leg and three main compartments in the forearm (see Figures 8-1 and 8-2). While these are the most common sites for compartment syndrome, it can also occur in other parts of the body such as the upper arm, the buttock, or the foot. A muscle compartment is enveloped by tough, inelastic fascial tissue. When swelling of the muscle inside the compartment occurs, the inelastic fascia does not expand. This increase in pressure from the swelling reduces capillary blood perfusion. When local blood flow is unable to meet the metabolic demands of the tissue, ischemia begins.

An ischemia-edema cycle represents the pathophysiology of compartment syndrome (Harvey, 2001). With the initial swelling and increased pressure within a compartment, the nerves and vessels are compressed. If the swelling is significant, the subsequent muscle ischemia will cause the release of histamine, which in turn leads to capillary dilation and increase in capillary permeability. The result is increased edema and further decreased perfusion and oxygenation of vital tissues. As fluid accumulates, hydrostatic pressure increases, further impeding drainage and reabsorption from the venous capillaries. If this cycle continues, the result will be irreversible tissue damage.

Compartment syndrome is caused by anything that increases the pressure within a compartment. It can result from either externally applied or internally expanding pressure forces (Hoover & Siefert, 2000). An internal pressure force causes increased compartment contents and can be caused from hemorrhage or edema. An external force causes decreased compartment size and can be caused by a splint, a cast, or prolonged compression to an extremity. Increased risk for development of compartment syndrome has been associated with distal long bone fractures, acute trauma, swelling, infection, and skin traction (McQueen, Gaston, & Court-Brown, 2000).

Clinical Manifestations

There are early and late signs of compartment syndrome. It is important to detect the early signs, as the late signs are indicative of irreversible damage. The onset of symptoms can occur as early as 30 minutes after ischemic injury (Harvey, 2001) or as late as one week after fracture reduction, necessitating continuous monitoring. If compartment

Figure 8-1
Compartments of the Lower Leg

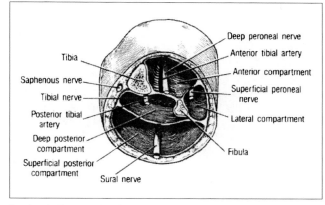

Reprinted with permission from Keating, E.M., & Meding, J.B. (2002). Perioperative blood management practice in elective orthopaedic surgery. *Journal of the American Academy of Orthopaedic Surgeons, 10,* 393-400.

Figure 8-2
Compartments of the Forearm

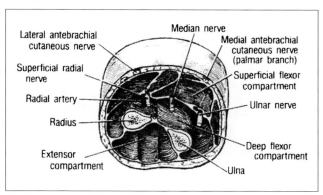

Reprinted with permission from the National Association of Orthopaedic Nurses (1990). Poster: *Neurovascular Assessment.* Pitman, NJ.

syndrome is not recognized and the pressure is not relieved, muscle damage will be irreversible after 4-6 hours of ischemia, and nerve damage will be irreversible after 12-24 hours (Janzing, Broos, & Rommens, 1996). The primary symptom of compartment syndrome is increasing pain or pain that is out of proportion to the injury. The pain is described as being unrelenting, not relieved by analgesic agents, loosening of a bandage, or bivalving/splitting of a cast. Specifically, pain with passive stretching of the muscles in a given compartment is one of the earliest clinical indicators; however, pain is not a reliable symptom in an insensate extremity due to prior injury or anesthesia, or for unconscious patients. Because nerve tissue is very sensitive to ischemia, sensory changes specifically associated with the nerve in the affected compartment also indicate the onset of decreased tissue perfusion (Tornetta & Templeman, 1997). Nerve paresthesias and a tense feeling can sometimes be felt as the pressure within the compartment increases (Hoover &

Siefert, 2000). If the intracompartmental pressure elevates to a level above systolic pressure, the pulse will be absent and capillary refill delayed, leading to pallor. The last sign of the very late stages of compartment syndrome is paralysis.

Although not specific to compartment syndrome, myoglobin in the urine and elevated serum CPK, LDH, and SGOT are indicative of muscle damage and can help to evaluate the extent of tissue necrosis. The only objective criterion for compartment syndrome is the measurement of intracompartmental pressures, which provides an indirect measurement of muscle and nerve ischemia. Normal compartment pressure is considered to be between 0-8 mm Hg (Tornetta & Templeman, 1997).

There are no guidelines that dictate definitive therapy when compartment pressures reach a specific level. Consensus is that, as long as the diastolic pressure remains high enough to perfuse the compartment, even absolute intracompartmental pressures of greater than 40 mm Hg do not require imminent surgical intervention (McQueen, Gaston, & Court-Brown, 2000). A differential pressure (the difference between blood pressure and compartment pressure) of 30 mm Hg is necessary to perfuse the compartment (McQueen, Gaston, & Court-Brown, 2000; Whitesides, Haney, Morimoto, & Harada, 1975).

Prevention and Nursing Interventions

Early recognition of the signs of compartment syndrome is important to prevent or minimize its negative consequences. The "6 P's of compartment syndrome" is a pneumonic to help remember key assessment parameters. While pain out of proportion to the injury and pressure may be noted prior to significant ischemia, pallor, paresthesia, pulselessness and paralysis are evident after vascular injury has occurred. The appearance of any signs or symptoms of compartment syndrome should prompt further evaluation, including measurement of the intracompartmental pressures.

Treatment

The primary treatment for compartment syndrome is to relieve the source of pressure. This may involve loosening an external constriction, such as removing a tight bandage or bivalving a cast. The extremity should be kept at heart level. Elevation above the heart decreases local arterial perfusion and may further compromise local blood flow. Adequate hydration should be provided to maintain mean arterial blood pressure. Appropriate pain management strategies should be initiated. If the relief of external pressure is not effective and the compartment pressures stay elevated or continue to rise, a fasciotomy may be necessary. Surgical incisions to open the involved compartments and fascial envelopes that surround the muscle compartments are necessary to provide adequate decompression. If one compartment is in danger, the other compartments are also at high risk (Harvey, 2001). Most often, multiple large incisions are required.

Early recognition is of utmost important for this complication. Nurses need to maintain a high suspicion for compartment syndrome in order to identify it early and implement measures to prevent negative outcomes.

Fat Embolism Syndrome

Fat embolism, a mechanical blockage of blood vessels by circulating fat particles, occurs most frequently following fractures. There are two predominant theories to explain the pathophysiology of fat embolism. The mechanical theory suggests that the increased intramedullary pressure that occurs following trauma causes fatty particles from the bone marrow to be released and travel to the lungs, blocking pulmonary capillaries. The biochemical theory suggests that hormonal changes secondary to trauma induce the systemic release of free fatty acids (Parisi, Koval, & Egol, 2002).

These fat droplets embolize primarily to the lung with smaller amounts traveling to other organs such as the brain. Severe fat embolism can lead to fat embolism syndrome (FES). The lungs respond to the fat droplets by secreting lipases that hydrolyze the fat into free fatty acids. The acids are chemically toxic to the lung parenchyma and cause a severe inflammatory reaction, eventually leading to adult respiratory distress syndrome (McDermott, Culpan, Clancy, & Dooley, 2002). Classic FES is characterized by pulmonary, cutaneous, and cerebral symptoms described below. Fat embolism occurs most frequently with fractures of the long bones, and the incidence increases with multiple fractures (Taviloglu & Yanar, 2007).

Pulmonary fat embolism is also directly related to the quantity of fat emboli resulting from operative manipulation of the bone during select surgical procedures. With a total hip arthroplasty, mechanical compression of the medullary canal during insertion of the stem causes an increase in the medullary pressure that is associated with the development of fat emboli. There is a significant relationship between the preoperative serum triglyceride level and fat embolization in patients having a total hip arthroplasty, suggesting lipid abnormalities may be an additional risk factor for this population (Kim, Oh, & Kim, 2002).

Clinical Manifestations and Assessment

The clinical presentation of FES varies widely. Some patients present with subtle signs and symptoms, and others present with significant respiratory failure. Characteristically, the clinical signs of FES do not appear until a symptom-free interval of at least 6-12 hours has elapsed from the time of injury (Taviloglu & Yanar, 2007). The primary symptoms of FES, which usually occur within 24-72 hours after the injury, are changes in mental status, increasing respiratory distress, and may include petechiae of the skin and mucosa (Schult, Frerichmann, Schiedel, Brug, & Joist, 2003). Petechiae are most often found in the axillae, on the anterior side of the chest and neck, around the navel, the conjunctivae, and the mucous membranes of the mouth. The rash results from occlusion of the dermal capillaries by fat causing increased capillary fragility (Taviloglu & Yanar, 2006). Initial mental status changes may include restlessness, somnolence, or confusion, which can then progress to complete loss of consciousness. Other signs and symptoms may include fever, tachycardia, retinal exudates and hemorrhage, jaundice, oliguria, proteinuria, hematuria, and unexplained anemia (Schult et al., 2003; Taviloglu & Yanar, 2007).

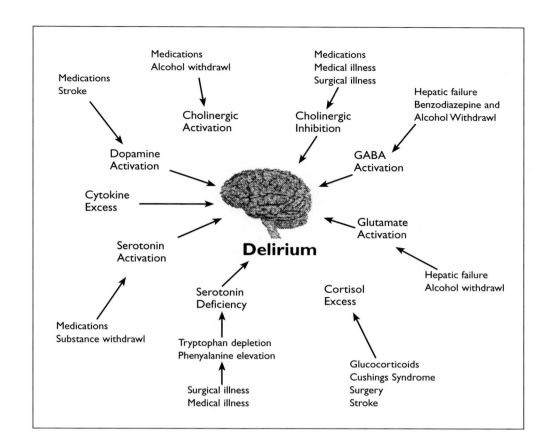

Figure 8-3
Proposed Mechanisms of Delirium

Medications
Stroke

Medications
Alcohol withdrawl

Medications
Medical illness
Surgical illness

Hepatic failure
Benzodiazepine and
Alcohol Withdrawl

Cholinergic
Activation

Cholinergic
Inhibition

Dopamine
Activation

GABA
Activation

Cytokine
Excess

Glutamate
Activation

Serotonin
Activation

Delirium

Hepatic failure
Alcohol withdrawl

Medications
Substance withdrawl

Serotonin
Deficiency

Cortisol
Excess

Tryptophan depletion
Phenyalanine elevation

Glucocorticoids
Cushings Syndrome
Surgery
Stroke

Surgical illness
Medical illness

Reprinted with permission from The Gerontological Society of America. Flacker, J.M., & Lipsitz, L.A. (1999). Neural mechanisms of delirium: Current hypotheses and evolving concepts. *Journal of Gerontology Series A - Biological Sciences Medical Sciences, 54*(6), 239-246.

There are no diagnostic tests specific for FES. Fat globules may be detected in the blood, urine, and sputum, and blood gas analysis may reveal a drop in PO2 to less than 50mm Hg (Kao, Yeh, & Chen, 2007). A chest x-ray is usually obtained to exclude other treatable causes of hypoxia such as pneumothorax, hemothorax, volume overload, pneumonia, and pulmonary embolus. A diffuse snowstorm pattern on a chest x-ray is characteristic of FES (Shaikh, 2009).

Treatment

Management of FES is primarily supportive, including intubation, ventilatory support, and ICU monitoring (White, Petrisor, & Bhandari, 2006). An awareness of risk factors and careful monitoring of patients at risk for developing FES are essential. The prognosis is good if supportive therapy is instituted early.

Recognition of symptoms is important in preventing morbidity and mortality associated with FES. Preventive measures include minimal movement of long-bone fractures with splinting and immobilization as soon as possible; operative bone stabilization within 24 hours of a major long-bone fracture; avoidance of hypovolemia; early drainage of fracture hematomas; administration of supplemental oxygen at the first sign of pulmonary distress, tachypnea, and dyspnea; and intubation and mechanical ventilation if pulmonary function deteriorates (White et al., 2006). There is evidence that aggressive rehydration, especially in the setting of possible dehydration, may also be a preventive measure (McDermott et al., 2002). Corticosteroids may be used to

prevent posttraumatic hypoxemia and may be beneficial in preventing FES, but not mortality in patients with isolated lower limb long-bone fractures, especially when early fracture stabilization is not possible (Babalis, Yiannakopoulos, Karliaftis, & Antonogiannakis, 2004; Bederman, Bhandari, McKee, & Schemitsch, 2009). Steroids are thought to limit the increase of free fatty acids, stabilize the membranes, and inhibit complement-mediated leukocyte aggregation. However, the use of steroids has not been proved by any large-scale prospective trials and given the side effect profile, its should only be used in select cases (Akhtar, 2009).

Delirium

Delirium, an acute confusional state with a decline in attention and cognition (Inouye), occurs in up to 87% of hospitalized patients (Demeure & Fain, 2006), with the orthopaedic population representing the higher end of the continuum. Postoperative delirium is associated with increased morbidity and mortality, longer hospitalization, functional disability, and increased health care costs (Demeure & Fain, 2006). Delirium presents as either hyperactive or hypoactive. Hyperactive delirium is characterized by a state of hyperarousal, hypervigilance, and agitation. Patients with hypoactive delirium are hypoalert and lethargic (Fricchione et al., 2008).

Pathophysiology

Multiple factors contribute to the development of delirium, yet the pathophysiology is not completely understood. The physiology of aging may explain some aspects of delirium

Table 8-2
Predisposing Factors for Delirium

Patient Characteristics
■ Age > 65 years
■ Male sex
■ Cognitive status: dementia, cognitive impairment, depression, history of delirium
■ Functional status: immobility, history of falls, functional dependence, sedentary
■ Sensory impairment: visual impairment, hearing impairment
■ Decreased oral intake: dehydration, malnutrition
■ Alcohol abuse
■ Polypharmacy
■ Multiple co-morbidities, fracture or trauma, terminal illness, HIV

Precipitating Factors
■ Medication use (sedative hypnotics, anticholinergics, narcotics)
■ Alcohol or drug withdrawal
■ Orthopedic surgery
■ Time in intensive care unit
■ Iatrogenic events
■ Infection
■ Hypoxia
■ Shock
■ Anemia
■ Dehydration
■ Poor nutritional status
■ Low serum albumin
■ Abnormal electrolytes, glucose, acid-base balance

Adapted form Dasgupta, M., & Dumbsrell, A.C. (2006). Preoperative risk assessment for delirium after non cardiac surgery: A systematic review. *Journal of the American Geriactric Society, 54*(10), 1578-1589.
and
Inouye, S.K., & Ferrucci, L. (2006). Elucidating the pathophysiology of delirium and the interrelationship of delirium and dementia. *Journal of Gerontology, Series A: Biological Sciences Medical Sciences, 61,* 1277-1280.
and
Robinson, T.N., Raeburn, C.D., Tran, Z.V., Angles, E.M., Brenner, L.A., & Moss M. (2009). Postoperative delirum in the elderly: Risk factors and outcomes. *Annals of Surgery, 249*(1), 173-178.

in the elderly if one considers the normal decline in cerebral blood flow, neuronal loss, and lower concentrations of brain neurotransmitters such as acetylcholine, dopamine, y-aminobutric acid (GABA), and norephinephrine. Deficits of any of the neurotransmitters might contribute to less physiologic reserve to handle the additional neurologic stress that occurs with metabolic disturbances or infection (Marcantonio et al., 2006; Roche, 2003). Impaired neurochemical tranmission systems are thought to play a role in the development of delirium (Roche, 2003; van der Mast & Fekkes, 2000). Figure 8-3 illustrates the proposed mechanisms of delirium and possible associated clinical conditions.

Risk Factors

Patient characteristics and events that occur during hospitalization have been identified as risk factors for delirium as shown in Table 8-2. The onset of delirium is directly related to the number of risk factors.

Clinical Manifestations and Assessment

The early detection of delirium enables the health care team to initiate interventions to minimize negative consequences. The initial assessment of cognitive status provides a baseline for comparison with subsequent assessments, which should be conducted in a systematic and comprehensive pattern throughout hospitalization. The American Psychiatric Association's criteria from the *Diagnostic and Statistical Manual of Mental Disorders,* 4th edition (2000) outline four essential features needed to make a diagnosis of delirium: inattention, change in cognition, acute onset and fluctuating pattern of disturbance, and identifiable medical cause (see Table 8-3). Assessment should focus on concentration, attention, orientation, and psychomotor behavior. The Mini-Mental State Examination (Folstein, Folstein, & McHugh, 1975), the Confusion Assessment Method Instrument (Inouye et al., 1990), the Memorial Delirium Assessment Scale (Casarett & Inouye, 2001), and the NEECHAM Confusion Scale (Neelon, Champagne, Carlson, & Funk, 1996) are all examples of instruments that help to identify changes in cognition. Measures of executive function such as the Digit Symbol Substitution subtest (Weschler, 1997) and the Trail Making Test (Ashendorf et al., 2008) have also been shown to predict delirium (Greene et al., 2009).

There are some easy bedside tests that measure attention. One is to ask the patient to recite the days of the week backward. The second is a Digit Span Test, asking the patient to repeat 5 numbers forward without error. Using an agreed-upon mental status questionnaire, measurement of attention, and a behavior rating scale can provide consistency over time and between evaluators. This will ultimately facilitate the monitoring of a patient's cognitive status.

Prevention and Nursing Interventions
Many of the risk factors for delirium can be addressed by

Table 8-3
Signs and Symptoms of Delirium

Inattention
■ Impaired ability to focus, sustain, or shift attention
■ Easily distracted
■ Gives the same answers to different questions
■ "Poor historian"

Change in Cognition
■ Disorientation to time or place
■ Mistinterpretations
■ Illusions
■ Hallucinations (visual, auditory, olfactory, gustatory, or tactile)

Acute and Fluctuating Change in Cognition
■ Onset over hours or days
■ Fluctuates during the course of the day
■ Medical Cause
■ Explanation for delirium identified (ie. medical condition, substance intoxication, substance withdrawal)

Reprinted with permission from the American Psychiatric Association (2000). *American Psychiatric Association: Diagnostic and statistical manual of mental disorders* (DSM-IV).

monitoring drug use; avoiding drugs with anticholinergic activity; maintaining hydration, perfusion, and oxygenation; meeting nutritional requirements; managing pain; enhancing sleep; and correcting metabolic imbalances (Inouye, 2006; Marcantonio, Flacker, Wright, & Resnick, 2001). Re-orienting patients in a consistent manner; minimizing disruption to the usual sleep patterns; providing social interaction; and ensuring access to glasses, hearing aids, and other mobility aids have been shown to prevent delirium but not impact its severity once it is established (Inouye et al., 1999). Table 8-4 lists strategies that can be used to minimize the risk of delirium (Inouye et al., 1999). These are also strategies that can be helpful in the management of delirium should it occur.

The actual management of delirium requires identification and treatment of the cause, environmental modification, and control of symptoms. The three most common causes of delirium are infection, metabolic disturbances, and medications (Roche, 2003). Environmental modification includes the strategies noted in Table 8-4 to minimize the risk of delirium. Drug therapy is indicated when agitation or behavior interferes with the evaluation or management of the patient. Control of symptoms often involves the use of drugs such as haloperidol or benzodiazepines. Haloperidol may be most effective in controlling hyperactivity, agitation, and mania; benzodiazepines are best for delirium caused by acute alcohol withdrawal (Bourne, Tahir, Borthwick, & Sampson, 2008). There is evidence that identifying high-risk patients upon admission and intervening early may prevent the development of delirium (Roche, 2003). Once delirium has occurred, however, options are limited to treating the identified cause and managing symptoms.

Hemorrhage, Significant Blood Loss, Anemia

Another complication that occurs with orthopaedic surgery is bleeding and anemia. Although surgery is inevitably associated with bleeding, select orthopaedic procedures have an increased likelihood of potential significant surgical blood loss. An understanding of hemostasis will help the nurse to understand the associated risk when hemostasis is interrupted and better anticipate patient care needs.

Hemostasis is a complex interaction between the vascular wall, platelets, coagulation factors and fibrinolysis. Primary hemostasis begins immediately after endothelial injury (Porte & Leebeek, 2002). This means that, at the moment of injury or with the initial incision during surgery, the formation of a platelet plug is the start of the hemostasis process. At the same time, the coagulation cascade is initiated. The conversion of fibrinogen to fibrin is the end stage of blood coagulation. The coagulation system is controlled at several levels by inhibitors. The balance between these procoagulant and anticoagulant factors is essential for hemostatic control. Disorders in the balanced system of coagulation and fibrinolysis may result in severe bleeding or thrombotic complications (Porte & Leebeek, 2002).

Risk Factors

Perioperative hemorrhage or excessive blood loss can be related to individual patient characteristics, the nature of the

Table 8-4
Minimizing the Risk for Delirium

1. Identify and use interventions to manage underlying medical condition.
2. Assess and meet personal hygiene needs.
3. Establish baseline mental status and reassess regularly.
4. Use prophylactic analgesics as indicated.
5. Assist with toileting as indicated.
6. Maintain an organized environment.
   (a) Provide name tags for health care workers.
   (b) Orient patient to room and unit.
   (c) Place familiar items within patient's view.
7. Provide meaningful sensory input.
   (a) Place clock and calendar within site.
   (b) Ensure lighting is appropriate to time of day.
   (c) Encourage visits by family and friends.
8. Maximize independence.
   (a) Incorporate patient's usual routines into hospital day.
   (b) Encourage active participation of the patient.

Adapted from Inouye, S.K., & Ferrucci, L. (2006). Elucidating the pathophysiology of delirium and the interrelationship of delirium and dementia. *Journal of Gerontology, Series A: Biological Sciences Medical Sciences, 61*, 1277-1280. and
Siddiqi, N., Stockdale, R., Britten, A.M., & Holmes, J. (2007). Interventions for preventing delirium in hospitalized patients. *The Cochrane Database Systematic Reviews, 2*, Art. No.: CD005563, doi: 1002/14651858. CD005563.pub2

injury or musculoskeletal condition, the specific surgical procedure, or postoperative complications. Patient characteristics that contribute to the risk of blood loss include coagulation disorders such as hemophilia and von Willebrand disease, vascular abnormalities like those seen with some connective tissue diseases, low platelet counts, and hypotension or hypertension. A fractured bone, a foreign body interrupting the blood vessel integrity, and tumor growth impinging blood vessels are all contributing factors to blood loss caused by the nature of the injury or the musculoskeletal condition. Surgical factors influencing blood loss are largely related to the anatomic and technical aspects of certain surgical procedures and the skill and experience of the surgical team (Porte & Leebeek, 2002). Postoperative complications that contribute to excessive blood loss include slipped ligatures, infection, and excessive anticoagulation.

Assessment of Risk

Increasingly, a preoperative assessment of estimated blood loss and transfusion risk is becoming more of a standard of care. If the estimated blood loss is anticipated to be high and the risk for needing a transfusion likely, blood management strategies should be utilized as anemia has an adverse effect on morbidity and mortality. Historically, allogenic blood transfusion has been the mainstay of perioperative blood management; however, more options are now available. The primary purpose of transfusion is to reduce the risks associated with anemia, which is common in patients undergoing elective orthopaedic surgery. Given the potential risk of transfusion reaction, immunosuppression, and

Figure 8-4
Use of Erythropoietin in Anemic Surgical Candidates

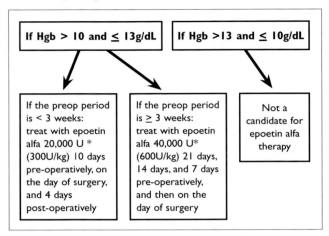

| If Hgb > 10 and ≤ 13g/dL | | If Hgb >13 and ≤ 10g/dL |

| If the preop period is < 3 weeks: treat with epoetin alfa 20,000 U * (300U/kg) 10 days pre-operatively, on the day of surgery, and 4 days post-operatively | If the preop period is ≥ 3 weeks: treat with epoetin alfa 40,000 U* (600U/kg) 21 days, 14 days, and 7 days pre-operatively, and then on the day of surgery | Not a candidate for epoetin alfa therapy |

Reprinted with permission from the National Association of Orthopaedic Nurses (1990). Poster: *Neurovascular Assessment*. Chicago, IL.

disease transmission associated with use of allogenic blood, prevention of the need for transfusion is preferred (Keating & Meding, 2002).

Blood Management Techniques

There are several approaches to blood conservation and minimizing blood loss during surgery. The primary initiatives include preoperative autologous donation, the use of erythropoietin, improvements in surgical practice, acute normovolemic hemodilution, perioperative blood salvage techniques, and the use of pharmacologic agents. Autologous transfusion, which reduces the need for allogenic transfusion, is often used in elective surgery (Vanderlinde, Heal, & Blumberg, 2002). This decreases the risk of transfusion transmitted diseases, however, preoperative autologous

donation has been associated with preoperative anemia (Ozawa, Shander, & Ochani, 2001) and ischemic events (Goodnough & Monk, 1996). The evidence for benefits of re-infusing autologous blood is lacking and warrants further study to determine if the benefits outweigh the risk (Carless, Moxey, O'Connell, & Henry, 2004). If employed, autologous blood donation generally should begin 3 to 5 weeks before scheduled surgery, and patients should receive supplemental oral iron therapy throughout this period (Keating & Meding, 2002).

A person's preoperative hemoglobin status will influence the perioperative course. Improving patients' preoperative hemoglobin levels can reduce the need for postoperative transfusion. The use of subcutaneous recombinant human erythropoietin has been safe and effective in select patients with anemia to increase hemoglobin levels (Ozawa et al., 2001). It also may reduce the need for transfusion in surgical patients (Feagan et al., 2000). It is important to note that concomitant use of exogenous iron is necessary even if the patient has normal iron stores (Ozawa et al., 2001). See the algorithm in Figure 8-4 for the use of erythropoietin in anemic surgical candidates.

Acute normovolemic hemodilution (ANH) involves simultaneous removal of whole blood from a patient immediately before beginning surgery and replacement with crystalloid or colloid fluids to maintain normovolemia (Bennett, Haynes, Torella, Grainger, & Mccollum, 2006). ANH is indicated in situations where at least 20% of blood volume is predicted to be lost. The blood that was drained preoperatively is anticoagulated, stored, and reinfused after any significant bleeding (Keating & Meding, 2002). The blood-sparing benefit of hemodilution is the result of reduced loss in red cell mass during surgical bleeding. The major limiting factor in choosing candidates for hemodilution is the patient's ability to tolerate a low volume of red blood cells (Vanderlinde et al., 2002), which is often a challenge for patients with advanced cardiac or pulmonary disease.

Table 8-5
CDC Criteria for Nosocomial Surgical Site Infections

Superficial Incisional SSI	Deep Incisional SSI	Organ/Space SSI
Infection occurs within 30 days after operative procedure, involves only skin or subcutaneous tissue.	Infection occurs within 30 days after the operative procedure (within one year if an implant is in place) and appears to be related to the operative procedure. Involves deep soft tissues.	Infection occurs within 30 days after the operative procedure (within one year if an implant is in place) and appears to be related to the operative procedure. Involves any part of the anatomy, other than the incision, opened or manipulated during the operative procedure.
Has purulent drainage from the skin or subcutaneous tissue, *or* positive aseptically obtained culture from the superficial incision, *And*, presence of pain/tenderness, localized swelling, or redness/heat, *And*, incision is deliberately opened by the MD, *Or*, diagnosis of superficial incisional SSI by MD.	Has purulent drainage from the deep incision (but not from the organ/space component of the surgical site), *or* spontaneous dehiscence or deliberate opening of a deep incision when the patient has either a fever > 38 degrees C or localized pain/tenderness unless the incision is culture-negative, *Or*, an abscess or evidence of infection is found on direct examination, during re-operation, or by histopathologic or radiologic examination, *Or*, diagnosis of a deep incisional SSI by MD.	Has purulent drainage from a drain that is placed through a stab wound into the organ/space, *Or*, positive aseptically obtained culture of fluid or tissue in the organ/space, *Or*, abscess or other evidence of infection found on direct examination, during re-operation, or by histopathologic or radiologic examination, *Or*, diagnosis of organ/space SSI by MD.

Reprinted with permission from Mangram, A.J., Horan, T.C., Pearson, M.L., Silver, L.C., & Jarvis, W.R. (1999). Guideline for prevention of surgical site infection, 1999. *Infection Control and Hospital Epidemiology, 20*(4), 247-278.

Blood salvage techniques can be used intraoperatively and postoperatively. Blood lost during surgery is collected by aspiration or drainage from the operative field. Citrate or heparin anticoagulant is added, and the contents are filtered to remove clots and debris. The blood is then centrifuged before being transfused back to the patient. Postoperative salvage refers to the process of recovering blood from wound drains and reinfusing the collected fluid with or without washing (Keating & Meding, 2002; Vanderlinde et al., 2002).

Pharmacologic options for blood conservation primarily consist of topical agents, antifibrinolytics, and agents that enhance platelet function and improve primary hemostasis (Levy, 2008). Two procoagulant drugs, recombinant factor VIIa (eptacog alfa) and desmopressin (DDAVP™) may be beneficial in blood conservation management with major orthopaedic surgical procedures. Topical agents are mainly used to control local capillary bleeding. Fibrin sealants are more effective in preventing rebleeding from a previously dry surgical wound surface than in achieving primary hemostasis at a continuously oozing surface (Carless, Henry, & Anthony, 2008).

Assessment

A strategy for managing perioperative blood loss can minimize or eliminate the need for allogenic blood transfusions. Ultimately, however, the need for a transfusion should be based on the nature and extent of the anemia and the patient's overall clinical status. Evaluation of clinical status in the postoperative period involves both subjective and objective data. Subjective data indicative of excessive blood loss include verbalization of actual bleeding, dizziness, weakness, and anxiety. Objective data include restlessness and confusion, tachycardia with a weak and irregular pulse, decreased blood pressure, a narrowed pulse pressure, rapid shallow breathing, pallor, cold moist skin, decreased urine output, and abnormal drainage from drains or wounds. Diagnostic testing includes serum laboratory studies such as a CBC and coagulation studies to determine the extent of blood loss and specific coagulation abnormalities that may be present. If the source of bleeding is difficult to determine, radiographic studies may be indicated.

Interventions

Astute nursing care will lead to early identification of excessive blood loss. If a direct source of bleeding is visible, direct pressure on the site is indicated. Depending on the cause of the bleeding, a return to the operating room or resuturing may be necessary. If excessive anticoagulation occurs, vitamin K or clotting factor replacement may be administered. With significant blood loss, volume replacement and blood transfusion are necessary. Oral iron supplementation should be considered to help restore lost reserves.

Surgical Site Infection

Infections related to surgery contribute to morbidity and are associated with longer hospitalizations and increased health care costs as well as mortality (Mangram, Horan, Pearson, Silver, & Jarvis, 1999). Antimicrobial-resistant pathogens and increased numbers of surgical patients who are elderly and/or have significant comorbidities may partially explain the incidence of surgical site infections. The Centers for Disease Control and Prevention (Mangram et al., 1999) provide criteria for nosocomial surgical site infections (SSIs) (see Table 8-5). The most frequently isolated pathogens from SSIs are Staphylococcus aureus, Staphylococcus epidermis, and Streptococcus species (Harkness & Daniels, 2003). Methicillin-resistant Staphylococcus aureus (MRSA) has become an increasingly more frequent cause of postoperative infections (Solomkin, 2001). The incidence of infection varies according to the site and extent of injury, the specific surgical procedure, and the general health of the patient.

When the integrity of the skin is interrupted from trauma or an incision, hemostasis begins immediately with activation of platelets and the coagulation cascade leading to vasoconstriction and clot formation (Teller & White, 2009). This is followed almost immediately with the onset of inflammation at the cellular level with vessel dilation, increased vascular permeability, and leukocyte transmission to the site of injury. Edema of the wound occurs as the intravascular fluid, protein, and cellular components move into the extravascular space. Restoration of the epithelium is important to the prevention of infection. Epithelial cells move and replicate in response

Table 8-6

Patient and Procedure-related Factors Related to the Risk of Surgical Site Infection Development

Patient
▪ Age
▪ Nutritional status (malnutrition)
▪ Diabetes
▪ Smoking
▪ Obesity
▪ Coexistent infections at a remote body site
▪ Colonization with microorganisms
▪ Altered immune response
▪ Length of preoperative stay

Operation
▪ Duration of surgical scrub
▪ Skin antisepsis
▪ Preoperative shaving
▪ Preoperative skin prep
▪ Duration of operation
▪ Antimicrobial prophylaxis
▪ Operating room ventilation
▪ Inadequate sterilization of instruments
▪ Foreign material in the surgical site
▪ Use of surgical drains and packings
▪ Surgical technique
• Poor hemostasis
• Failure to obliterate dead space
• Tissue trauma

Adapted from Cheadle, W.G. (2006). Risk factors for surgical site infection. *Surgical Infections, 7*(1), S7-S11.
and
Mangram, A.J., Horan, T.C., Pearson, M.L., Silver, L.C., & Jarvis, W.R. (1999). Guideline for prevention of surgical site infection, 1999. *Infection Control and Hospital Epidemiology, 20*(4), 247-278.

Table 8-7
Strategies to Prevent Surgical Site Infections

Preoperative	■ Encourage tobacco cessation
	■ Optimize cardiopulmonary function
	■ Control hypertension
	■ Prevent sympathetically induced peripheral vasoconstriction by maintaining blood volume, controlling pain, alleviating anxiety, and keeping the patient warm
	■ Replenish nutritional deficits
	■ Minimize unnecessary movement of fractured bones
	■ Treat any existing infection
	■ Improve or maintain blood sugar control to avoid hyperglycemia
	■ Do not remove/shave hair around the operation site
	■ Have patients bathe with an antiseptic agent the night before the operation
Intraoperative	■ Antimicrobial prophylaxis
	■ Strict aseptic techniques
	■ Gentle handling of the soft tissues
	■ Meticulous debridement of devitalized bone and soft tissues
	■ Stable fixation of fractures
	■ Keep patient warm to avoid vasoconstriction
	■ Elevate PaO2
	■ Wound closure without excessive tension and with use of appropriate sutures (multifilament nylon instead of silk), skin tapes, and dressings
	■ Minimally invasive procedures when possible
Postoperative	■ Provide adequate analgesia
	■ Keep patient warm to avoid vasoconstriction
	■ Assess capillary refill
	■ Maintain hydration
	■ Control blood pressure and hyperglycemia
	■ Assess and provide for nutritional needs
	■ Aseptic technique with dressing changes
	■ Microbial therapy as indicated
	■ Thorough hand washing

Adapted from Boni, L., Benrento, A., Rovera, F., Dionigi, G., DiGiuseppe, M., Bertoglio, C., & Dionigi, R. (2006). Infective complications in laproscopic surgery. *Surgical Infections, 7*(S), 109-111.
and
Dronge, A.S., Perkal, M.F., Kancir, S., Concato, J., Aslan, M., & Rosenthal, R.A. (2006). Long-term glycemic control and postoperative infectious complications. *Archives of Surgery, 141,* 375-380.
and
Hoover, T.J., & Siefert, J.A. (2000). Soft tissue complications of orthopaedic emergencies. *Emergency Medicine Clinics of North America, 18,* 115-139.
and
Managram, A.J., Horan, T.C., Pearson, M.L., Silver, L.C., & Jarvis, W.R. (1999). Guideline for prevention of surgical site infection, 1999. *Infection Control and Hospital Epidemiology, 20*(4), 247-278.
and
Sessler, D.I., & Akca, O. (2002). Nonpharmacological prevention of surgical wound infections. *Clinical Infectious Diseases, 35*(11), 1397-1404.
and
Webster, J. & Osbourne, S. (2007). Preoperative bathing or showering with skin antiseptics to prevent surgical site infection. *The Cochrane Database of Systemic Review, 2,* Art. No.: CD004985. doi: 10.1002/14651858. CD004985

to growth factors and oxygen tension. This begins early in healing, but it is not obvious for several days. Epithelialization reestablishes the external barrier that minimizes fluid losses and bacterial invasion (Teller & White, 2009).

Risk Factors

Recognition of risk factors or characteristics that increase the likelihood of developing a surgical site infection enable the nurse to initiate preventive strategies and identify infection in its early stages. Table 8-6 lists patient and procedure-related factors that may influence the risk of SSI development.

Clinical Manifestations

The signs and symptoms of surgical site infections are related to the inflammatory response that accompanies an initial infection. These may include verbalization of a new or higher level of pain, increased warmth and/or odor beneath a bandage or cast, and fever or chills. Objective findings include erythema, edema, warmth, malodor, and purulent exudate from the incision or wound, fever, and poor wound healing.

Diagnostic indicators of a surgical site infection may be an elevated white blood cell (WBC) count, an elevated erythrocyte sedimentation rate (ESR), and an elevated C-reactive protein. A culture indicates a specific organism present within the incision or wound, and quantitative microbiology attempts to indicate colonization versus invasion; however, even if 105 organisms per gram of tissue are found in a wound, a definitive diagnosis of infection cannot be made without considering the nature of the wound and the organism involved (Thomson & Smith, 1994).

Prevention and Nursing Interventions

Interventions to reduce the risk of wound infection involve all members of the health care team. Adherence to standard precautions, aseptic technique, and appropriate hand washing will help to prevent infection. Postoperative host defenses, however, are a major factor that determines whether a surgical patient becomes infected (Sessler & Akca, 2002). Select interventions, as described in Table 8-7, should be instituted during the preoperative, intraoperative, and postoperative periods to promote timely healing with the lowest risk of infection. Maintenance of normothermia and provision of supplemental oxygen in the immediate postoperative period have been shown to improve immunity (Sessler & Akca, 2002). Ischemic tissue can easily become infected and generally does not heal well. Therefore, it is important to promote adequate local perfusion and oxygenation to improve healing and resistance to infection.

Elevated glucose levels have also been linked with potential infectious outcomes. Normal physiologic processes to fight foreign agents are potentially impaired during periods of hyperglycemia. Outcomes are improved when tighter glycemic control is achieved (Aragon, Ring, & Covelli, 2003).

Antimicrobial prophylaxis can decrease the incidence of incisional wound infection. Current recommendations include using appropriate prophylactic antibiotics at the start of any procedure in which infection is highly probable or

Table 8- 8
Risk Factors for Hospital-Acquired Pneumonia

Patient-Related Risk Factors	■ Older age ■ Aspiration ■ Malnutrition ■ Hypotension ■ Tobacco use ■ Metabolic acidosis ■ Immunosuppression ■ Decreased consciousness ■ Severe or chronic illness including CHF, diabetes, chronic liver and renal disease, COPD, sleep apnea, obesity, or chronic neurologic disease ■ Prolonged hospitalized preoperative period ■ Hospitalization greater than 3 days ■ Intraoperative blood loss exceeding 1,200 mL
Infection Control-Related Factors	■ Inadequate hand washing ■ Contaminated respiratory therapy devices and equipment
Intervention-Related Factors	■ Supine positioning ■ Medications: proton pump inhibitors, sedatives, corticosteroids ■ Endotracheal tubes ■ Nasogastric tubes/enteral feeding ■ Recent prior antibiotic use

Adapted from American Thoracic Society (2005). Guidelines for the management of adults with hospital-acquired, ventilator-assisted, and health care-associated pneumonia. *American Journal of Respiratory Critical Care Medicine, 171,* 388-416.
and
Dupont, H., Montravers, P., Gauzit, R., Veber, B., Pouriat, J.L., & Martin, C. (2003). Outcome of postoperative pneumonia in the Eole study. *Intensive Care Medicine, 29*(2), 179-188.

has significant consequences. A single antibiotic dose given 30 minutes before the skin incision provides therapeutic drug levels in the wound and surrounding tissues during the operation. If surgery is longer than 3 hours, major blood loss occurs, or an antimicrobial with a short half-life is used, one or more additional antibiotic doses are advisable during the procedure (Abramowicz, 2009).

Because of their complexity, treating infected wounds may require systemic antibiotics as well as local wound care. In addition, attention to the factors that promote wound healing—adequate perfusion, oxygenation, and optimal nutritional intake—is critical. Decisions about antimicrobial therapy should be determined after reviewing the results of a microbiologic culture. Ultimately, determination of the value of antibiotic therapy should be made in conjunction with the clinical evaluation of the patient and the characteristics of the wound.

Prevention of infection is important to avoid increased discomfort for the patient, the possibility of additional surgical procedures, prolonged hospitalization and rehabilitation, the necessity of broad spectrum antibiotics, and possible long-term negative consequences. Thorough assessment and a high index of suspicion help the nurse

identify those patients at risk for infection and allow for interventions to limit infection. Interventions target the reduction of bacterial contamination of the surgical incision and enhance the patient's defenses against infection.

Hospital Acquired Pneumonia (HAP)

Hospital-acquired pneumonia (HAP), pneumonia occurring 48 or more hours after admission excluding any infection that is incubating at the time of admission (American Thoracic Society, 2005), is a severe nosocomial infection that requires early recognition and adequate and timely antimicrobial therapy to reduce mortality.

Risk Factors

There are multiple risk factors for HAP (see Table 8-8) and nursing can play a role in prevention as well as early recognition.

Clinical Manifestations

A new onset of fever, leukocytosis, purulent sputum, and a decline in oxygenation are all signs of pneumonia. A radiographic infiltrate that is new or progressive, along with clinical findings suggesting infection, confirms the diagnosis (American Thoracic Society, 2005). Patients with suspected pneumonia should have a chest x-ray and blood cultures. Arterial blood gas or oximetry can help determine the severity of illness and the need for supplemental oxygen. A complete blood count (CBC), serum electrolytes, and determination of renal and liver function can indicate multiple organ dysfunction, helping to define the severity of the illness. The culture of expectorated sputum is neither sensitive nor specific for identifying the etiologic pathogen of HAP, thus limiting the value of Gram's stain and sputum culturing (American Thoracic Society, 2005).

Prevention and Interventions

Prevention of HAP is the best way of decreasing the associated morbidity and mortality. Use of pneumococcal and influenza vaccination, handwashing, alcohol-based hand disinfection by healthcare professionals, early removal of invasive devices, avoiding supine positions by keeping the patient in a semi-recumbent position with the head of the bed at 30-45 degrees when possible, and isolating patients with multiple resistant respiratory tract pathogens have all been shown to be efficacious (Alcon, Fabregas, & Torres, 2003; American Thoracic Society, 2005).

Appropriate antibiotic therapy is the primary treatment for HAP. Empirical drug therapy that is initiated promptly is effective in reducing the mortality and morbidity of HAP. Consideration should be given to severity of illness, comorbid conditions that can lead to infection with specific pathogens, and length of hospitalization when determining appropriate monotherapy or combination therapy. Response to antibiotic therapy should be evident in 48-72 hours (American Thoracic Society, 2005). Additional supportive therapy such as supplemental oxygen, nutritional support, and chest physical therapy should be used as appropriate.

Postoperative Nausea and Vomiting (PONV)

Postoperative nausea and vomiting is a common complication after anesthesia and surgery. It usually occurs in the first 24 hours after surgery, with the highest incidence during the first 2 hours, however it can extend throughout the 72-hour postsurgical period (Wender, 2009). Persistent or severe nausea and vomiting not only cause generalized discomfort but can contribute to dehydration, electrolyte imbalance, increased discomfort, and delay in discharge (Golembiewski & O'Brien, 2002).

Risk Factors for PONV

The cause of postoperative nausea and vomiting is multifactorial. The primary predictors of PONV and additional factors that increase the risk are shown in Table 8-9.

Mechanisms of PONV

Stimulation of the vomiting center can come from vagal afferent nerves, the cerebral cortex, the vestibular apparatus, the chemoreceptor trigger zone, and the endocrine environment (Golembiewski & O'Brien, 2002). Activation of dopamine, serotonin, histamine, acetylcholine, and opioid receptors play an important role in producing nausea and vomiting. Antiemetic drugs that block these receptors are indicated to reduce PONV (Golembiewski & Tokumaru, 2007).

Prevention of PONV

Prevention and early intervention can minimize the discomfort and risks associated with PONV and potentially result in cost savings if discharge is not delayed. Specifically, successful PONV prevention and management can result in positive patient outcomes such as increased well-being, decreased lengths of stay due to improved surgical recovery, improved mobility, and improved nutritional intake. If patients are not experiencing PONV, they can more easily participate in postoperative care such as use of an incentive spirometer, coughing and deep breathing, and earlier participation in physical therapy.

If a patient has one to two risk factors for PONV, a single antiemetic agent is recommended. If they have three to four risk factors, a combination of antiemetic agents that work by different mechanisms of action is recommended for both prevention and treatment of PONV in adults (Golembiewski & Tokumaru, 2007). The antiemetic effect of glucocorticoids has been demonstrated with a single dose of dexamethasone given preoperatively (Fujii & Nakayama, 2005) however concerns about potential side effects has limited use. Although many patients may benefit from preoperative antiemetic treatment, prophylaxis is costly, and antiemetics, like any drugs, have the potential risks of adverse drug reactions (Tramer, 2001). The numbers of risk factors for PONV, and subsequent consequences for the patient should PONV occur, are key when determining whether or not to use prophylactic antiemetics (Gan et al., 2007).

Treatment and Nursing Interventions

Attempts to manage PONV involve pharmacologic and nonpharmacologic measures. There are five neurotransmitter receptors found within the chemoreceptor trigger zone. Drugs that block these receptors are most useful. No single antiemetic medication has been found to be 100% effective (Nelson, 2002). This is likely due to the multifactorial nature of PONV; if one drug isn't effective, it is often helpful to add a second drug from a different class (see Table 8-10). Prophylactic drug therapy is likely to be useful only for patients at moderate to high risk for PONV (Golembiewski & Tokumaru, 2007). Drugs with different mechanisms of action should be used in combination to optimize efficacy for prophylaxis (Gan et al., 2007).

There are alternatives to pharmacologic therapy for PONV. The administration of supplemental oxygen has been found helpful in preventing PONV in some studies (Couture, Maye, O'Brien, & Smith, 2007). Intraoperative colloid administration reduces postoperative nausea and vomiting and is associated with an improvement in the quality of postoperative recovery (Moretti, Robertson, El-Moalem, & Gan, 2003). Isopropyl alcohol inhalation is reported to be an effective, low-cost treatment for PONV, although the length of effectiveness, standard dose required, and mode of inhalation are not clear (Merritt, Okyere, & Jasinski, 2002; Winston, Rinehart, Riley, Vaccinhiano, & Pelligrini, 2003). Aromatherapy with peppermint, isopropyl alcohol, and placebo are all equally effective in relieving postoperative nausea (Anderson & Gross, 2004). Ginger, taken orally, has also demonstrated effectiveness in minimizing PONV (Chaiyakunapruk, Kitikannakorn, Nathisuwan, Leeprakobbon, & Leelasettagool, 2006). Acupressure, acupuncture, transcutaneous electrical stimulation (TENS), and acupoint stimulation are all alternatives, with varying

Table 8-9
Risk Factors for Postoperative Nausea and Vomiting

Primary Risk Factors	■ Female gender ■ History of PONV ■ History of motion sickness ■ Nonsmoking status
Additional Risk Factors	■ Surgery > 60 minutes ■ Use of opioids postoperatively ■ General anesthesia ■ Younger age ■ Shoulder surgery ■ History of delayed gastric emptying ■ Preoperative anxiety ■ Preoperative orthostatic dysfunction ■ Postoperative hypotension

Adapted from Golembiewski, J.A., & O'Brien, D. (2002). A systematic approach to the management of postoperative nausea and vomiting. *Journal of PeriAnesthesia Nursing, 17*(6), 364-376. doi: 10.1053/jpan.202.36596
and
Golembiewski, J.A. & Tokumaru, S. (2007). Pharmacological prophylaxis and management of adult postoperative/postdischarge nausea and vomiting. *Journal of PeriAnesthesia Nursing, 21*(7), 385-397.
and
Nelson, T.P. (2002). Postoperative nausea and vomiting: Understanding the enigma. *Journal of PeriAnesthesia Nursing, 17*(3), 178-189.
and
Stadler, M., Bardiau, F., Seidel, L., Albert, A., & Boogaerts, J.G. (2003). Difference in risk factors for postoperative nausea and vomiting. *Anesthesiology, 98*, 46-52.

Table 8-10
Antiemetic Drugs

Class	Examples	Key Points
Antidopaminergic	– metoclopramide (Reglan®) – prochlorperazine (Compazine®)	Helpful in reducing nausea and vomiting
Selective 5-HT3 receptor antagonist	– ondansetron (Zofran®) – dolasetron (Anzemet®)	Highly specific for nausea and vomiting, superior to the traditional antiemetic agents but more costly
Antihistamine	– diphendydramine (Benadryl®) – hydroxyzine (Vistaril®)	Drug of choice to prevent and manage PONV after middle ear surgery, in patients with a history of motion sickness, and possible PONV caused by opioids
Anticholinergic	– scopolamine (Transderm Scop®) – atropine	Block cholinergic transmission in the vomiting center of the CNS

Golembiewski, J.A., & O'Brien, D. (2002). A systematic approach to the management of postoperative nausea and vomiting. *Journal of PeriAnesthesia Nursing, 17*(6), 364-376. doi: 10.1053.jpan.2002.36596

degrees of success, to antiemetic therapy (Lee & Done, 2004). Appropriate pain control; adequate hydration; the encouragement of slow, deep breaths; minimizing abrupt movements with the patient; and avoidance of hypotension, tight-fitting oxygen masks, overuse of oral airways, and suctioning all can be helpful (Borgeat, Ekatodramis, & Schenker, 2003).

Given the distress of PONV and the risk of increased complications and cost, assessment and early intervention for PONV is warranted for high risk patients. In particular, attention should be paid to nonsmoking women with a prior history of PONV or motion sickness who are undergoing surgery lasting longer than 1-2 hours in duration.

Constipation

Constipation, a decrease in frequency of defecation accompanied by difficult or incomplete passage of hard, dry stool (Gordon, 2007), is a common postoperative complication. Table 8-11 lists the diagnostic and supporting signs of constipation as described by the North American Nursing Diagnosis Association.

Early detection of constipation allows for the initiation of interventions to minimize any negative consequences. In addition to assessing usual bowel patterns, it is essential to monitor bowel elimination on a daily basis. Systematic recording of bowel function will facilitate communication between nurses, allowing for easy recognition of bowel patterns. In addition, it is important to note the use of constipating medications and the ingestion of binding foods. The abdomen should be examined for tenderness, masses, and gaseous or fluid distention. Determining fluid intake

and evaluating skin turgor provides information regarding risk for, or actual, dehydration. A digital rectal exam is indicated to rule out fecal impaction. Additional diagnostic testing is usually not necessary in the hospitalized patient who presents with constipation and has no prior history of elimination problems.

Risk Factors

There are many contributing factors to the development of constipation. Hospitalized patients in particular encounter immobility, decreased dietary fiber, changes in regular dietary intake, dehydration, side effects of medications (especially opioids), change in environment and routine, stress, and situations causing one to ignore the gastrocolic reflex, the urge to defecate.

Assessment and Prevention

Assessing usual bowel patterns enables the nurse to determine any changes from baseline that warrant intervention. Daily evaluation of bowel function allows for early intervention and potentially prevents the negative consequences associated with constipation or impaction. Patients should be encouraged to follow the same defecation routine they have at home. For example, encourage efforts to defecate daily after breakfast if that is consistent with a patient's home pattern. Provide privacy and promote the use of a toilet or commode instead of a bedpan when possible. Warm fluids can help to initiate the gastrocolic reflex. Encourage physical activity and mobility. Support dietary selections of foods high in fiber, and urge an adequate intake of fluids, generally 6-8 glasses per day. Sufficient fluid intake will promote adequate hydration of stools, especially if the fiber intake is increased. Emollient laxatives result in a softening of stools within 1-3 days and are generally used to prevent constipation (Dipiro et al., 2005).

Table 8-11
Diagnostic and Supporting Signs and Symptoms of Constipation

Diagnostic Signs and Symptoms	Supporting Signs and Symptoms
– Decreased frequency of stool – Decreased volume of stool – Inability to pass stool – Dry, hard, formed stool – Report of rectal fullness or pressure	– Straining with defecation – Abdominal tenderness – Abdominal pain – Distended abdomen – Palpable rectal or abdominal mass – Increased abdominal pressure – Abdominal dullness on percussion – Hyperactive or hypoactive bowel sounds – Severe flatus – Presence of soft paste-like stool in the rectum – Anorexia – Headache – Indigestion – Nausea or vomiting – Bright red blood with defecation – Black or tarry stool

Reprinted with permission from Gordon, M. (2007). *Manual of nursing diagnosis* (11th ed., p. 132). Sudbury, MA: Jones & Bartlett.

Treatment

If the efforts to maintain usual bowel patterns are not successful, laxative agents can be used safely on an intermittent basis. There are three primary categories of laxative agents used for the treatment of constipation: bulk laxatives, osmotic agents, and stimulant laxatives. Efforts to optimize bowel function generally begin with bulk agents; osmotic agents are added as second-line therapy if necessary; and stimulant agents are used only on an as needed basis. Fiber and bulk agents are useful to increase stool weight and reduce colonic transit time, with the goal being a soft, formed stool. The amount of fiber or bulk agent necessary is individualized and based on patient response. Because failure to balance fiber with fluid can worsen constipation, adequate intake of fluids is essential (Doughty, 2002). Osmotic agents work by pulling fluid into the colon, which distends the bowel and stimulates contractions. Their rapid onset and action (30 minutes to 3 hours) makes them preferable for acute constipation, and they are generally safe and effective (American Gastroenterological Association, 2000). Stimulant laxatives cause water retention and stimulate peristalsis. They typically produce a bowel movement within 6 to 8 hours after ingestion and are not recommended for regular daily use (Dipiro et al., 2005). Enemas are indicated for fecal impaction and acute constipation. Suppositories may be used to empty the lower bowel.

The choice of drug therapy depends on the specific circumstances. Dietary changes and increased fluid intake are the initial interventions recommended in most situations. Stimulant laxatives are generally helpful when constipation is related to prolonged immobility, as is frequently seen after orthopaedic surgical procedures.

Constipation is a common problem encountered in nursing. Implementing a systematic approach to help patients maintain or establish normal bowel functioning with minimal reliance on medication is an important aspect to consider. The goal is to promote regular defecation such that patients avoid the discomfort associated with constipation.

Urinary Retention

In adults, typical voiding patterns are every 2-6 hours; the frequency varies according to bladder capacity, fluid consumption, availability of a toilet, and the amount of insensible fluid losses (Gray, 2000b). Postoperative urinary retention is a relatively common problem after surgery. It occurs as a direct result of the type of anesthetic, advanced age, the total amount of fluid replacement over a 24-hour postoperative period, the types and amounts of analgesics, and a history of postoperative urinary problems (Wynd, Wallace, & Smith, 1996). Opioids and anesthetic agents are specifically associated with impaired detrusor contractility. The patient with acute urinary retention presents with an inability to void despite the presence of urine in the bladder and the desire to urinate (Gray, 2000a; Lau & Lam, 2004). Often, the patient will also complain of suprapubic pressure or pain.

Protuberance of the midline of the abdomen may be visible, and percussion of the suprapubic area will be dull if the bladder is full of urine. Dullness of the bladder to the level

Table 8-12
Risk Factors for Pressure Ulcers

- Impaired mobility
- Increased age
- Moisture/Incontinence
- Dehydration
- Compromised nutrition (obesity and malnutrition)
- Altered tissue perfusion
- Altered level of consciousness
- Altered sensory perception
- Use of sedatives and analgesics

Adapted from Baharestani, M.M., Ratliff C., & the National Pressure Ulcer Advisory Panel (2007). Pressure ulcers in neonates & children: An NPUAP White Paper. *Advances in Skin and Wound Care, 20*(4): 208-220.
and
Baumgarten, M., Margolis, D. J., Localio, A. R., Kagan, S. H., Lowe, R. A., Kinosian, B., ...Mehari, T. (2008). Extrinsic risk factors for pressure ulcers early in the hospital stay: A nested case-control study. *Journal of Gerontology, Series A, Biological Sciences Medical Sciences, 63*(4), 408-413.
and
Reddy, M., Gill, S. S., & Rochon, P. A. (2006). Preventing pressure ulcers: A systematic review. *Journal of the American Medical Association, 296*(8), 974-984.
and
Redelings, D., Lee, N. E., & Sorvillo, F. (2005). Pressure ulcers: More lethal than we thought? *Advances in Skin & Wound Care, 18*(7), 367-372.

of the umbilicus indicates at least 500 mL of urine in the bladder (Gray, 2000b). Light palpation will also reveal an enlarged bladder. Clinical examination of the abdomen by abdominal palpation and suprapubic percussion, however, is dependent on the skill of the practitioner (Weatherall & Harwood, 2002). Bladder ultrasonography with a portable bladder scanner has been shown to be more effective than manual palpation in the assessment of postoperative bladder distention (Rosseland, Stubhaug, & Breivik, 2002).

Prevention and Nursing Interventions

Catheterization can be done to drain the urine and evaluate the degree of urinary retention (Lau & Lam, 2004). Prompt bladder drainage and the prevention of tissue trauma and infection associated with catheterization are important. Warm beverages with a relatively high dose of caffeine per fluid ounce, such as coffee or tea, may be helpful because caffeine has been shown to stimulate both the urge to urinate and smooth muscle contractility (Gray, 2000b). Postoperative urinary retention is generally time-limited: with each postoperative day, the effects of the anesthetic and analgesics decrease, and the volume of intravenous fluid replacement is usually less.

In-out intermittent catheterization is recommended when the bladder volume (as measured with ultrasound) is greater than 600ml over a minimum period of 2 hours. This is done to prevent bladder distention that can lead to voiding dysfunction (Baldini, Bagry, Aprikian, & Carli, 2009). Appropriate technique is necessary to avoid the complications of infection, urethral trauma, and patient discomfort.

Urinary retention is a common postoperative occurrence. The nursing management of the patient focuses on timely recognition of urinary retention, emptying the bladder of retained urine, recognition and reduction or elimination of

Table 8-13

Support Surfaces Used in the Prevention and Treatment of Pressure Ulcers

Group	Characteristics	Options	Indications
1	– Static – Do not require electricity	– Air overlay/mattress – Foam overlay/ mattress – Gel overlay/mattress – Water overlay/mattress	Patient at low risk for pressure ulcer development
2	– Dynamic – Powered by electricity or pump	– Alternating pressure overlays or mattress – Low-air loss mattress	– If reactive hyperemia is noted on bony prominences – Patients at moderate to high risk for pressure ulcers – Patients who already have a full thickness pressure ulcer
3	– Electric – Contain silicon-coated beads that become liquefied when air is pumped through the bed	– Air fluidized beds	Patients with non-healing full thickness pressure ulcers

Adapted from de Laat, E. H., Pickkers, P., Schoonhoven, L., Verbeek, A. L., Feuth, T., & van Achterberg, T. (2007). Guideline implementation results in a decrease of pressure ulcer incidence in critically ill patients. *Critical Care Medicine, 35*(3), 815-820.
and
Duncan, K. D. (2007). Preventing pressure ulcers: The goal is zero. *The Joint Commission Journal on Quality and Patient Safety, 33*(10), 605-610.
and
McInnes, E., Bell-Syer, S. E. M., Dumville, J. C., Legood, R., & Cullum N. A. (2008). Support surfaces for pressure ulcer prevention. *The Cochrane Database of Systematic Reviews, 4*, Art. No.: CD001735. doi: 10.1002/14651858. CD001735.pub3.
and
Vanderwee, K., Grypdonck, M. & Defloor, T. (2008). Alternating pressure air mattresses as prevention for pressure ulcers: A literature review. *International Journal of Nursing Studies, 45*(5), 784-801.

factors contributing to the risk for urinary retention, and prevention of recurrent episodes (Gray, 2000b; Lau & Lam, 2004).

Pressure Ulcers

Pressure ulcers are a high-frequency problem in many health care settings. The decreased mobility associated with many orthopaedic procedures places patients undergoing orthopaedic surgical procedures at a greater risk for pressure ulcers. Pressure ulcers develop from persistent pressure on a bony site significant enough to impede healthy capillary flow, leading to tissue necrosis. Pressure ulcers, "localized injury to the skin and/or underlying tissue usually over a bony prominence, as a result of pressure, or pressure in combination with shear and/or friction" (Black et al., 2007) affect a significant number of patients every year. Damage to the skin occurs when external pressure exceeds capillary closing pressure obstructing blood flow to tissue and causing local ischemia. When this pressure is sustained for 2 hours, it can lead to tissue death (Barton, 2006; Bouten, Oomens, Baaijens, & Bader, 2003). A patient's severity of illness and comorbidity may change the physiology enough that less pressure is required to actually obstruct capillary blood flow. Disruption of the microvasculature by shearing forces can also reduce tissue oxygenation. A pressure ulcer can develop within 2-6 hours, making risk assessment critical in order for preventive measures to be put into place in a timely manner (Barton, 2006; Lyder, 2003).

Risk Factors

Numerous risk factors for pressure ulcers have been identified. Many of these are related to medical conditions that negatively impact microcirculation such as diabetes, peripheral vascular disease, and hypotension (Lyder, 2003). Table 8-12 describes other conditions that increase the risk for pressure ulcers. Every patient should be assessed upon admission, and daily thereafter, to identify risk for and early signs of pressure ulcer development (Garcia & Thomas, 2006). Risk assessment can be accomplished by using a validated assessment tool, such as the Braden Scale and the Norton Scale, which provide the nurse with an efficient and systematic means of identifying patients at high risk for pressure ulcer development. Elements of a risk assessment include evaluation of nutrition, mobility, elimination, sensation, and the skin itself with an emphasis on temperature, turgor, color, integrity, moisture and capillary refill (Duncan, 2007; Hommel, Biorkelund, Thorngren, & Ulander, 2007; Nixon, Cranny, & Bond, 2007; Stratton et al., 2005). Determination of blood pressure as well as serum glucose, albumin, and blood count all contribute to risk assessment.

Prevention and Nursing Interventions

Once a patient's risk for pressure ulcer development has been determined, it is important to put appropriate interventions in place. A multidisciplinary panel (Panel for the Prediction and Prevention of Pressure Ulcers in Adults, 1992) developed evidence-based clinical practice guidelines related to pressure ulcer prediction and prevention in adults that focus on the following goals: 1) identifying at-risk individuals and the specific factors placing them at risk; 2) maintaining and improving tissue tolerance to pressure to prevent injury; 3) protecting against adverse effects of external mechanical forces (pressure, friction, and shear); and 4) reducing the incidence of pressure ulcers through educational programs. The primary emphasis should be on removing or redistributing the pressure to sensitive areas of the body. Table 8-13 describes three types of support surfaces frequently used in hospitals to prevent injury by redistributing pressure, and Table 8-14 notes additional measures to reduce the development of pressure ulcers.

Table 8-14
Measures to Reduce the Development of Pressure Ulcers

- Assess skin daily with attention to areas at high risk - sacrum, back, buttocks, heels, and elbows

- Manage moisture due to incontinence, perspiration or wound drainage
  - Keep skin clean with mild cleansing agent to minimize irritation and dryness of the skin
  - Minimize skin exposure to moisture with use of topical agents that work as moisture barriers
  - Use underpads made of materials that absorb moisture and provide a quick-drying surface to the skin

- Optimize nutrition and hydration
  - Consider a consult to a clinical dietician
  - Correct fluid and nutritional deficiencies
  - Nutritional supplements or support may be needed if dietary intake is insufficient

- Minimize pressure/shearing forces
  - Increase mobility; establish a repositioning schedule every 2-hours for all patients at risk
  - Avoid positioning patient directly on a pressure ulcer
  - Maintain the head of the bed at the lowest degree of elevation consistent with medical conditions and other restrictions to minimize shear and friction forces between the skin and the bed
  - Use positioning devices to keep bony prominences from direct contact with one another
  - If completely immobile, totally relieve pressure on the heels
  - Use a pressure-reducing surface (mattress overlays, low air loss bed, air fluidized bed) in those patients at risk
  - Use lifting devices such as a trapeze or bed linen to move immobile patient in bed
  - Avoid massage over bony prominences
  - Minimize friction and shear forces by proper position, transferring, and turning techniques - lubricants, protective films, dressings, and padding can also be used

Adapted from Bouten, C. V., Oomens, C. W., Baaijens, F. P., & Bader, D. L. (2003). The etiology of pressure ulcers; skin deep or muscle bound? *Archives of Physical Medicine and Rehabilitation, 84*(4), 616-619.
and
de Laat, E. H., Pickkers, P., Schoonhoven, L., Verbeek, A. L., Feuth, T., & van Achterberg, T. (2007). Guideline implementation results in a decrease of pressure ulcer incidence in critically ill patients. *Critical Care Medicine, 35*(3), 815-820.
and
Dini, V., Bertone, M. S., & Romanelli, M. (2006). Prevention and management of pressure ulcers. *Dermatologic Therapy, 19*, 356-364.
and
Duncan, K. D. (2007). Preventing pressure ulcers: The goal is zero. *The Joint Commission Journal on Quality and Patient Safety, 33*(10), 605-610.
and
Reddy, M., Gill, S. S., & Rochon, P. A. (2006). Preventing pressure ulcers: A systematic review. *Journal of the American Medical Association, 296*(8), 974-984.

Table 8-15
National Pressure Ulcer Advisory Panel Pressure Ulcer Staging System

Pressure Ulcer Stages
Stage I: Intact skin with non-blanchable redness of a localized area usually over a bony prominence. Darkly pigmented skin may not have visible blanching; its color may differ from the surrounding area. *This area may be painful, firm, soft, warmer or cooler as compared to adjacent tissue.*
Stage II: Partial thickness loss of dermis presenting as a shallow open ulcer with a reddened wound bed, without slough. May also present as an intact or open/rupture serum-filled blister. *Presents as a shiny or dry shallow ulcer without slough or bruising.*
Stage III: Full thickness tissue loss. Subcutaneous fat may be visible but bone, tendon or muscle are not exposed. Slough may be present but does not obscure the depth of tissue loss. May include undermining and tunneling. *The depth of a Stage III pressure ulcer varies by anatomical location. Bone/tendon is not visible or directly palpable.*
Stage IV: Full thickness tissue loss with exposed bone, tendon or muscle. Slough or eschar may be present on some parts of the wound bed. Often include undermining and tunneling. *The depth of a Stage IV pressure ulcer varies by anatomical location.*
(Suspected) Deep Tissue Injury
Purple or maroon localized area of discolored intact skin or blood-filled blister due to damage of underlying soft tissue from pressure and/or shear. The area may be preceded by tissue that is painful, firm, mushy boggy, warmer or cooler as compared to adjacent tissue. (This may rapidly deteriorate to a deeper injury despite the best preventative measures taken.)
Unstageable
Full thickness tissue loss in which the base of the ulcer is covered by slough and /or eschar in the wound bed. *Until enough slough and/or eschar is removed to expose the base of the wound, the true depth, and therefore stage, cannot be determined. Stable (dry, adherent, intact without erythema or fluctuance) eschar on the heels serves as "the body's natural (biological) cover" and should not be removed.*

Adapted from Black, J., Baharestani, M. M., Cuddigan, J., Dorner, B., Edsberg, L., Langemo, D., ... The National Pressure Ulcer Advisory Panel. (2007). National Pressure Ulcer Advisory Panel's updated pressure ulcer staging system. *Advances in Skin and Wound Care, 20*(3), 269-274.

Clinical Manifestations and Treatment Approach

The evaluation of a pressure ulcer should include the wound stage, and characteristics such as length, width and depth; tissue color; granulation versus eschar tissue; odor; drainage; undermining; and pain (Garcia & Thomas, 2006). The Stages of Pressure Ulcers (Table 8-15) improve care planning and communication about the amount of anatomical tissue loss in a pressure ulcer. This staging system should be used only to describe pressure ulcers. The first step in treating pressure ulcers is to remove the pressure. Further intervention depends on the stage of the ulcer and the specific condition of the patient as illustrated in Table 8-16.

Table 8-16
Interventions for Pressure Ulcers

Stage I	Stage II	Stage III and IV
– Remove the pressure – Increase mobility – Correct nutritional deficiencies – Avoid hypotension – Ensure adequate oxygenation – Eliminate excess moisture – Avoid shearing forces	– Interventions noted for Stage I Pressure Ulcer – Appropriate dressing (want to maintain moist wound environment; use wet-to-dry gauze dressing only if there is poor granulation tissue and debridement is necessary) – Determination of the most appropriate type of dressing is based upon staging of the pressure ulcer and amount of drainage • Transparent films • Hydrocolloids • Alginates • Foams • Hydrogels • Hydrofibers • Gauze dressing	– Interventions noted for Stage I and II pressure ulcer – Debride necrotic tissue – Appropriate dressing changes – Correction of underlying medical problems – Consider consultation with a skin care/wound specialist

Adapted from Dini, V., Bertone, M. S., & Romanelli, M. (2006). Prevention and management of pressure ulcers. *Dermatologic Therapy, 19*, 356-364.
and
Garcia, A. D., & Thomas, D. R. (2006). Assessment and management of chronic pressure ulcers in the elderly. *Medical Clinics of North America, 90*(5), 925-944.
and
Lyder, C. H. (2003). Pressure ulcer prevention and management. *Journal of the American Medical Association, 289*, 223-26.

Summary

There are many potential complications that can occur related to orthopaedic conditions and surgeries. Knowing the risk factors and intervention methods to prevent the occurrence of complications associated with orthopaedic conditions and surgical procedures will contribute to positive outcomes. Prevention is key to the most favorable patient outcomes, regardless of the type of complication. Orthopaedic nurses are challenged to recognize and anticipate the risk for complications, initiate appropriate interventions, and decrease the likelihood of undesirable patient outcomes.

References

Abramowicz, M. (Ed.) (2009). Antimicrobial prophylaxis in surgery. *Medical Letters and Drug Therapy, 82*, 47-53.

Akhtar, S. (2009). Fat embolism. *Anesthesiologist Clinics, 27*(3), 533-550.

Alcon, A., Fabregas, N., & Torres, A. (2003). Hospital-acquired pneumonia: Etiologic considerations. *Infectious Disease Clinics of North America, 17* (4), 679-695.

American Gastroenterological Association (2000). American Gastroenterological Association medical position statement: Guidelines on constipation. *Gastroenterology, 119*, 1776-1778.

American Psychiatric Association (2000). *American Psychiatric Association: Diagnostic and statistical manual of mental disorders* (4th ed., DSM-IV, pp. 135-136). Washington, DC: American Psychiatric Association.

American Thoracic Society (2005). Guidelines for the management of adults with hospital-acquired, ventilator-associated, and health care-associated pneumonia. *American Journal of Respiratory Critical Care Medicine, 171*, 388-416.

Anderson, D.R., Kahn, S.R., Rodger, M.A., & Wells, P. S. (2007). Computed tomographic pulmonary angiography vs. ventilation-perfusion lung scanning in patients with suspected pulmonary embolism: A randomized controlled trial. *Journal of the American Medical Association, 298*, 2743-2753.

Anderson, L. A., & Gross, J. B. (2004). Aromotherapy with peppermint, isopropyl alcohol, and placebo are all equally effective in relieving postoperative nausea. *Journal of Perianesthia Nursing, 19*, 29-35.

Aragon, D., Ring, C. A., & Covelli, M. (2003). The influence of diabetes mellitus on postoperative infections. *Critical Care Nursing Clinics of North America, 15*, 125-135.

Ashendorf, L., Jefferson, A. L., O'Connor, M. K., Chaaisson, C., Green, R. C., & Stern, R. A. (2008). Trial making test errors in normal aging, mild cognitive impairment, and dementia. *Archives in Clinical Neuropsychology, 23*, 129-137.

Babalis, G. A., Yiannakopoulos, C. K., Karliaftis, K., & Antonogiannakis, E. (2004). Prevention of posttraumatic hypoxemia in isolated lower limb long bone fractures with a minimal prophylactic dose of corticosteroids. *Injury, 35*(3). 309–317.

Baharestani, M.M., Ratliff, C., and the National Pressure Ulcer Advisory Panel. (2007). Pressure ulcers in neonates & children: An NPUAP White Paper. *Advances in Skin and Wound Care, 20*(4), 208-220.

Baldini, G., Bagry, H., Aprikian, A., & Carli, F. (2009). Postoperative urinary retention: Anesthetic and perioperative considerations. *Anesthesiology, 110*, (5), 1139-1157. doi: 10.1097/ALN.0b013e31819f7aea

Barton, A. A. (2006). The pathogenesis of skin wounds due to pressure. *Journal of Tissue Viability, 16*(3), 12-15.

Baumgarten, M., Margolis, D. J., Localio, A. R., Kagan, S. H., Lowe, R. A., Kinosian, B., ...Mehari, T. (2008). Extrinsic risk factors for pressure ulcers early in the hospital stay: A nested case-control study. *Journal of Gerontology, Series A, Biological Sciences Medical Sciences, 63*(4), 408-413.

Bederman, S. S., Bhandari, M., McKee, M. D., & Schemitsch, E. H. (2009). Do corticosteroids reduce the risk of fat embolism syndrome in patients with long-bone fractures? A meta-analysis. *Canadian Journal of Surgery, 52*(5), 386-393.

Bennett, J., Haynes, S., Torella, R., Grainger, H., & Mccollum, C. (2006). Acute normovolemic hemodilution in moderate blood loss surgery: A randomized controlled trial. *Transfusion, 46*(7), 1097-1103.

Black, J., Baharestani, M. M., Cuddigan, J., Dorner, B., Edsberg, L., Langemo, D., ...The National Pressure Ulcer Advisory Panel (2007). National Pressure Ulcer Advisory Panel's updated pressure ulcer staging system. *Advances in Skin and Wound Care, 20*(3), 269-274.

Boni, L., Benevento, A., Rovera, F., Dionigi, G., DiGiuseppe, M., Bertoglio, C., & Dionigi, R. (2006). Infective complications in laparoscopic surgery. *Surgical Infections, 7*(S), 109-111.

Borgeat, A., Ekatodramis, G., & Schenker, C. A. (2003). Postoperative nausea and vomiting in regional anesthesia: A review. *Anesthesiology, 98*, 530-547.

Bourne, R. S., Tahir, T. A., Borthwick, M. & Sampson, E. L. (2008). Drug treatment of delirium: Past, present and future. *Journal of Psychosomatic Research, 65*, 273-282.

Bouten, C. V., Oomens, C. W., Baaijens, F. P., & Bader, D. L. (2003). The etiology of pressure ulcers; skin deep or muscle bound? *Archives of Physical Medicine and Rehabilitation, 84*(4), 616-619.

Bulger, E. M., Smith, D. G., Maier, R. V., & Jurkovich, G. J. (1997). Fat embolism syndrome, a 10-year review. *Archives of Surgery, 132*, 435-439.

Carless P.A., Henry, D.A., & Anthony, D.M. (2008). Fibrin sealant use for minimizing peri-operative allogeneic blood transfusion. *The Cochrane Database of Systematic Reviews, 1.* doi: 10.1002/14651858.CD004171

Carless, P., Moxey, A., O'Connell, D., & Henry, D. (2004). Autologous transfusion techniques: A systematic review of their efficacy. *Transfusion Medicine, 14* (2), 123-144.

Carter, C. J. (1994). The pathophysiology of venous thrombosis. *Progress in Cardiovascular Diseases, 36*, 439-446.

Casarett, D. J. & Inouye, S. K. (2001). Diagnosis and management of delirium near the end of life. *Annals of Internal Medicine, 135*, 32-40.

Chaiyakunapruk, N., Kitikannakorn, N., Nathisuwan, S., Leeprakobbon, K., & Leelasettagool, C. (2006). The efficacy of ginger for the prevention of postoperative nausea and vomiting: A meta-analysis. *American Journal of Obstetrics and Gynecology, 194*(1), 95-99.

Cheadle, W. G. (2006). Risk factors for surgical site infection. *Surgical Infections, 7*(1), S7-S11.

Couture, D. J., Maye, J. P., O'Brien, D., & Smith, A. B. (2007). Therapeutic modalities for the prophylactic management of postoperative nausea and vomiting. *Journal of PeriAnesthesia Nursing, 21*(7), 398-403.

Dasgupta, M., & Dumbrell, A. C. (2006). Preoperative risk assessment for delirium after non cardiac surgery: A systematic review. *Journal of the American Geriatric Society, 54*(10), 1578-1589.

de Laat, E. H., Pickkers, P., Schoonhoven, L., Verbeek, A. L., Feuth, T., & van Achterberg, T. (2007). Guideline implementation results in a decrease of pressure ulcer incidence in critically ill patients. *Critical Care Medicine, 35*(3), 815-820.

Demeure, M. J., & Fain, M. J. (2006). The elderly surgical patient and postoperative delirium. *Journal of the American College of Surgeons, 203*, 752-757.

Dini, V., Bertone, M. S., & Romanelli, M. (2006). Prevention and management of pressure ulcers. *Dermatologic Therapy, 19*, 356-364.

Dipiro, J. T., Talbert, R. L., Yee, G. C., Matzke, G. R., Wells, B. G., & Posey, L. M. (Eds.) (2005). *Pharmacotherapy, A pathophysiologic approach* (6th ed, pp. 687-689). New York: McGraw Hill.

Doughty, D. B. (2002). When fiber is not enough: Current thinking on constipation management. *Ostomy Wound Management, 48,*(12), 30-41.

Dronge, A. S., Perkal, M. F., Kancir, S., Concato, J., Aslan, M., & Rosenthal, R. A. (2006). Long-term glycemic control and postoperative infectious complications. *Archives of Surgery, 141*, 375-380.

Duncan, K. D. (2007). Preventing pressure ulcers: The goal is zero. *The Joint Commission Journal on Quality and Patient Safety, 33* (10), 605-610.

Dupont, H., Montravers, P., Gauzit, R., Veber, B., Pouriat, J. L., & Martin, C. (2003). Outcome of postoperative pneumonia in the Eole study. *Intensive Care Medicine, 29*(2), 179-188.

Feagan, B. G., Wong, C. J., Kirkley, A., Johnston, D. W. C., Smith, F. C, Whitsitt, P., ...Lau, C. Y. (2000). Erythropoietin with iron supplementation to prevent allogeneic blood transfusion in total hip joint arthroplasty- A randomized, controlled trial. *Annals of Internal Medicine, 133*, 845-854.

Finlayson, E., & Birkmeyer, J. D. (2009). Surgical outcomes. In J.B. Halter, J.G. Ouslander, M.E. Tinetti, S. Studenski, K.P. High, & S. Asthana (Eds.), *Hazzard's Geriatric Medicine and Gerontology, 6e.* Retrieved on March 5, 2010, from http://www.accessmedicine.com/content.aspx?aID=5114872

Flacker, J.M., & Lipsitz, L.A. (1999). Neural mechanisms of delirium: Current hypotheses and evolving concepts. *Journals of Gerontology Series A – Biological Sciences & Medical Sciences, 54*(6):B239-246.

Fleisher, L.A., Beckman, J. A., Brown, K. A., Calkins, H., Chaikof, E. L., Fleischmann, K. E.,...Robb, J.F. (2007). ACC/AHA 2007 Guidelines on perioperative cardiovascular evaluation and care for noncardiac surgery: A report of the American College of Cardiology/American Heart Association task force on practice guidelines. *Journal of the American College of Cardiology, 50*, 1707-1732. doi: 10.1161/CIRCULATIONAHA.107.185699

Folstein, M. F., Folstein, S. E., & McHugh, P. R. (1975). Mini-mental state: A practical guide for grading the cognitive state of patients for clinicians. *Journal of Psychiatric Research, 12*, 189-198.

Fricchione, G. L., Nejad, S. H., Esses, J. A., Cummings, T. J., Quesques, J., Cassem, N. H., ...Murray, G. B. (2008). Postoperative delirium. *American Journal of Psychiatry, 165*(7), 803-812.

Fujii, Y., & Nakayama, M. (2005). Effects of dexamethasone in preventing postoperative emetic symptoms after total knee replacement surgery: A prospective, randomized, double-blind, vehicle-controlled trial in adult Japanese patients. *Clinical Therapeutics, 27*, 740-745.

Gan, T. J., Meyer, T. A., Apfel, C. C., Chung, F., Davis, P. J., Habib, A.S., ...Watcha, M. (2007). Society of Ambulatory Anesthesia Guidelines for the management of postoperative nausea and vomiting. *Anesthesia Analog, 105*, 1615-1628.

Gangireddy, C., Rectenwald, J. R., Upchurch, G. R., Wakefield, T. W., Khuri, S., Henderson, W., ...Henke, P. K. (2007). Risk factors and clinical impact of postoperative symptomatic venous thromboembolism. *Society for Vascular Surgery, 45*, 335-342.

Garcia, A. D., & Thomas, D. R. (2006). Assessment and management of chronic pressure ulcers in the elderly. *Medical Clinics of North America, 90*(5), 925-944.

Geerts, W. H., Bergqvist, D., Pineo, G. R., Heit, J. A., Samama, C. M., Lassen, M. R., ...Colwell, C. W. (2008). Prevention of venous thromboembolism. *Chest, 133* (1S), 381S-453S.

Gibson, N.S., Schellong, S.M., El Kheir, D.Y., Beyer-Westendorf, J., Gallus, A. S., McRae, S., ... Buller, H.R. (2009). Safety and sensitivity of two ultrasound strategies in patients with clinically suspected deep venous thrombosis: A prospective management study. *Journal of Thromobsis and Haemostasis, 7*(12), 2035–2041.

Golembiewski, J. A., & O'Brien, D. (2002). A systematic approach to the management of postoperative nausea and vomiting. *Journal of PeriAnesthesia Nursing, 17*(6), 364-376. doi: 10.1053/jpan.2002.36596

Golembiewski, J. A., & Tokumaru, S. (2007). Pharmacological prophylaxis and management of adult postoperative/postdischarge nausea and vomiting. *Journal of PeriAnesthesia Nursing, 21*(7), 385-397.

Goodnough, L. T., & Monk, T. G. (1996). Evolving concepts in autologous blood procurement and transfusion: Case reports of perisurgical anemia complicated by myocardial infarction. *American Journal of Medicine, 101*, 33S-37S.

Gordon, M. (2007). *Manual of Nursing Diagnosis* (11th ed., p. 132). Sudbury, MA: Jones & Bartlett.

Gray, M. (2000a). Urinary retention, management in the acute care setting. Part 1. *American Journal of Nursing, 100*(7), 40-47.

Gray, M. (2000b). Urinary retention, management in the acute care setting. Part 2. *American Journal of Nursing, 100*(8), 36-43.

Green, R. M. (2003). The role of prophylactic anticoagulation in the surgical patient. *Current Problems in Surgery, 40*(2), 92-130.

Greene, N. H., Attix, D. K., Weldon, B. C., Smith, P. J., McDonagh, D. L., & Monk, T. G. (2009). Measures of executive function and depression identify patients at risk for postoperative delirium. *Anesthesiology, 110*, 788-795.

Harkness, J.W., & Daniels, A.U. (2003). Introduction and overview. In S.T. Canale, K. Daugherty, & L. Jones (Eds.), *Campbell's operative orthopaedics* (pp. 223-242). St. Louis: Mosby.

Harvey, C. (2001). Compartment syndrome: When it is least expected. *Orthopaedic Nursing, 20*(3), 15-23.

Hemker, H.C., AlDieri, R., & Beguin, S. (2005). Laboratory monitoring of low-molecular-weight heparin therapy – part II. *Journal of Thrombosis and Haemostasis, 3*(3), 571-573. doi: 10.1111/j.1538-7836.2005.01206.x

Holzer, P. (2008). New approaches to the treatment of opoid-induced constipation. *European Review for Medical and Pharmacological Sciences, 12*(S1), 119-127.

Hommel, A., Bjorkeuland, K.B., Thorngren, K.G., & Ulander, K. (2007). Nutritional status among patients with hip fracture in relation to pressure ulcers. *Clinical Nutrition, 26*(5), 589-596.

Hoover, T. J., & Siefert, J. A. (2000). Soft tissue complications of orthopaedic emergencies. *Emergency Medicine Clinics of North America, 18*, 115-139.

Hshieh, T. T., Fong, T. G., Marcantonio, E. R., & Inouye, S. K. (2008). Cholinergic deficiency hypothesis in delirium: A synthesis of current evidence. *Journal of Gerontology, Series A: Biological Sciences Medical Sciences, 63*(7), 764-772.

Inouye, S. K. (2006). Delirium in older persons. *The New England Journal of Medicine, 354*(11), 1157-1165.

Inouye, S. K., Bogardus, S. T., Charpentier, P. A., Leo-Summers, L., Acampora, D., Holford, T R., ...Cooney, L. M. (1999). A multicomponent intervention to prevent delirium in hospitalized older patients. *New England Journal of Medicine, 340*, 669-676.

Inouye, S. K., & Ferrucci, L. (2006). Elucidating the pathophysiology of delirium and the interrelationship of delirium and dementia. *Journal of Gerontology, Series A: Biological Sciences Medical Sciences, 61*, 1277-1280.

Inouye, S.K., van Dyck, C., Alessi, C., Balkin, S., Siegal, A., & Horwitz, R. (1990). Clarifying confusion: The confusion assessment method. *Annals of Internal Medicine, 113*(12), 941-948.

Janzing, H., Broos, P., & Rommens, P. (1996). Compartment syndrome as a complication of skin traction in children with femoral fractures. *The Journal of Trauma: Injury, Infection, and Critical Care, 41*, 156-158.

Kaboli, P., Henderson, M. C., & White, R. H. (2003). DVT prophylaxis and anticoagulation in the surgical patient. *The Medical Clinics of North America, 87*, 77-110.

Kao, S. J., Yeh, D. Y., & Chen, H. I. (2007). Clinical and pathological features of fat embolism with acute respiratory distress syndrome. *Clinical Science (London), 113*(6), 279-285.

Kearon, C., Kahn, S. R., Agnelli, G., Goldhaver, S. Z., Raskob, G. E., & Comerota, J. A. (2008). Antithrombotic therapy for venous thromboembolic disease. American College of Chest Physicians Evidence-Based Clinical Practice Guidelines, *Chest, 133*, 454S-545S.

Keating, E. M., & Meding, J. B. (2002). Perioperative blood management practices in elective orthopaedic surgery. *Journal of the American Academy of Orthopaedic Surgeons, 10*, 393-400.

Kim, Y.H., Oh, S.W., & Kim, S.S. (2002). Prevalence of fat embolism following bilateral simultaneous and unilateral total hip arthroplasty performed with or without cement. *The Journal of Bone and Joint Surgery, 84A*, 1372-1379.

Kim, H. J., Walcott-Sapp, S., Leggett, K., Bass, A., Adler, R. S., Pavlov, H., ...Westrich, G. H. (2008). The use of spiral computed tomography scans for the detection of pulmonary embolism. *The Journal of Arthoplasty, 23*(S1), 31-35.

Lau, H., & Lam, B. (2004). Management of postoperative urinary retention; a randomized trial of in-out versus overnight catheterization. *ANZ Journal of Surgery, 74*(8), 658-661.

Lee, A., & Done, M. L. (2004). Stimulation of the wrist acupuncture point p6 for preventing postoperative nausea and vomiting. *Cochrane Database Systematic Review, 3*. doi: 10.1002/14651858. CD003281.pub2

Levy, J. H. (2008). Pharmacologic methods to reduce perioperative bleeding. *Transfusion, 48*(S1), 31S-38S.

Lidegaard, O., Lokkegaar, E., Svendsen, A. L., & Agger, C. (2009). Hormonal contraception and risk of venous thromboembolism; National follow-up study. *British Medical Journal, 339*, b2890. doi: 10.1136/bmj.b2890

Lyder, C. H. (2003). Pressure ulcer prevention and management. *Journal of the American Medical Association, 289*, 223-226.

Mangram, A. J., Horan, T. C., Pearson, M. L, Silver, L. C., & Jarvis, W. R. (1999). Guideline for prevention of surgical site infection, 1999. *Infection Control and Hospital Epidemiology, 20*(4), 247-278.

Marcantonio, E. R., Flacker, J. M., Wright, R. J., & Resnick, N. M. (2001). Reducing delirium after hip fracture: A randomized trial. *Journal of the American Geriatrics Society, 49*(5), 516-522.

Marcantonio, E. R., Rudolph, J. L, Culley, D., Crosby, G., Alsop, D., & Inouye, S. K. (2006). Interrelationship of delirium and dementia, Review article: Serum biomarkers for delirium. *Journal of Gerontology, Series A: Biological Sciences Medical Sciences, 61*, 1281-1286.

McInnes, E., Bell-Syer, S. E. M., Dumville, J. C., Legood, R., & Cullum N. A. (2008). Support surfaces for pressure ulcer prevention. *The Cochrane Database of Systematic Reviews, 4*, Art. No.: CD001735. doi: 10.1002/14651858. CD001735.pub3

McDermott, I. D., Culpan, P., Clancy, M., & Dooley, J. F. (2002). The role of rehydration in the prevention of fat embolism syndrome. *Injury, 33*, 757-759.

McQueen, M. M., Gaston, P., & Court-Brown, C. M. (2000). Acute compartment syndrome. *The Journal of Bone and Joint Surgery, 82B*, 200-203.

Merritt, B. A., Okyere, C. P., & Jasinski, D. M. (2002). Isopropyl alcohol inhalation: Alternative treatment of postoperative nausea and vomiting. *Nursing Research, 51*, 125-128.

Moretti, E. W., Robertson, K. M., El-Moalem, H., & Gan, T. J. (2003). Intraoperative colloid administration reduces postoperative nausea and vomiting and improves postoperative outcomes compared with crystalloid administration. *Anesthesia & Analgesia, 96*, 611-617.

Murphy, M. J., Hooper, V. D., Sullivan, E., Clifford, T., & Apfel, C. C. (2007). Identification of risk factors for postoperative nausea and vomiting in the perianesthesia adult patient. *Journal of PeriAnesthesia Nursing, 21*(6), 377-384.

Neelon, V., Champagne, M., Carlson, J., & Funk, S. (1996). The NEECHAM confusion scale: Construction, validation, and clinical testing. *Nursing Research, 45*, 324-330.

Nelson, T. P. (2002). Postoperative nausea and vomiting: Understanding the enigma. *Journal of PeriAnesthesia Nursing, 17*(3), 178-189.

Nixon, J., Cranny, G., & Bond, S. (2007). Skin alterations of intact skin and risk factors associated with pressure ulcer development in surgical patients: A cohort study. *International Journal of Nursing Studies, 44*, 655-663.

Ozawa, S., Shander, A., & Ochani, T. D. (2001). A practical approach to achieving bloodless surgery. *Association of Operating Room Nurses Journal, 74*(1), 34-47.

Panel for the Prediction and Prevention of Pressure Ulcers in Adults (1992). *Pressure ulcers in adults: Prediction and prevention. Clinical practice guideline, Number 2.* AHCPR Publication No. 92-0047. Rockville, MD: Agency for Health Care Policy and Research, Public Health Service, U. S. Department of Health and Human Services.

Parisi, D. M., Koval, K., & Egol, D. (2002). Fat embolism syndrome. *American Journal of Orthopedics, 31*(9), 507-512.

Porte, R. J., & Leebeek, F. W. G. (2002). Pharmacological strategies to decrease transfusion requirements in patients undergoing surgery. *Drugs, 62*, 2193-2211.

Reddy, M., Gill, S. S., & Rochon, P. A. (2006). Preventing pressure ulcers: A systematic review. *Journal of the American Medical Association, 296*(8), 974-984.

Redelings, D., Lee, N. E., & Sorvillo, F. (2005). Pressure ulcers: More lethal than we thought? *Advances in Skin & Wound Care, 18*(7), 367-372.

Robinson, T. N., Raeburn, C. D., Tran, Z. V., Angles, E. M., Brenner, L. A., & Moss, M. (2009). Postoperative delirium in the elderly: Risk factors and outcomes. *Annals of Surgery, 249*(1), 173-178.

Roche, V. (2003). Etiology and management of delirium. Kaplan, N. M., & Palmer, B. F. (Eds.). *The American Journal of the Medical Sciences, 325*(1), 20-30.

Rosseland, L. A., Stubhaug, A., & Breivik, H. (2002). Detecting postoperative urinary retention with an ultrasound scanner. *Acta Anaesthesiologica Scandinavica, 46*(3), 279-282.

Schult, M., Frerichmann, U., Schiedel, F., Brug, E., & Joist, A. (2003). Pathophysiology of fat embolism after intramedullary reaming. *European Journal of Trauma, 29*, 68-73.

Sessler, D. I., & Akca, O. (2002). Nonpharmacological prevention of surgical wound infections. *Clinical Infectious Diseases, 35*(11), 1397-1404.

Shaikh N. (2009).Emergency management of fat embolism syndrome. *Journal of Emergencies, Trauma and Shock, 2*, 29-33.

Schellong, S. M., Beyer, J., Kakkar, A. K., Halbritter, K.,Eriksson, B. I., Turpie, A. G. G., ...Kalebo, P. (2007). Ultrasound screening for asymptomatic deep vein thrombosis after major orthopaedic surgery: The VENUS study. *Journal of Thrombosis and Haemostasis, 5*, 1431–1437.

Siddiqi, N., Stockdale, R., Britton, A. M., & Holmes, J. (2007). Interventions for preventing delirium in hospitalized patients. *The Cochrane Database Systematic Reviews, 2*, Art. No.: CD005563. doi:1002/14651858. CD005563.pub2

Solomkin, J. S. (2001). Antibiotic resistance in postoperative infections (supplement). *Critical Care Medicine, 29*, N97-N99.

Stadler, M., Bardiau, F., Seidel, L., Albert, A., & Boogaerts, J. G. (2003). Difference in risk factors for postoperative nausea and vomiting. *Anesthesiology, 98*, 46-52.

Stratton, R. J., Ek, A. C., Engfer, M., Moore, Z., Rigby, P., Wolfe, R., ... Elia, M. (2005). Enteral nutritional support in prevention and treatment of pressure ulcers: A systematic review and meta-analysis. *Aging Research Reviews, 4*(3), 422-450.

Tapson, V. G., & Witty, L.A. (1995). Massive pulmonary embolism, diagnostic and therapeutic strategies. *Clinics in Chest Medicine, 16*, 329-340.

Taviloglu, K., & Yanar, H. (2007). Fat embolism syndrome. *Surgery Today, 37*(1), 5-8. doi: 10.1007/s00595-006-3307-5

Teller, P., & White, (2009). The physiology of wound healing: Injury through maturation. *Surgical Clinics of North America, 89*(3), 599-610.

ten Cate-Hoek, A.J., & Prins, M.H. (2005). Management studies using a combination of D-dimer test results and clinical probability to rule out venous thromboembolism: A systematic review. *Journal of Thrombosis Haemostasis, 3*, 2465–2470.

Thomson, P. W., & Smith, D. J. (1994). What is infection? *The American Journal of Surgery, 167*(1A), 7S-11S.

Tramer, M. R. (2001). A rational approach to the control of postoperative nausea and vomiting: Evidence from systematic reviews. Part I. Efficacy and harm of antiemetic interventions, and methodological issues. *Acta Anaesthesiology Scandinavica, 45*, 4-13.

Turkoski, B. (2000). Preventing DVT in orthopaedic patients. *Orthopaedic Nursing, 19*, 93-99.

van der Mast, R. C., & Fekkes, D. (2000). Serotonin and amino acids: Partners in delirium pathophysiology? *Seminars in Clinical Neuropsychiatry, 5*, 125-131.

Vanderwee, K., Grypdonck, M., & Defloor, T. (2008). Alternating pressure air mattresses as prevention for pressure ulcers: A literature review. *International Journal of Nursing Studies, 45* (5), 784-801.

Vanderlinde, E. S., Heal, J. M., & Blumberg, N. (2002). Autologous transfusion. *British Medical Journal, 324*, 772-775.

Wallvik, J., Själander, A., Johansson, L., Bjuhr, O., & Jansson, J.H. (2007). Bleeding complications during warfarin treatment in primary healthcare centers compared with anticoagulation clinics. *Scandanavian Journal of Primary Health Care,25*(2), 123-128. doi: 10.1080/02813430601183108

Weatherall, M., & Harwood, M. (2002). The accuracy of clinical assessment of bladder volume. *Archives of Physical Medicine & Rehabilitation, 83*(9), 1300-1302.

Webster, J., & Osborne, S. (2007). Preoperative bathing or showering with skin antiseptics to prevent surgical site infection. *The Cochrane Database of Systematic Review, 2*, Art. No: CD004985.doi: 10.1002/14651858.CD004985.

Wender, R. H. (2009). Do current antiemetic practices result in positive patient outcomes? Results of a new study. *American Journal of Health System Pharmacy, 1*(66, S1), S3-S10.

Weschler, D. (1997). Wechsler Adult Intelligence Scale-III. Administration and scoring manual (3rd ed., pp. 1-10). San Antonio: Psychological Corporation.

White, T., Petrisor, B. A., & Bhandari, M. (2006). Prevention of fat embolism syndrome. *Injury, 37S*, S59-S67.

Whitesides, T. E.J., Haney, T. C., Morimoto, K. & Harada, H. (1975). Tissue pressure measurements as a determinant for the need of fasciotomy. *Clinical Orthopaedics, 11*, 43-51.

Winston, A. W., Rinehart, R. S., Riley, G. P, Vaccinhiano, C. A., & Pelligrini, J. E., (2003). Comparison of inhaled isopropyl alcohol and intravenous ondansetron for treatment of postoperative nausea. *Journal of the American Association of Nurse Anesthetists, 71*(2), 127-132.

Chapter 9

Body Mechanics, Mobility Techniques, and Post-Surgical Precautions

Anita Summerville, BS, PTA, PAS, CSCS

Objectives

- Identify proper body mechanics in caring for post-surgical orthopaedic patients.

- Apply appropriate postoperative precautions when caring for orthopaedic patients.

- Apply knowledge of proper assistive devices when mobilizing patients.

Key Terms

Adaptive equipment: equipment used to assist the patient with activities of daily living such as a reacher, sock aid, long handled shoehorn, and dressing stick.

Assistive devices: equipment that aids in ambulation.

Body mechanics: the positioning of the body through the use of muscle contractions.

Extensor lag: a decrease in the amount of extension a joint can achieve.

Gait belt: a belt-like device used to assist the patient in moving from one place to another.

Lateral thrust: an excessive sideways movement of the body.

Lordosis: anterior curvature of the spine as seen in the cervical and lumbar regions; if curvature is exaggerated, it is considered a spinal deformity.

Shearing forces: forces that are applied parallel to or along the surface of an object.

Stance: the position of standing.

The proper care of the orthopaedic patient depends on the ability to transfer and ambulate in the most safe and effective manner. By learning methods to mobilize patients while maintaining proper body mechanics, optimum patient outcomes can be achieved. The nurse should be familiar with effective mobilization strategies that will assist the patient in achieving the highest functional level.

Body Mechanics

In caring for the orthopaedic patient, it is essential for caregivers to use proper posture and body mechanics. Failure to do so can increase the risk of personal injury. In fact, 8 out of 10 people will be affected by back pain at some point during their lives (National Institute of Arthritis and Musculoskeletal and Skin Diseases (NIAMS), 2009). Back pain is one of the leading causes of disability among adults in the United States (Center for Disease Control (CDC), 2009) and accounts for productivity losses of almost $28 billion per year (Wheeler, 2009). Risk factors for back pain include smoking, obesity, physically strenuous work, stressful jobs, and female gender (Mayo Clinic, 2008). Orthopaedic nurses, as well as other health care workers, commonly suffer from work-related musculoskeletal disorders (MSDs) due to the frequent handling of high risk patients (Sedlak, Doheny, Nelson, & Waters, 2009).

Posture is defined as the relative position or attitude of the body at any one period of time (Kolber, 2008). When evaluating an individual's posture, a comparison should be made to standard posture (Hall & Brody, 2005). The ideal standard posture is a mechanically efficient alignment of the body in which positioning is centered, joints are relaxed, and muscles are free of unnecessary tension (Asher, 2005). Posture is usually evaluated in the standing position. It is important when standing to avoid slouching with the head protruded forward. This position puts pressure on the lumbar discs and can increase the chance of back injury (Figure 9-1). A plumb line can be useful in evaluating proper standing posture (Figure 9-2).

A good sitting posture can help prevent back injuries. The proper sitting position is with the shoulders back, feet on the floor, and hips level with the knees (Figure 9-3). A lumbar roll behind the back can provide good support to the lumbar lordotic curve.

Lying positions are also important to maintain body mechanics. When lying on the back, it is best to keep a pillow under the knees. Side lying can be comfortable with a pillow between the legs (Figure 9-4). It is best to use one pillow under the head to maintain proper neck posture.

Proper lifting techniques are crucial in preventing back injuries. It is important to begin with proper posture and head alignment, keeping the feet spaced shoulder width apart and objects close to the body. Bending should take place at the knees, never at the back, and the abdominal

Figure 9-1
Lumbar Disc Pressures

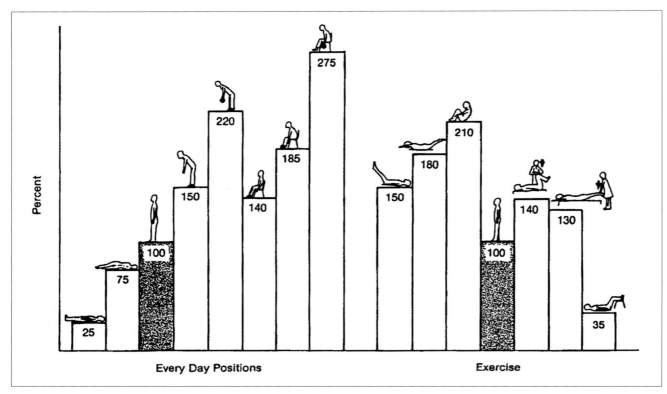

Reprinted with permission of the Saunders Group, Inc.

Figure 9-2
Proper Posture

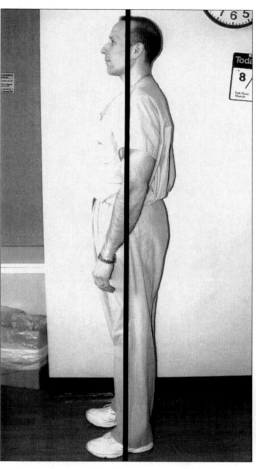

Photogaphy by Mark Nuytten.

Figure 9-3
Proper Sitting Posture

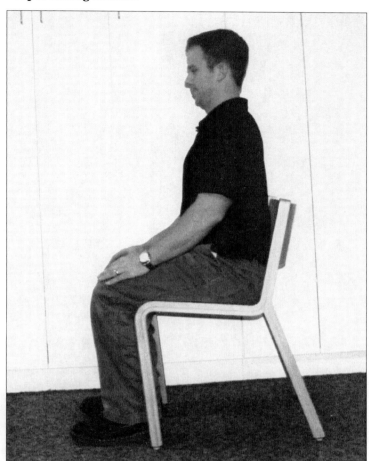

Photogaphy by Mark Nuytten.

Figure 9-4
Side Lying
Positioning

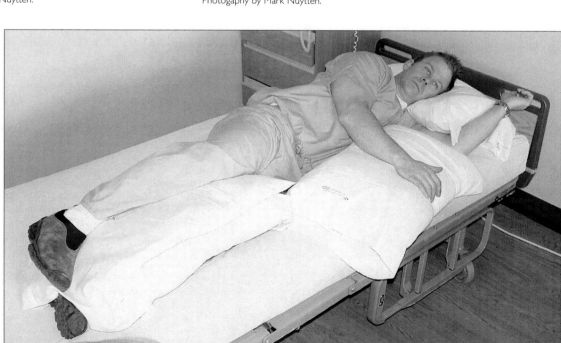

Photogaphy by
Mark Nuytten.

Figure 9-5
Proper Lifting Mechanics

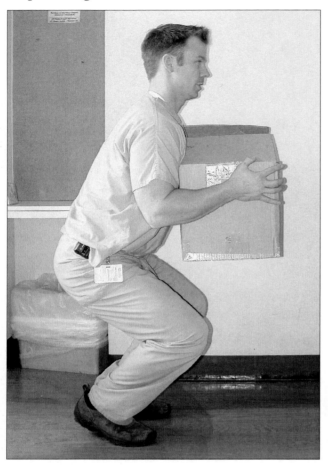

Photography by Mark Nuytten.

muscles should be contracted. Twisting at the waist and pulling the object should be avoided. If possible, the object to be lifted should be brought to waist height (see Figure 9-5). When lifting a patient in bed, the bed should be raised. See Table 9-1 for proper lifting techniques.

If good judgment is used in conjunction with proper body mechanics, the risk of injury to both the patient and caregiver is decreased. It is critical not to rush procedures when transferring or lifting patients. In addition, the patient should be instructed to assist during the transfer to achieve a successful outcome.

Transfer Techniques

Proper transfer techniques are important in the safe and effective movement of all patients, particularly orthopaedic patients. Most orthopaedic patients have a traumatic or surgical insult to their body that can impede them from achieving their maximum mobility. When transferring a patient, the caregiver must assess the ability of the patient to participate in the transfer in order to avoid injury to the patient and self. If the caregiver must lift more than 35 pounds of the patient's weight, then the patient is considered fully dependent and

an assistive device should be used (Waters, 2007). A grading system can be used to communicate the amount of transfer assistance a patient requires to move (see Table 9-2). Familiarity with this system allows unambiguous and consistent communication of the patient's ability to transfer (O'Sullivan & Schmitz, 2007).

Bed Mobility

Bed mobility enables the patient to move in bed and consists of scooting, rolling, and/or moving from a supine or side-lying to a sitting position. The bed should be positioned at elbow height. Scooting is very helpful in moving the patient toward the head of the bed. It can be performed by having the patient bend one knee and hold an overhead trapeze with two hands, and lift the trunk to slide up in bed. If the patient is having difficulty performing this activity, a draw sheet can be placed under the trunk and hips to slide the patient to the middle or head of the bed. If the patient is at risk for pressure ulcers, a friction-reducing device should be used to eliminate shearing forces (Guldmann, 2009).

Patients who are able to move well in bed and participate in a transfer can be assisted to a bedside chair or wheelchair. The logroll maneuver should be used when moving from the supine to the sitting position. With the logroll movement, the patient turns the entire body as one unit, then rolls to the side, lowers the legs off the bed, and uses the arms to push up to a sitting position (Figures 9-6a, b, and c). Depending on the condition of the patient, the nurse may assist at the shoulder, remembering never to pull on the arm or neck. The patient should be encouraged to provide partial or full assistance by using a repositioning aid, such as a trapeze, to facilitate bed mobility , thus reducing the risk of musculoskeletal injury to both the nurse and the patient (Gonzalez, Howe, Waters, & Nelson, 2009).

Patients who are physically compromised and unable to either attain a sitting position on the side of the bed or participate in a transfer should initially be seated in a cardiac chair, which allows gradual movement to an upright position with less disruption of the patient's hemodynamic status. A draw sheet or polyethylene slide board can be used to perform a safe and effective transfer to the cardiac chair (Figure 9-7). Mechanical lifts are available for difficult transfers including larger patients or individuals with very limited mobility. There are various types of mechanical lifts,

Table 9-1
Proper Lifting Techniques

- Bend at the knees and avoid bending the back when lifting
- Feet should be kept shoulder width apart when possible
- Keep objects to be moved close to body and avoid twisting
- Strong core muscles, through exercise, can prevent injuries while lifting
- Proper attire and footwear are critical for safe lifting
- Raise bed to waist level for patient care to avoid bending at the waist
- Heavy objects may require two or more people to move safely

Created by author.

Table 9-2
Levels of Assistance

Types of transfer assistance	Definition
Independent	Patient is able to perform the transfer without any help.
Supervision	Patient is able to perform the transfer without help but someone is standing nearby.
Contact Guard assist	Patient performs transfer with the caregiver touching the patient for support.
Minimal assist	Patient performs the majority of the transfer. The caregiver contributes approximately 10-25% assist.
Moderate assist	The caregiver gives approximately 25-50% assist to the patient.
Maximal assist	The caregiver gives greater than 50% assist to the patient.
Dependent transfer	The caregiver performs the transfer. The patient is completely dependent on the caregiver.

Adapted from O'Sullivan, S., & Schmitz, T. (2007). *Physical rehabilitation: Assessment and treatment* (5th ed., pp. 379-380, 541, 548). Philadelphia: Davis.

the most common of which is the hydraulic full-body lift (Hegner & Caldwell, 2004).

Chair Transfers

It is important to assess the patient's surroundings prior to attempting a chair transfer. The room should be well-organized, with all furniture moved out of the way. Organizing the environment will allow a smooth transfer process. Blankets or pillows can be used to increase the height of the chair seat if hip precautions are in place or the chair is uncomfortably low. The chair should be positioned on the patient's unaffected side to use the stronger leg to assist in the transfer. Attention must be paid to foley catheters, IVs, and any other devices while the patient is being transferred.

A gait belt is highly recommended to assist the patient to a standing position or balance them once sitting or standing. The gait belt is applied around the waist and over the patient's clothing. If abdominal surgery was performed or the patient has a large abdominal girth, the belt can be applied under the patient's axillae. The Occupational Safety and Health Administration (U.S. Department of Labor, 2009) specifies contraindications for the use of the gait belt including abdominal or spine surgery, abdominal aneurysm, and colostomy.

Before attempting to stand, the patient must edge forward so both feet are planted evenly on the floor. If the patient has difficulty moving to the edge of the sitting surface, assistance should be provided to enable the patient to scoot one buttock at a time to move forward. To assist the patient to plant their feet, the positioning of "nose over toes" can be used. The patient is instructed to push off the bed or chair using upper extremity strength. Both hands should remain on the bed until the patient has reached a full standing position and is fully balanced. Once in this position, the

Figure 9-6a, 6b, 6c
Log Rolling

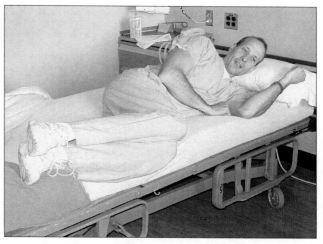

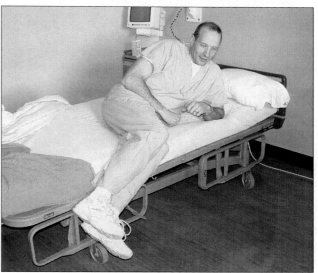

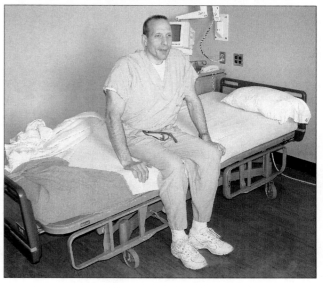

Photography by Mark Nuytten.

Table 9-3
Types of Transfers

Standing Pivot	Caregiver stands in front of the patient using a gait belt, assists the patient into standing position and guides them toward the chair. The patient must be able to weight bear to accomplish the transfer.
Sitting Pivot	The patient is positioned at the edge of the bed. They are pivoted from the bed to a chair. This is sometimes performed with a sliding board. The patient is usually moved toward the stronger or unaffected side.
Modified Pivot	The patient is able to bear some weight on the lower legs but still requires significant assist with the transfer. The patient is usually able to stand while the caregiver pivots them to a chair.
Two Man Lift	A dependent transfer performed by the caregiver. The patient is unable to assist.

Reprinted with permission from *An introduction to orthopaedic nursing* (2004). C. Mosher (Ed.), (3rd ed., p.91). Chicago, IL: National Association of Orthopaedic Nurses.

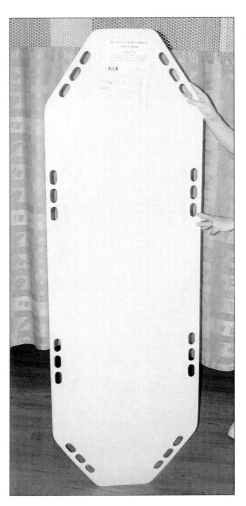

Photogaphy by Mark Nuytten.

Figure 9-7
Polyethylene Slide Board

patient can safely place both hands on a walker, if one is needed. The patient should never pull on the walker or caregiver to rise to the standing position. Depending on the patient's strength, a pivot transfer or stand-by assist transfer can be used (see Table 9-3). If the patient is transferring to or from a wheelchair, the wheels must be locked and the legs and arm rests removed.

With the chair behind, the patient should be instructed to reach one hand back and place it on the arm of the chair. Before lowering to the chair, the second hand can be removed from the walker and used to reach behind to the chair for support. If the patient has an affected lower extremity, such as a total hip or knee arthroplasty, placing the affected leg out in front of the body is best while lowering to the chair.

When transferring from the chair back to bed, it is helpful to move the chair so the unaffected leg is closest to the bed. The patient is instructed to place their hands on the arms of the chair and using upper body strength, push up to a standing position. Once balanced, the patient can place both hands on the walker, if using one. The patient is instructed to turn their back to the bed using a pivot or stand-by transfer. Once the backs of their legs touch the bed, the patient should reach one hand back toward the mattress. While lowering to the bed, the second hand should reach back for the mattress. Again, if the patient has an affected lower extremity, the leg should be positioned out straight in front of the body while lowering to the bed.

Toilet Transfer

A more difficult transfer to perform is between a toilet and a wheelchair. The bathroom is usually a very small transfer space. It is best to use a shower chair for a toilet transfer, since these chairs have wheels and can easily be moved (Figure 9-8). It is important to lock the wheels on the shower chair when moving the patient. See the above discussion regarding chair transfers for proper hand placement and positioning of the leg if the patient has an affected lower

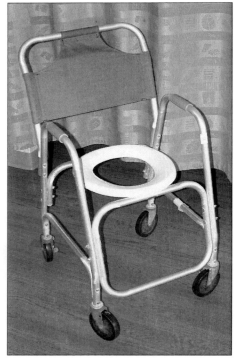

Figure 9-8
Shower Chair with Wheels

Photogaphy by Mark Nuytten.

extremity. When the patient is transferring directly onto the toilet, it is best to reach behind and use the toilet for support, grab bars if they have been installed, or the arms of a raised toilet seat. If there is doubt about the patient's ability to actively participate in a transfer, assistance should be sought from additional caregivers. It is important for all staff and the patient to be confident about the transfer in order to ensure a safe outcome.

Assistive Devices

The need for an assistive device occurs mainly because of a change in a patient's gait pattern. Table 9-4 describes a number of common gait disturbances that the nurse may encounter. Following surgery or other events which change a patient's ability to ambulate, an assessment must be made to determine the need for an assistive device. Assistive devices allow a degree of mobility while increasing the stability of the patient when moving. The physical therapist determines the proper assistive device for the patient, considering certain factors including age, balance, upper extremity strength, weight-bearing status of the lower extremities, joint stability, and patient goals (O'Sullivan & Schmitz, 2007). It is important that the orthopaedic nurse be aware of all the assistive devices available and how to properly use them.

All assistive devices should be in good working order. Patients need to be instructed on the correct use of their assistive device. When returning home, the home environment should be checked for hazards such as electrical wires, pets, throw rugs, clothing, or bedspreads that might cause tripping. Good lighting in the home is important to prevent falls. Consideration should also be made for patient safety and accessibility with activities such as stair climbing or ambulating on uneven surfaces as well as maneuverability throughout the home.

Walkers

Many patients use a walker as an assistive device. Walkers are effective in unloading weight from the affected lower extremity. There are several styles of walkers available, and most are foldable. A standard walker has 4 legs and is the most common type used postoperatively (Figure 9-9). Pediatric-size, wide, and tall walkers are also available (Figure 9-10). It is important that the height of the walker is measured accurately for each individual patient. In the standing position, the handles of the walker should be in line with the patient's wrist. This allows for a 30-degree bend in the elbow and gives the patient a mechanical advantage when bearing weight through their upper extremities.

A rolling walker has two wheels at the front end (Figure 9-11). Although rolling walkers are not as stable as the standard walker, they require less energy expenditure to move. Some wheels rotate to allow an easy change of direction, while others remain locked. Sometimes, the rear legs of a rolling walker are fitted with tennis balls or rear skis so that the walker glides more easily. A Winnie walker has three or four wheels, with a seat and brakes as safety features (Figure 9-12). Rolling walkers work well for

Table 9-4
Gait Disturbances

Antalgic (Painful) Gait	Stance phase on the affected leg is decreased and step length on the unaffected leg is shorter. *Cause:* Injury or condition of the pelvis, hip, knee, ankle, or foot.
Arthrogenic (Stiff Legged) Gait	Minimal movement is seen in the affected hip or knee and it may be painful or pain free. *Cause:* Results from stiffness, laxity, or deformity in the knee or hip.
Ataxic Gait	A wide based gait in which difficulty or inability to tandem walk (heel to toe walking) is present with possible veering to one side and incoordination of the upper extremities. *Cause:* central nervous system dysfunction.
Drop Foot (or Steppage) Gait	Excessive hip flexion occurs so the affected foot will clear the floor as the leg is advanced. *Cause:* Weak ankle dorsiflexors (tibialis anterior).
Parkinsonian Gait	Short, shuffling steps that accelerate as the patient advances. *Cause:* Parkinson's disease.
Trendelenburg Gait	Extensive lateral thrust of the thorax over the unaffected leg and hip when the patient bears weight on the weak side. *Cause:* Weak hip abductor muscles.

Adapted from Masle, D. (2008). *Orthopaedic physical assessment* (5th ed., p. 960). St. Louis: W.B. Saunders.

Figure 9-9
Standard Folding Walker

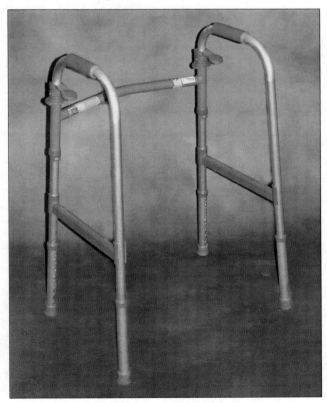

Photography by Mark Nuytten.

Figure 9-10
Wide Non-folding Walker

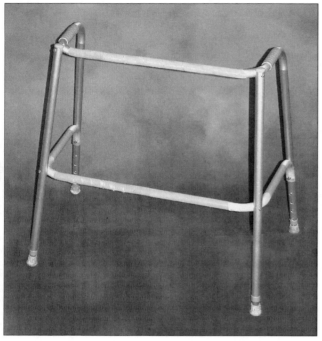

Photogaphy by Mark Nuytten.

patients with decreased balance and unrestricted weight bearing precautions of their lower extremities. After lumbar surgery, some patients may benefit from a rolling walker to stabilize their gait.

Another type of rolling walker is a knee walker. This walker is beneficial for patients who have limited to no use of one lower extremity. This may be due to weight bearing limitations, paresis, paralysis, or various injuries below the knee (i.e., fractures, dislocations, amputations, diabetic ulcers, heel spurs, foot surgery, etc.). The patient places the affected limb on the walker and uses the unaffected leg to propel forward, steering the handle bars like on a bicycle (Figure 9-13).

Platform walkers accommodate the patient with compromised upper extremities (Figure 9-14). An attachment allows the affected arm to rest on a platform while the walker is advanced. Patients with wrist fractures combined with lower extremity afflictions benefit from a platform walker.

The patient should be instructed to place their hands in the center of the hand grips. They are taught to first move the walker forward, followed by the affected extremity, and finally advancing the unaffected extremity. This technique allows the patient's upper body strength to support the involved leg. When a patient moves backward, the walker technique is the opposite: the unaffected extremity moves

Figure 9-11
Rolling Walker

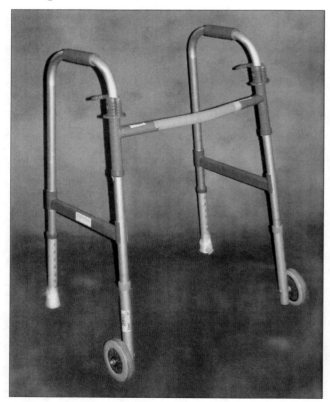

Photogaphy by Mark Nuytten.

Figure 9-12
Winne Walker

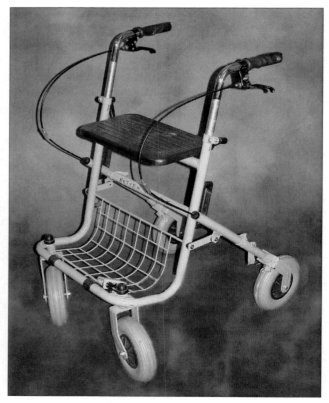

Photogaphy by Mark Nuytten.

Figure 9-13
Knee Walker

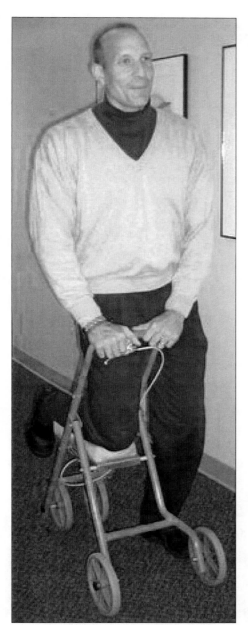

Photogaphy by
Cindi Mosher.

can be used on curbs and stairs. Stair-climbing walkers are available if more stability is needed. Until comfortable and strong enough to climb stairs alone, the patient must be accompanied by another person. Patients are instructed to use the handrail to provide support as they negotiate stair climbing. Although the physical therapist will instruct the patient in the correct technique, the nurse is typically the person who answers final questions upon discharge. It is imperative to be familiar with stair climbing: the unaffected leg goes up the step first, and the affected leg comes down first. Patients may be taught the familiar phrase, "up with the good, down with the bad". For patients who have weight bearing restrictions, assistive devices play a significant role in helping to unweight the affected leg. Sometimes, patients who have stability issues maneuvering stairs despite using assistive devices, handrails, and support from another person, can be taught to bump up and down the stairs while sitting down, extending the affected leg out in front of them, and using the unaffected leg to propel their movement.

Crutches

Crutches are another assistive device commonly used by patients with good coordination and balance. There are two types of crutches: axillary and Lofstrand (Figure 9-15).

Figure 9-14
Platform Walker

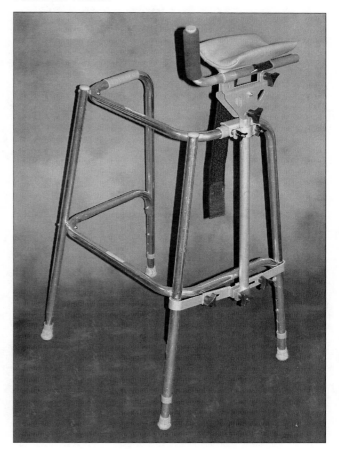

Photography by Mark Nuytten.

first, followed by the affected extremity, and then the walker. The walker should be advanced a comfortable distance, usually an arm's length away, and the patient should be reminded not to step too close to the walker as this can cause loss of balance (Ohio State University Medical Center, 2006). The patient should be reminded to always keep all walker legs on the floor when ambulating. When weight-bearing restrictions are in place, it is important for the patient to use their upper extremity strength to keep weight off the affected leg. Walker-assisted gait can be very fatiguing, and patients may need rest breaks. A patient who is non-weight-bearing on the affected leg expends the most energy because the upper extremities must maintain balance.

The patient must learn the proper technique for negotiating stairs and curbs before being discharged home. Most walkers

Figure 9-15
Left: Lofstrand Crutches; Right: Axillary Crutches

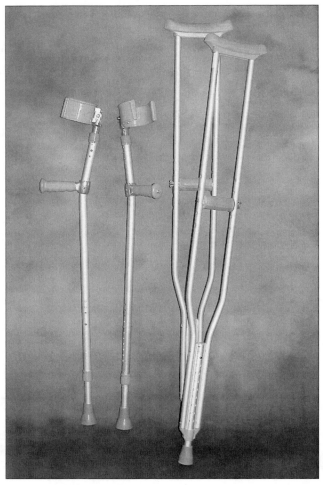

Photogaphy by Mark Nuytten.

Axillary crutches are available in wood or aluminum, in sizes from pediatric to adult. Newer crutches have the crutch height printed on the legs; however, they still must be accurately measured to the patient, with two inches between the axilla (armpit) and the top of the crutch. A slight bend should be apparent at the patient's elbow, and the crutch tips should be placed approximately six inches in front of and two inches lateral to the patient's foot (Dreeben, 2007). When measuring crutch size, the patient should have shoes on in order to get an accurate length. The patient must be taught to avoid leaning on the crutches, since this can compromise circulation to the axilla and cause nerve damage. High quality crutch tips, hand grips, and axillary grips can be utilized to maximize patient safety and comfort.

Lofstrand or forearm crutches have an attachment that cups around the forearm. The patient must use their upper body strength to move the crutches. Lofstrand crutches are not as tall as axillary crutches and are sometimes difficult to remove from the forearms; however, they work well on stairs, and the patient can easily mobilize their hands.

When transferring to a chair using crutches, the patient should be taught to place both crutches on the affected side before sitting down. This gives added balance to the weaker side. Different gait patterns can be used when ambulating with crutches, depending on the patient's weight-bearing restrictions, balance, coordination, and strength. The physical therapist will determine and instruct the patient in the appropriate gait technique using crutches. There are four typical crutch gait patterns that are used after orthopaedic surgery. Three-point gait involves advancing both crutches and the affected leg together, followed by the unaffected leg. With two-point gait, the patient advances the left crutch with the right leg and the right crutch with the left leg. The swing-through pattern requires the advancement of both crutches together followed by swinging both legs together past the crutches. Finally, the swing-to gait pattern involves advancing both crutches together, as in the swing-through pattern, but followed by swinging of both legs together only to the level of the crutches (O'Sullivan & Schmitz, 2007).

Canes

Canes are often helpful assistive devices, particularly if a patient's balance is slightly compromised. The cane is placed on the opposite side of the affected extremity. When measuring cane size, the handle should be in line with the patient's wrist when the arm is bent 30 degrees at the elbow. The bottom of the cane should be positioned 6 inches away from the patient's foot.

Figure 9-16
Canes (left to right): Standard Cane, Large Base Quad Cane, Small Base Quad Cane, and Hemi Cane

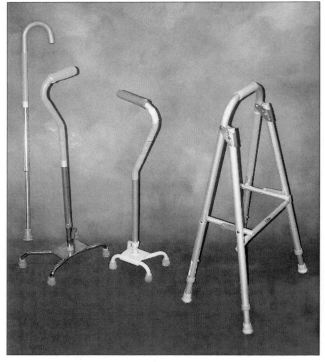

Photography by Mark Nuytten.

The standard cane comes in both wood and aluminum with curved and straight handles to accommodate various patient needs and comfort. A quality rubber cane tip is recommended to provide maximum stability and minimize slipping of the cane. The quadruped cane consists of both a large and a small base. Quadruped canes provide more balance than a standard cane because of the increased base of support. However, if all four legs of the quadruped cane are not on the floor, the patient might feel unsteady, increasing risk for fall. For this reason, standard canes are preferred for postoperative patients. Hemi or walking canes are also available, providing the largest base of support, but they are difficult to use on stairs (Figure 9-16).

When using a cane on stairs, the patient should follow the same rule as for walkers: up with the unaffected leg and down with the affected leg. When ascending stairs, the unaffected leg should be placed on the step. The cane can also be placed on the step or can be left with the affected leg for extra support, depending on patient preference. When descending stairs, the affected leg and cane go down first. A cane is very useful when there is only one stair handrail, as it gives the patient support. Postoperatively, the patient holds the cane in the opposite hand from the affected limb. As the affected leg is moved forward, the cane is advanced simultaneously. If the patient has no differences in lower extremity function, the cane should be used on the side most comfortable to the patient. Many patients prefer the cane in their dominant hand.

Body Alignment Following Surgery

Total Hip Arthroplasty

Certain body alignment precautions must be in place following specific orthopaedic procedures. Patients undergoing total hip arthroplasty (THA), in particular, must take specific protective precautions to avoid hip dislocation (see Figures 9-17a, b, and c). These precautions require that patients:

- Avoid crossing legs or ankles; while in bed, the patient should keep pillows between legs as a reminder;

- Avoid bending at the hip or exceeding 90 degrees of hip flexion;

- Avoid reaching across affected side;

- Avoid twisting motions; and

- Avoid rotating the toes inward;

- Maintain instructed weight bearing restriction.

Hip dislocation is the most common complication of total hip arthroplasty, occurring in 4% of first time surgeries and up to 15% of total hip revisions (Cluett, 2008). If a dislocation occurs, it is most common within the first 8 weeks after surgery (Harris & Candando, 1998). Hip dislocation precautions are surgeon-dependent and usually adhered to for an average of 12 weeks following surgery.

Patients must follow hip precautions when transferring in and out of bed. It is helpful to keep the head of the bed flat.

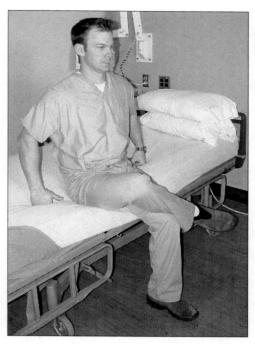

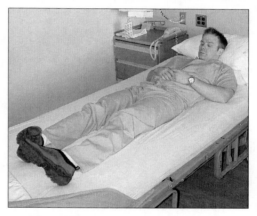

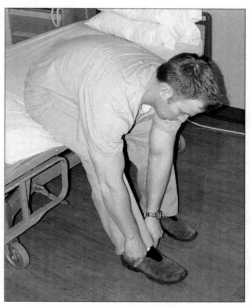

Figures 9-17a, 9-17b, 9-17c Post Surgical Total Hip Positions to Avoid

Photography by Mark Nuytten.

**Figure 9-18
Shower Bench**

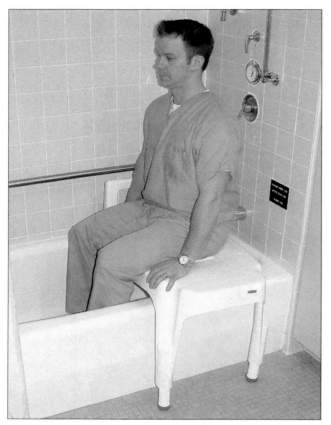

Photography by Mark Nuytten.

The patient must remember not to lean forward while in bed to reach for covers; instead, a reacher should be used. When transferring from a supine to sitting position, the patient can bend the unaffected leg and scoot toward the edge of the bed using upper body strength to rise to a sitting position. Patients should not rely on side rails or the trapeze to assist in the transfer unless rails and a trapeze are available at home.

To maintain dislocation precautions after a total hip arthroplasty, it is important to sit on high surfaces. It is helpful to keep the affected leg forward when performing sit-to-stand transfers to decrease the pressure at the hip joint and maintain hip flexion at less than 90 degrees. Depending on the patient's weight-bearing status, it may be beneficial to limit stair climbing because this increases hip contact pressure. Patients are generally instructed to limit stair climbing to once a day in the first postoperative month. The use of a knee immobilizer can be helpful to prevent hip flexion, especially in confused patients (Colwell, 2009).

Weight-bearing precautions need to be addressed postoperatively for most orthopaedic patients undergoing surgery of the lower extremity. The surgeon will determine how much weight can be placed on the affected extremity. It is important to be aware of the patient's weight bearing status during all transfers and when mobilizing the patient

to avoid injury and promote healing. See Table 9-5 for the various types of weight-bearing statuses.

When a total hip patient transfers in and out of a car, hip precautions must also be observed. When getting into a car, it is best to place the passenger seat as far back as possible and have it slightly reclined. Blankets or pillows can be placed on the seat to elevate the sitting surface. When entering the car, the patient should back into the seat, with the affected leg extended out of the car, and then scoot far enough back in the seat while leaning back so the affected leg can clear the car as it is brought in. Patients are usually allowed to resume driving 4-6 weeks postoperatively.

Prior to discharge, the patient is instructed on the use of a tub transfer bench if they have a tub at home. A tub transfer bench is placed half-in and half-out of the tub (Figure 9-18). With a tub transfer bench, the patient has no need to perform a standing transfer. A walk-in shower is another option that increases the ease and safety with which the patient can bathe and eliminates the need for a standing transfer. It is helpful to have grab bars and a hand-held showerhead for safety.

The patient must be reminded of the importance of continued use of their assistive device until the surgeon advises them to stop. Following total hip arthroplasty, it is especially important to rely on the assistive device because the hip abductor muscles are weakened. Weakness of these muscles results in a trendelenburg gait, whereby the patient exhibits a lateral thrust over the stance leg when taking a step (Magee, 2008). The gluteus medius muscle needs to be strengthened through physical therapy in order to prevent a long term limp (Harris & Candando, 1998).

Hip Fracture

Following a hip fracture, postoperative precautions are dependent on the type of surgery performed. In the case of a hemiarthroplasty, some surgeons prefer that total hip precautions be followed. Depending on the stability of the joint, the hip can still be at risk for dislocation. In the case of an open reduction internal fixation (ORIF) repair, there are no necessary hip precautions but there may be weight-

**Table 9-5
Types of Weight Bearing**

Full Weight Bearing (FWB)	Full weight on lower extremities.
Weight Bear as Tolerated (WBAT)	As much weight as tolerated can be applied to the lower extremity.
Partial Weight Bearing (PWB)	Only a percentage of weight can be applied to the affected lower extremity, usually specified by the physician.
Toe Touch Weight Bearing (TTWB)	Toes can be placed on the ground for balance only; no weight on the leg.
Non-Weight Bearing (NWB)	No weight on affected lower extremity.

Reprinted with permission from *An introduction to orthopaedic nursing* (2004). C. Mosher (Ed.), (3rd ed., p.96). Chicago, IL: National Association of Orthopaedic Nurses.

bearing restrictions dependent on surgeon preference or satisfactory level of surgical fixation achieved. Raised surfaces are often preferred when sitting in the bathroom and on chairs for comfort reasons. After a hip fracture, it is critical for the patient to follow a physical therapy routine to increase strength, normalize gait, and ensure safety. Patients who receive an increased number of physical therapy sessions in the first few days following surgery have improved outcomes (Penrod et al., 2004). Driving restrictions are similar to those of total hip arthroplasty.

Total Knee Arthroplasty

After total knee arthroplasty surgery, there are also precautions the patient must adhere to. The surgeon will determine any weight-bearing precautions the patient might have, although the majority of total knee patients can full weight-bear after surgery. However, the patient should not stand, bend knees, and twist at the same time. The patient with a total knee arthroplasty should not place a pillow directly under the knee because it may cause excessive knee flexion. Prolonged knee flexion can prevent obtainment of full knee extension. Even an extensor lag as minimal as 15 degrees can cause knee pain and difficulty with walking (Harris & Candando, 1998). However, a pillow under the lower leg can promote extension and avoid a flexion contracture. Normal range of motion of the knee can vary between 0-130 degrees of flexion and 0-15 degrees of extension (Upham, 2007). Postoperatively, patients who achieve between 128 and 132 degrees of knee flexion experience less pain and have better overall results (Ritter, Lutgring, Davis, & Berend, 2008). Preoperative range of motion is a good predictor of what the patient might achieve following surgery.

Exercises are an important part of the recovery process for both total hip and knee patients. The physical therapist will instruct the patient in specific exercises to strengthen their muscles and improve overall function. Some of the exercises include ankle pumps, quadriceps and gluteal sets, straight leg raises, heel slides, and short arc quads. The nurse, along with the physical therapist, will encourage the patient to continue these exercises while they are in the hospital. Once discharged to home, exercises are continued and progressed with the assistance of a home health or outpatient physical therapist. Exercises are continued for a specific time frame, prescribed usually for several months but dependent upon the patient's progress and functional needs. Ambulation goals also are set in increasing distances and with specific instructions regarding weight bearing restrictions and the use of a gait aid. Once the patient is recovered, they can usually resume driving 4-6 weeks postoperatively.

Shoulder Surgery

Patients who have rotator cuff shoulder surgery must adhere to postoperative precautions. Precautions will depend on the age of the patient, surgical technique, size of the cuff tear, tissue quality, and systemic disease process (Leggin & Kelley, 2000). The surgeon will prescribe appropriate precautions and review general guidelines with the patient. The patient should avoid lifting with the operated arm, leaning on the elbow of the affected arm, lying on the operated side,

reaching behind the back (internal rotation of the shoulder), and pushing or pulling. The patient is typically instructed in pendulum exercises in the hospital. The exercises are performed by bending forward and allowing gravity to move the shoulder joint in a swinging motion. If the patient must wear a sling or brace for a prolonged period of time, an occupational therapist may discuss activities of daily living (ADL) issues and instruct the patient on donning and doffing of the sling or brace if needed. Depending on the surgical procedure, physical therapy may begin immediately or be delayed until the surgeon deems it appropriate. Resumption of driving is also determined by the surgeon and may be 2-6 weeks or more postoperatively.

A patient with a total shoulder arthroplasty must also follow certain precautions, much like a total hip arthroplasty patient. The patient must avoid external rotation and abduction, external rotation and extension, lying on the affected arm, pushing, pulling, or lifting. Some surgeons may also limit raising the shoulder up over the head for 6 weeks. A sling is worn for 2-6 weeks postoperatively. When applying or taking off the sling, it must be slipped between the arm and the body to avoid abducting the arm. An occupational therapist may discuss activities of daily living (ADL) issues and instruct the patient on donning and doffing of the sling or brace if needed. The patient cannot drive until allowed to lift the affected arm overhead, usually about 6 weeks postoperatively.

Spine Surgery

Patients undergoing lumbar laminectomy or discectomy surgery have specific postoperative precautions to avoid: bending or twisting of the spine, lifting more than 10 pounds, and sitting longer than 20-30 minutes. Precautions are usually followed for 6 weeks. Patients should not drive until given permission by the surgeon. Patients undergoing laminectomy or discectomy procedures are generally allowed to drive 2-3 weeks postoperatively while those undergoing more extensive procedures such as multi-level fusions can drive 4-6 weeks after surgery. Some patients may be required to wear a brace postoperatively (AAOS, 2009). If so, the brace will be prescribed by the surgeon.

Following lumbar surgery, the patient's initial exercise program consists mainly of walking short distances on a frequent basis. Some patients might require assistive devices to ambulate safely. A physical therapist can assist in the evaluation and recommendation of the appropriate assistive device to meet the patient's needs as well as devise a suitable exercise program that accommodates any requirements or precautions that the surgeon deems necessary.

Other Musculoskeletal Conditions or Surgery

Although there are many conditions and surgeries relative to the orthopaedic patient, the aforementioned list provides an overview of some common conditions or surgeries. It is essential that coordination of care be considered from a multidisciplinary care model when assisting the orthopaedic patient population regardless of the specific condition or surgery.

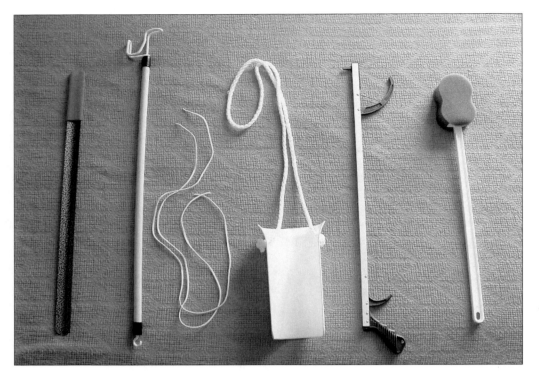

Figure 9-19
Adaptive Equipment (left to right): Long Handled Shoe Horn, Dressing Stick, Elastic Shoelaces, Sock Aid, Reacher, and Long Handled Sponge

Photography by Mark Nuytten.

Activities of Daily Living

There are several types of adaptive equipment to assist a patient following surgery with activities of daily living (ADLs). An occupational therapist can assess the patient to determine their individual ADL needs, based on their current and prior level of function as well as postoperative precautions. Adaptive equipment can be recommended by the occupational therapist to facilitate safe self-care. See Table 9-6 and Figure 9-19 for examples of common adaptive equipment. Occupational therapy can assist patients with work simplification and energy conservation as well.

Durable medical equipment (DME) is essential for most patients following surgery. There are several types of equipment including walkers, wheelchairs, hospital beds, shower chairs or tub transfer benches, bedside commodes, and elevated toilet seats. Depending on specific postoperative precautions, certain types of equipment may be necessary to allow the patient to return home safely.

Summary

It is important for all health care providers to be aware of proper body mechanics, transfer techniques, use of assistive devices, and precautions following orthopaedic surgeries. An educated and informed nurse projects confidence and generates trust. This is crucial when treating patients, in order to create a safe environment that allows the patient to return to optimal functional status.

References

American Academy of Orthopaedic Surgeons, (2009). Lumbar spinal stenosis. Retrieved March 5, 2010 from http://orthoinfo.aaos.org/topic.cfm?topic=A00329

Table 9-6
ADL Equipment and Uses

Reacher	Long handled device that will allow the patient to retrieve items off the floor or out of reach. The patient can also use a reacher to dress the lower body. Hip and spine patients most commonly require a reacher.
Long handled sponge	Allows the patient to wash the lower body when mobility precautions limit the ability to bend forward.
Long handled shoe horn and sock aide	Allow the patient to don\doff socks and shoes without bending forward.
Elastic shoe laces	Eliminates the task of bending forward to tie shoes. Shoes can be slipped on.

Reprinted with permission from *An introduction to orthopaedic nursing* (2004). C. Mosher (Ed.), (3rd ed., p.98). Chicago, IL: National Association of Orthopaedic Nurses.

Asher, A. (2005). *Back & neck pain*. Retrieved June 15, 2009, from http://backandneck.aboutcom/od/i/g/idealalignment.htlm

Centers for Disease Control and Prevention (2009). *Morbidity and mortality weekly report, 58*(16), 421-426.

Cluett, J. (2008). *Hip replacement dislocation: Complication of hip replacement surgery*. Retrieved July 8, 2009, from http://orthopedics.about.com/od/hipkneereplacement/a/dislocation.html

Colwell Jr., C. (2009). Instability after total hip arthroplasty. *Current Orthopedic Practice, 20*(1), 8-14.

Dreeben, O. (2007). *Introduction to physical therapy for physical therapist assistants*. Sudbury: Jones & Bartlett.

Gonzalez, C., Howe, C., Waters, T., & Nelson, A., (2009). Recommendations for turning patients with orthopaedic impairments. *Orthopaedic Nursing: The Leader in Practice and Education, 28*(2S), S9-S12.

Guldmann, Inc. (2009). Safe patient handling in orthopaedic nursing. *Supplement to Orthopaedic Nursing, The Leader in Practice and Education 28*(2S).

Hall, C., & Brody, L. (2005). *Therapeutic exercise: Moving toward function* (2nd ed., p. 168). Baltimore: Lippincott, Williams, & Wilkins.

Harris, M., & Candando, P. (1998). The physical therapist as a member of the home health team. *Home Healthcare Nurse, 16*(3), 153-156.

Hegner, B., & Caldwell, E. (2004). *Nursing assistant: A nursing process approach* (p. 260). Toronto: Delmar Learning.

Kolber, M. (2008). *Posture: what about it?* Retrieved March 5, 2010, from http://www.spineuniverse.com/wellness/ergonomics/posture-what-about

Leggin, B., & Kelley, M. (2000). Rehabilitation of the shoulder following rotator cuff surgery. *The University of Pennsylvania Orthopaedic Journal, 13*, 10-17.

Magee, D. (2008). *Orthopaedic physical assessment* (5th ed., p.960). St. Louis: W.B. Saunders.

Mayo Clinic (2008). *Back pain: risk factors.* Retrieved July 8, 2009, from http://www.mayoclinic.com/health/back-pain/DS00171

Moffat, M., & Vickery, S. (1999). *Book of body mechanics and repair.* New York: Round Stone.

National Institute of Arthritis and Musculoskeletal and Skin Diseases (2009). *Back pain.* Retrieved July 17, 2009, from http://www.niams.nih.gov/Health_Info/Back_Pain/default.asp#2

O'Sullivan, S., & Schmitz, T. (2007). *Physical rehabilitation: Assessment and treatment* (5th ed., pp. 379-380, 541-548). Philadelphia: Davis.

Ohio State University Medical Center, Mount Carmel Health and Ohio Health (2006). *Using a walker.* Retrieved July 19, 2009, from http://www.healthinfotranslations.com/pdfDocs/Using_a_Walker.pdf

Penrod, J., Boockvar, K., Litke, A., Magaziner, J., Hannan, E., Halm, E., … Siu, A., (2004). Physical therapy and mobility 2 and 6 months after hip fracture. *Journal of the American Geriatrics Society, 52*(7), 1114-1120.

Ritter, M., Lutgring, J., Davis, K., & Berend, M. (2008). The effect of postoperative range of motion on functional activities after posterior cruciate-retaining total knee arthroplasty. *Journal of Bone and Joint Surgery, 90*, 777-784.

Scherokman, B., & Alguire, P. (2009). American Academy of Neurology. *Gait disturbances.* Retrieved July 8, 2009, from http://www.aan.com/go/education/curricula/internal/chapter8

Sedlak, C., Doheny, M., Nelson, A., & Waters, T. (2009). Development of the National Association of Orthopaedic Nurses guidance statement on safe patient handling and movement in the orthopaedic setting. *Orthopaedic Nursing: The Leader in Practice and Education, 28*(2S), S2-S8.

Upham, K. (2007). Musculoskeletal assessment. In National Association of Orthopaedic Nurses, *NAON Core curriculum for orthopaedic nursing* (6th ed., p.44). Boston: Pearson.

U.S. Department of Labor (2009). *Ergonomics for the prevention of musculoskeletal disorders: Guidelines for nursing homes.* Retrieved March 2, 2010, from http://www.osha.gov/SLTC/healthcarefacilities/training/activity/_6.html

Waters, T. (2007). When is it safe to manually lift a patient? *American Journal of Nursing, 107*(8), 53-58.

Wheeler, A. (2009). *Pathophysiology of chronic back pain.* Retrieved March 9, 2010, from http://emedicine.medscape.com/article/1144130-overview